PSYCHIATRIC ASPECTS
OF NEUROLOGIC DISEASE

SEMINARS IN PSYCHIATRY

Series Editor

Milton Greenblatt, M.D.
Chief, Psychiatry Service
Veterans Administration Hospital
Sepulveda, California, and
Professor of Psychiatry
University of California, Los Angeles

Other Books in Series:

PSYCHIATRIC ASPECTS OF NEUROLOGICAL DISEASE

Edited by

D. Frank Benson, M.D.
Director, Neurobehavioral Center
Boston Veterans Administration Hospital
and
Professor of Neurology
Boston University School of Medicine
Boston, Massachusetts

Dietrich Blumer, M.D.
Associate Psychiatrist
McLean Hospital
Belmont, Massachusetts
and
Associate Professor of Psychiatry
Harvard Medical School
Boston, Massachusetts

GRUNE & STRATTON
A Subsidiary of Harcourt Brace Jovanovich, Publishers
New York   San Francisco   London

Library of Congress Cataloging in Publication Data
Main entry under title:

Psychiatric aspects of neurologic disease.

Includes bibliographies.
1. Psychological manifestation of general diseases.
2. Neuropsychiatry. I. Benson, David Frank, 1928-
II. Blumer, Dietrich. [DNLM: 1. Mental disorders.
2. Nervous system diseases. WL100 B474p]
RC341.P89   616.8   75-6521
ISBN 0-8089-0860-X

Grune & Stratton, Inc.
111 Fifth Avenue
New York, New York 10003

Library of Congress Catalog Card Number 75-6521
International Standard Book Number 0-8089-0860-X
Printed in the United States of America

Contents

Contributors

Martin Albert, M.D.
Director, Neurobehavioral Section
Department of Neurology
Hadassah Medical Organization
Jerusalem, Israel

Ross J. Baldessarini, M.D.
Associate Professor of Psychiatry
Psychiatric Research Laboratories
Massachusetts General Hospital
and
Harvard Medical School
Boston, Massachusetts

D. Frank Benson, M.D.
Director, Neurobehavioral Center
Boston Veterans Administration Hospital
and
Professor of Neurology
Boston University School of Medicine
Boston, Massachusetts

Manfred Bleuler, M.D.
Professor of Psychiatry
University of Zurich
Zurich, Switzerland

Dietrich Blumer, M.D.
Associate Professor of Psychiatry
Harvard Medical School
Boston, Massachusetts
and
Associate Psychiatrist
McLean Hospital
Belmont, Massachusetts

Marshal F. Folstein, M.D.
Assistant Professor of Psychiatry
Cornell University Medical School
The New York Hospital
Westchester Division
White Plains, New York

Norman Geschwind, M.D.
James Jackson Putnam Professor of Neurology
Harvard Medical School
Boston, Massachusetts

Richard N. Harner, M.D.
Associate Professor of Neurology
University of Pennsylvania Graduate Hospital
Philadelphia, Pennsylvania

Professor Henry Hecaen
Directeur d'Études à l'École
Pratique des Hautes Études
Unité de Recherches Neuropsychologiques et Neurolinguistiques
Paris, France

Zbigniew J. Lipowski, M.D.
Professor of Psychiatry
Dartmouth Medical School
Hanover, New Hampshire
Former Consultant in Psychiatry, Montreal Neurological Institute

Nathan Malamud, M.D.
Professor of Neuropathology in Residence, Emeritus, University of California
Chief, Neuropathology Service
Langley Porter Neuropsychiatric Institute
San Francisco, California

C. David Marsden, M.Sc., M.R.C.P.
Professor of Neurology
University Department of Neurology
Institute of Psychiatry
The Maudsley Hospital, London
and
King's College Hospital, London

Paul R. McHugh, M.D.
Professor and Chairman
Department of Psychiatry
University of Oregon Medical School
Portland, Oregon

Felix Post, M.D., F.R.C.P., F.R.C. Psych.
Consultant Psychiatrist
The Bethlem Royal Hospital
and
The Maudsley Hospital
London, England

Daniel Tarsy, M.D.
Assistant Professor, Neurology
Department of Neurology
Boston Veterans Administration Hospital
and
Boston University School of Medicine
Boston, Massachusetts

A. Earl Walker, M.D.
Professor of Neuro-Surgery
The University of New Mexico
School of Medicine
Albuquerque, New Mexico

Preface

Between psychiatry and neurology lies a vast borderland. Some have said that this borderland is no longer, no more important than the borderland between psychiatry and medicine, or between psychiatry and the law. There is probably much truth there. Nevertheless, the fact remains that psychiatry and neurology are wedded together by history and tradition, by the philosophically and scientifically valid assumption that much of human behavior can be explained by what happens in the brain, and by the clinical reality that many of our patients suffer from disease located in that particular territory. In the borderland may be found the dementias and pseudodementias, many depressions and schizophreniform psychoses, acute and chronic confusional states, disorders of speech and language, the more specific aphasias, many epileptiform states, a legion of senile and arteriosclerotic changes, and a very wide variety of psychiatric manifestations of drug intoxication, physical disease, and gross and subtle genetic abnormalities affecting brain and mind.

Topic Editors Benson and Blumer have done a valiant job of bringing together an internationally distinguished group of experts to teach us what we, as practicing psychiatrists and as eternal students in the school of continuing education, must know.

Seminars in Psychiatry has just finished five years as a professional journal recognized for its high scientific quality and for its effectiveness as an educational vehicle. Both assets are needed more than ever for continuing education is rapidly being accepted as a necessity for all physicians in our country, as in other nations. Self-assessment, re-examination, recertification, and even mandatory statutory relicensure are becoming the motif of the day. Thus our publisher, Grune & Stratton, has encouraged us to move from journals to books. Not only can books be beamed to a wider and more specialized audience, but in fact those journal issues that have also been reproduced as books have enjoyed an enthusiastic acceptance by a new and larger audience.

Thus, *Psychiatric Aspects of Neurologic Disease* by D. Frank Benson and Dietrich Blumer marks the first of this new *book* series. We will be issuing several more such up-to-date volumes in the near future. For example: *Borderline States,* edited by John E. Mack; *Topics in Psychoendocrinology,* edited by Edward J. Sachar; and *Drugs in Combination with Other Therapies,* edited by Milton Greenblatt.

We are enormously indebted to the Editorial Board of *Seminars in Psychiatry* for seeing us through our first epoch as a journal. Our gratitude, therefore, to Ernest Hartmann, Associate Editor; Evelyn M. Stone, Managing Editor; and to Board members Jonathan O. Cole, Jack R. Ewalt, Seymour Fisher, Myron R. Sharaf, George Vaillant, and Stanley Walzer.

Now, in a series of books, pursuing the same path of excellence, we look forward to continuing useful service to our professional public.

Milton Greenblatt, M.D.
Series Editor

Introduction

For most practicing psychiatrists, the problems of organic mental disease occupy only a small portion of their practice. These, however, are very real problems and almost invariably are difficult to handle. One reason for this difficulty is that training in the diagnosis and treatment of neuropsychiatric disorders has been minimal in the past few decades. At most, there are a few lectures on organic mental problems in medical schools; few books or journal articles cover these topics (and many of these are published in foreign languages), and there is little exposure to organic mental problems during specialty training. Responsibility for the care of such patients has been dispersed among general physicians, internists, neurologists, neurosurgeons, and psychiatrists, and frequently there is no interested physician. With little exception, there is a substantial gap between the quality of care given to organic mental problems and to other medical disorders.

The abnormal behaviors traditionally called psychiatric disease can result from abnormality in three separate spheres: the organism itself, the environment influencing the organism, and physical disease affecting the organism. To say that psychiatric disease often results from trouble in two or even all three of these spheres is merely to state the obvious. Yet, in the contemporary practice of psychiatry, the importance of one of these factors, environmental influence, has been placed so high as to almost totally eclipse the other two. This is particularly true in America where a combination of behaviorist psychological and Freudian influenced psychodynamic theories have strongly dominated psychiatric thinking. Consequently, many psychiatrists tend to overlook both the genetic factors and the presence of physical disease when evaluating their patients. The emphasis on psychodynamic patterns has been so strong that the existence of specific psychiatric, and particularly neuropsychiatric, syndromes has often been overlooked. This same bias has led to an erroneous belief that the organic mental syndromes are intractable and can be safely ignored.

Much so-called organic psychiatry, unfortunately, has been characterized by a very restricted viewpoint which has failed to recognize the extreme complexity of human personality and behavior. Understandably, serious students of modern psychiatry have been unable to accept such a simplistic approach. Even when formal investigation has been directed toward these problems the approach has not been adequate. Most such efforts have been ultraacademic, tending toward elegantly designed psychological testing, intricate biochemical or physiologic experimentation, or complex statistical studies. Almost invariably these studies lack a foundation based on sound clinical diagnosis and are thus invalidated.

Recent years have seen an increasing awareness by all psychiatrists of both the genetic and physical facets of psychiatric disease. Several excellent reviews documenting the genetic basis of psychiatric disorders have appeared recently (see especially Slater and Cowie, *The Genetics of Mental Disorder*, London, Oxford, 1971). There is, however, comparatively little literature which attempts to explore the vast borderland of psychiatry and neurology. This volume attempts to point out and discuss a number of the psychiatric problems seen in neurologic disease.

In order to present as much expert opinion as possible, we have asked a number of our colleagues to contribute chapters from their own domain. As always, the multi-author approach produces an unevenness in presentation; some chapters offer overviews of major areas while others focus sharply on limited topics. This volume cannot be considered a textbook of clinical neuro-psychiatry; nonetheless, it does contain much practical clinical information of value to the psychiatrist and neurologist.

A separate chapter on amnesia has not been included. While amnesia is, without doubt, a topic of importance to both neurology and psychiatry, in recent years memory and memory disorders have received a great deal of attention. There are excellent books, monographs, and papers which discuss the phenomenology of amnesia from the neurologic and psychiatric stand-points, others which discuss the psychologic and physiologic bases of memory, and there is even a neuropathology of amnesia. While not yet widely recognized, an understanding of the clinical and scientific correlates of amnesia is available. Discussion of and references to amnesia are included in Chapter 10.

Similarly, we have made no attempt to cover the many clinical neuro-psychiatric problems of childhood. This topic is vast and sufficiently important to warrant a volume of its own. Finally, we have not presented an up-to-date report on the status of the many neuropsychologic studies bearing on organic mental disorders. Neuropsychology is a comparatively new and potentially important discipline which is actively investigating many aspects of the disorders discussed in this book. Unfortunately, contemporary neuropsychologic research is hindered by the same lack of a solid diagnostic foundation that has weakened psychiatric research.

The emphasis in this volume is toward the clinical characterization of the mental disorders occurring in neurologic disease and their treatment. In the opening chapter, Norman Geschwind explores some of the basic problems that exist in the field and outlines some of the major misconceptions held by both psychiatrists and neurologists concerning these problems.

D. Frank Benson
Dietrich Blumer

PSYCHIATRIC ASPECTS OF NEUROLOGIC DISEASE

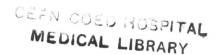

Norman Geschwind, M.D.

1

The Borderland of Neurology and Psychiatry: Some Common Misconceptions

While it has become fashionable to acknowledge the existence of an area of overlap between neurology and psychiatry, this common ground unfortunately bears more resemblance to a no-man's-land than to an open border. While neurologists tend to mutter darkly about the failure of psychiatrists to be aware of the brain as the organ of the mind, psychiatrists, perhaps somewhat defensively, have stressed their awareness of the whole man, biologic as well as psychologic. Unfortunately, few members of either group have in fact really interested themselves in the borderland area, and too frequently interactions between them are educationally disappointing, whether at the level of mutual consultation or in the interchange of residents for training. Hopefully, this situation will be corrected in the next few years, but until then, both psychiatrists and neurologists will often have to acquire the necessary knowledge themselves.

It is obviously important first to be aware of the magnitude and the difficulties of the problem. There are some who would like to believe that neurologic causes of psychiatric disorder are rare. Neurologic disorders, however, account for at least 30 percent of all first admissions to mental hospitals.[3] Furthermore, even if neurologic causes of psychiatric disorder were uncommon, this would still not justify their neglect, since some of these conditions are treatable. Because of the general lack of interest in this area,

Some of the work reported here was supported by Grant NS-06209 National Institute of Neurological Diseases and Blindness to the Boston University School of Medicine.

misdiagnoses are common. These errors include not only the failure to diagnose neurologic disease causing psychiatric symptoms, but also, far more often than is appreciated, the mistaken diagnosis of untreatable neurologic disorder in patients with reversible psychiatric disease, particularly the late-life depressions. It is not surprising that both types of mistakes are made, since a differential diagnosis can be carried out successfully only if one is aware of both groups of conditions.

Over the years, psychiatric residents occasionally have asked me whether they could not avoid such errors in diagnosis by referring all cases for a neurologic consultation. There are major objections to this policy. First, at this time, too few neurologists are themselves adequately trained in the psychiatric aspects of neurologic disease. Second, it would be a serious error in the management of many psychiatric patients to refer them routinely for neurologic examination, a fact that should not need further emphasis. Just as the psychiatrist must have enough experience and knowledge to decide which patients with somatic complaints need referral to nonpsychiatrists, so he must acquire enough expertise to pick up the signals that make neurologic referral useful. Since this type of referral requires diagnostic skill and medical knowledge, the decision for neurologic referral cannot be delegated to medically untrained personnel, as is sometimes the practice. The psychiatrist also must learn, like any other physician, how to choose and evaluate his consultants, and must be prepared for interchange of ideas with them. He will soon learn that some neurologists will be only too happy to find neurologic disorder in every case referred, while others will be more interested in proving themselves more "psychiatric" than the psychiatrist. He will learn that, in a large number of cases, the neurologist will be as uncertain as he himself as to the presence of organic causation. In other words, the neurologist cannot be expected in every case magically to "rule in" or "rule out" organic disorder with absolute certainty.

It is sometimes argued that psychiatric patients may suffer from physical disorders involving the heart, the lungs, the skin, indeed any organ system. The argument often follows that the brain can simply be regarded as one of a large list of organs that may be affected, and there is no reason why the psychiatrist need be any more expert on the brain than he is on, let us say, gynecologic disorders. I believe, however, that there are reasons why the brain has a very special importance for the psychiatrist. It is, of course, true that many disorders of the nervous system are not different in their psychiatric implications from nonneurologic disorders. One would hardly argue that the behavioral responses of a patient to a peripheral neuropathy would be *directly* affected by the neurologic lesion, and it would be reasonable in such a case to place major emphasis on the past experience of the patient. It may well be reasonable in such a case to speak of "a psychiatric overlay," i.e., the response of the patient to the illness. As we shall see, however, many lesions of the brain directly affect the parts of the nervous system that are involved in emotional behavior and may cause primary behavior disorder. To speak of "overlay" in such a case is misleading.

It must be realized that every behavior has an anatomy. This applies to both elementary and higher-level behaviors. We would accept that, when someone moves his arm, the impulses eventually leading to the movement will be transmitted over delimited, even if multiple, pathways in the nervous system. The same is true if someone speaks and is also true when someone gets angry. There is often the temptation to assume that emotion must be a function of the whole brain. This is, however, not supported by experimental facts. The parts of the brain from which emotional behavior is elicited are limited in extent. One need only cite the extensive physiologic work of Flynn[2] on the regions in which stimulation elicits or inhibits aggression. Thus, stimulation of the lateral hypothalamus leads to aggressive behavior, and its bilateral destruction leads to tameness. When a normal animal learns to respond aggressively to some stimulus, he must carry on this learning by modification of a pathway that eventually will fire the lateral hypothalamus or a small number of related structures. If these structures are destroyed, the animal will not become angry, regardless of his previous life experience. Similarly, destruction of the region of the ventromedial hypothalamus will lead to aggression, regardless of previous experience.

It is clear, therefore, that certain organic lesions can lead to changes in behavior, which in many instances are uninfluenced by the past experience of the animal. Furthermore one can place lesions so that different emotional responses can be elicited from different parts of the brain[1] which are not connected to each other. Hence, the strategy of "looking at the whole patient," which is often so useful to the psychiatrist in other circumstances, may be actively misleading when certain discharging or destructive lesions of the brain are present.

Neglect of the fact that every behavior has an anatomy may lead in some cases to incorrect psychodynamic explanations of changes in behavior that are not dependent on past experience. One should not, however, make the equally serious error of concluding that, since all behavior takes place in the brain, all disorders of behavior must be organic, a view sometimes expressed in the vivid, but, in my opinion, erroneous aphorism that "behind the crooked thought lies the crooked molecule." No one can deny that learning is one of the major functions of the brain, and it is reasonable to assume that normal learning processes can lead to difficulties in adjustment. To pick a naive example, the child who is taught that dogs are dangerous will have difficulties in ordinary life, but this disadvantageous learning occurs by the same normal mechanism by which he advantageously learns that tigers are dangerous.

Some have argued, as noted above, that since all behavior is a function of the brain, one cannot draw a distinction between "organic" and "functional" disorders. I believe, however, that the organic-functional distinction is valid. A behavior disorder is "functional" if it is learning that has modified the brain by normal physiologic mechanisms; in theory, the functional disorder can be reversed by learning. On the other hand, the organic disorder is one in which the brain structures mediating behavior undergo alterations that reduce partially, or completely, the effects of past experience or new learning. These alterations may consist of destructive or discharing lesions or may consist of biochemical changes affecting impulse transmission or propagation.

It is worth mentioning that, in theory, any behavior disorder, whether organic or functional, can be treated by organic means. On the other hand, many organic disorders cannot be treated by learning methods (in which, of course, I include psychotherapy). Thus, an animal who responds with rage to certain stimuli will lose this response if drugs or surgery put the appropriate regions out of action. But learning cannot affect the activity of areas that are themselves destroyed, or whose necessary afferent pathways are cut off. The fact that organic methods can be used to treat behavior disorders of any etiology is, of course, widely reflected in clinical practice. Perhaps the most widely used form of psychiatric treatment is drug therapy. Each drug probably acts at a limited number of sites in the nervous system, and the use of drugs is in effect chemical, and usually reversible, neurosurgery. The very fact that so much treatment depends on the use of neurally acting agents is another reason for the psychiatrist to be especially aware of the nervous system.

Once the importance of organic causation of a significant minority of psychiatric cases is accepted, the request often follows for some simple method to establish or exclude organic causation. There are, however, no simple methods. If one were to ask a cardiologist for a rule of thumb by which one might diagnose all organic causes of chest pain, he would almost certainly decline to supply it. One must simply learn the clinical pictures of angina, myocardial infarction, dissecting aneurysm, acute pericarditis, rupture of the esophagus, and so on. If simple rules work poorly in the diagnosis of chest or abdominal pain, they must surely be less applicable to that organ of the body that is capable of the widest variety of responses.

Organic causes of behavior disorders are not excluded by a normal elementary neurologic examination. A normal EEG similarly fails to exclude neurologic disease. In fact, in some disorders with striking behavioral change—for example, Alzheimer's disease—the EEG usually remains fully normal. Furthermore, even repeated normal EEGs do not necessarily exclude epilepsy, since the epileptogenic focus may simply be too deep or too distant from the recording electrodes. The lumbar puncture is an extremely useful tool and in general seriously underused in psychiatric circles. I have seen several patients with psychiatric disorders in whom only the presence of abnormalities on lumbar puncture gave away the organic causation. But a normal lumbar puncture does not exclude organic disease. Indeed, even a normal postmortem examination of the brain does not exclude organic causation. One need think not only of obvious disorders, such as drug intoxications, but even of such conditions as Sydenham's chorea, in which most investigators argue that no characteristic pathology has been found.

Another major source of error is the tendency to lump organic disorders into the categories of acute and chronic brain syndromes. These categories are as acceptable for the brain as would be the diagnosis of chronic myocardiopathy for all forms of chronic heart disease. It is obvious that some patients with chronic heart disease have large hearts, while others do not; some are hypertensive, while others have low blood pressure; some have rhythm disorders, while others do not. *Similarly, there is no single feature common to all forms of organic brain disease with behavior disorder.* Memory disorder may be prominent in some cases, but lacking in others. Some patients may be hypomanic, while others are apathetic. The patient with frontal lobe disorder tends to have short-lived shallow anger, which usually disappears rapidly, while the temporal lobe epileptic is likely to justify his anger with elaborate moral arguments and is frequently very slow to forget.

Other sources of error stem from failures on even more elementary levels. There are some psychiatric institutions in which histories are taken by nonmedical personnel, so that certain information is missed. Thus, one patient I saw had a history of episodes of depersonalization, but only slight effort was needed to bring out the fact that these were ushered in by an intense smell of burning rubber. This had been overlooked in a psychiatric hospital where the physician did not take a history, and only later in another hospital, when this information was obtained, was the presumption of temporal lobe epilepsy raised, and confirmed.

Another common failure in taking histories or examining patients, even when done by a physician, is the tendency by some to make dynamic interpretations of the patient's behavior right from the initial contact. The possibility of organic diagnosis is almost excluded when the patient is approached in so closed-minded a fashion. It should furthermore be kept in mind that the mere fact that a patient's behavior is concordant with his personality dynamics does not mean that the disorder is psychogenic.

The impression often exists that when organic mental disorder is present, there must be failures in intellectual functioning. This belief is subject to pitfalls in more than one direction. While the presence of true intellectual deficit is an excellent sign of organic behavior disorder, its absence fails to rule it out, and patients with organic disorder may be missed. Patients with frontal lesions, particularly in the early stages, may have striking changes in behavior with no intellectual deficit. Temporal lobe epilepsy with behavioral change is compatible with a distinctly superior level of intellectual performance.

There exists, however, a much greater danger, that of incorrectly diagnosing incurable organic disorder when treatable functional disorder is present. Many patients with functional disorder present with apparent intellectual deficit. This can occur as hysterical pseudodementia, which is not very common. On the other hand, a number of patients suffering from *depression* will present with apparent intellectual failure. English psychiatrists are apparently well aware of this and are more likely to diagnose depression in the aged than many of their American counterparts.[4] The failure to consider this diagnosis is a serious error, since it results in failure to treat a usually reversible disorder. The argument is sometimes advanced that, although some of these patients are depressed, they are also intellectually impaired, and indeed it is often stated that depression itself is the first sign of dementia. My own view, however, is that this is not usually the case and that in general the apparent dementia disappears when the depression is reversed. I recently saw a 75-year-old woman who had been diagnosed as having a progressive dementia because of her gross failures in mental examination; after treatment for depression, she showed perfectly preserved intellectual capacities and she is representative of many such cases.

Psychological testing is, of course, a tremendously useful tool, but the desire of many people for a simple means of diagnosing organicity often leads to a mistaken confidence in such test findings. Patients with gross organic behavioral disorders may lack any of the so-called signs of organicity. On the other hand, some patients with pseudodementias can be incorrectly diagnosed as showing organic disorder. Psychologic test results are most useful in the context of the entire clinical picture.

There are a few rules that may be helpful. There are patients who may be thought to be cases of manic psychosis who turn out to have disease of the frontal lobe. This occurs classically in general paresis but can occur with other disorders, such as multiple sclerosis or frontal tumors. On the other hand, the ability to maintain a fully classical *agitated* depression almost always excludes organic disease. Apathy is, however, an important feature of many organic disorders and is very frequently misinterpreted as depression. Incontinence of urine or feces is a major danger signal, since it almost never occurs in functional disorders. Neglect of this simple sign has led in my experience to diagnoses that were missed over several months. On the other hand, this sign may lose its usefulness if the patient has been placed on large doses of psychotropic drugs or has recently received electroconvulsive therapy. Another common error is that of misinterpreting the abnormality of emotional expression in patients with bilateral pyramidal disease (so-called pseudobulbar paralysis) as a change in subjective affect, so that the patient may be incorrectly thought to be depressed or euphoric.

The behavioral changes of temporal lobe epilepsy are relevant here. Some physicians have the idea that behavior disorders typically occur only during seizures, and that the patient is amnesic for the episode. The absence of amnesia is often thought to rule out epileptic behavior disorder. This is, however, a misleading rule. The behavioral changes associated with epilepsy are usually present *between* seizures and behavior disorder occurring only *during* a seizure is rare. Furthermore, in my experience the patient usually remembers acute episodes of anger quite distinctly. The claim of amnesia is often undertandably made by the patient when there is a threat of retribution.

The diagnostic difficulties of this borderland area between neurology and psychiatry should not be underestimated. Even expert observers can be misled for months or years. Let me cite only a few illustrative cases.

An atomic physicist on a mission abroad began to develop paranoid ideas about the stealing of atomic secrets. He was returned home, diagnosed as schizophrenic and hospitalized. After several months he suffered a grand mal seizure. He was seen again in consultation by an expert psychiatrist who felt that the clinical picture was so characteristically schizophrenic that organic causes could be dismissed as the cause of the psychosis. Within a short time, however, when severe headaches developed, the patient was referred for study and a temporal lobe glioblastoma was found.

A hard-driving and very successful business man in his thirties stopped sleeping with his wife shortly after his promotion to vice-president of his company. At his wife's insistence, he went into psychotherapy. It was only several months later that his work performance began to decline, followed by a deterioration in personal cleanliness. These were interpreted as signs of depression, for which the patient was eventaully hospitalized. Although he then developed incontinence, the possibility of organic disorder was still not considered until he became stuporous. He was found to have a large subfrontal tumor.

A previously highly successful young officer in the diplomatic corps was returned home because of a loss of interest in his work and a decline in his performance. Despite psychiatric help, he became increasingly apathetic about his work and he was dismissed. He took on a series of successively less attractive jobs and was finally employed keeping pigs. He was repeatedly diagnosed as a character disorder. He eventually developed severe headaches and was found to have a large craniopharyngioma that had compressed the undersurface of his frontal lobe.

A college student sought help because he was afraid that he might attack one of the girls in his classes. He was thought to be preschizophrenic and placed in psychotherapy. Within a year, he had become obviously paranoid and was hospitalized. It was not until about 2 years later that a movement disorder was noticed, although he had not been treated with phenothiazines. He was found to have Huntington's chorea.

The purpose of this chapter has been, to a great extent, a negative one. It has been my intention to point out that disease of the brain is an important and often treatable cause of behavior disorders, which occupies a special place in psychiatry, in terms of both practice and theoretical understanding. I have tried to discourage the notion that simple rules of thumb enable one to separate the organic from the functional. I have also attempted to show that not only is the organic disease erroneously diagnosed as functional, but it is also common to misdiagnose treatable functional disorders as irreversible organic disease. Above all, I have tried to convince the reader that in order to be an effective diagnostician, one must learn the natural course and clinical pictures of the different syndromes, just as one would have to do in any branch of medicine. One must be aware of the different clinical pictures of frontal lobe disorders and temporal lobe epilepsy, of the behavior disorders with which Huntington's chorea may present, or organic causes of tics, of the distinctive behavioral changes in different types of aphasia, of the characteristic pictures of hysterical pseudo-dementia on the one hand, and of depressive pseudo-dementia on the other, of the psychoses associated with various endocrine diseases. This is only a partial list. The following chapters should provide a useful beginning.

REFERENCES

1. Downer, J L de C: Interhemispheric Integration in the Visual Systems, in Mountcastle, V B (ed): Interhemispheric Relations and Cerebral Dominance. Baltimore, Johns Hopkins Press, 1962, pp. 87–100.
2. Flynn, J P: The Neural Basis of Aggression in Cats, in Glass, D C (ed): Neurophysiology and Emotion. New York, Rockefeller Univ., 1967, pp 40–59.
3. Malzberg, B: Important Statistical Data About Mental Illness, in Arieti, S (ed): American Handbook of Psychiatry, vol 1. New York, Basic Books, 1959, pp 161–174.
4. Roth, M: Ageing and Mental Diseases of the Aged, in Slater, E, Roth, M (eds): Clinical Psychiatry. London, Bailliéne, Tindall and Cassell, 1969, pp. 533–629.

Commentary

While providing a picture of the misconceptions concerning organic mental disorders that currently plague medical practice, Dr. Geschwind has also directed our attention to several of the more important problem areas. Several of these problems will be topics of discussion later in this volume. For instance, Dr. Geschwind has emphasized that depression may be mistaken for organic mental disorder. While depressed patients may appear demented, demented patients may also appear depressed. The interrelationship and differentiation of depression, dementia, and pseudodementia in the elderly will be discussed in detail in Chapter 6.

One of the foremost problems facing the individual interested in the borderland between neurology and psychiatry concerns nomenclature and the classification of organic mental disorders. It goes without saying that the present Standard Psychiatric Nomenclature is, at best, inadequate for the discussion of the organic mental syndromes. While it is easy to criticize the standard nomenclature, it is difficult to present a reasonable and rational alternative. The following presentation will attempt to do exactly that. At first reading, the proposed alterations may appear sweeping, and readers may be unwilling to accept many of the changes. The problem is very real, however, and these suggestions are worthy of consideration.

Zbigniew J. Lipowski, M.D.

2
Organic Brain Syndromes: Overview and Classification

The area of psychopathology causally related to physical, and especially cerebral, disease has been relatively neglected in the past several decades. This neglect has resulted partly from a reaction against the narrow viewpoint of the old-fashioned neuropsychiatry, which attempted to account for all mental illness in terms of neuropathology. Failure of this one-sided approach to the etiology of disorders of mental function and behavior provoked a swing to other extreme positions and led to an equally restricting focus on purely psychologic explanatory hypotheses as the chief concern of psychopathology. Somatic factors came to be largely disregarded and their etiologic role in psychiatric disorders ignored. The main directions in American psychiatry over the past several decades have tended to bypass the psychopathologic consequences of cerebral dysfunction and disease. The latter have remained a no-man's-land straddling the boundaries of psychiatry, neurology, and neuropsychology.

As a result, no area of psychiatry is so riddled with conceptual and semantic confusion, so poorly taught and full of obsolete views. Recent developments in the neurosciences, as well as growing appreciation that all psychiatric syndromes are multidetermined, have stimulated a renewed interest in the role of physical illness in general, and cerebral disorders in particular, as etiologic factors in psychologic dysfunction. Psychiatrists working as consultants on the medical, neurologic, and surgical wards have had ample opportunity in recent years to observe psychopathologic effects of organic diseases of all kinds[20,22]. The accumulated descriptive material allows a more balanced delineation of organic brain syndromes, their natural history and variants. Such study is of both theoretical and practical importance. It promotes further advances in the understanding of brain–behavior relationships in health and disease. On the practical side, development of this area of psychopathology is essential for improved methods of diagnosis, treatment, and prevention of behavior disorders caused by degenerative, vascular, toxic, and other diseases of the brain. Increased longevity, with the related frequency of chronic diseases, alcoholism, drug intoxication, and head trauma is chiefly responsible for the increasing incidence of organic brain syndromes. It is worth noting, for example, that 34.6 percent of patients 65 years of age and older discharged from general hospital psychiatric units in the United States between September 1970 and August 1971 were given the diagnosis of organic brain syndrome.[36]

The purpose of this chapter is to outline an organizing schema for the diagnosis and study of organic brain syndromes. This task includes a new classification, definitions of the syndromes, and a general discussion of the etiologic factors and pathogenic mechanisms involved in the psychopathology of cerebral disorders.

CLASSIFICATION

One may distinguish three major classes of psychiatric disorders causally related to organic disease:

1. Organic brain syndromes, that is, various constellations of psychopathologic symptoms resulting from brain damage or temporary metabolic derangement involving the brain as a whole or one of its parts.
2. Reactive syndromes, that is, psychoses, neuroses, personality, and behavioral disorders representing maladaptive modes of coping with a given somatic, including cerebral, disease and its subjectively distressing psychologic and social consequences.
3. Deviant illness behavior, such as self-destructive lack of compliance with or avoidance of medical management, massive denial of illness, regressive dependence, and other forms of behavior that do not fit into the current classification of psychiatric syndromes but that result in psychogenic invalidism or even death.

At the basis of these general groupings lies the assumption that some psychopathologic complications of organic illness are a direct effect of demonstrable cerebral damage or transient dysfunction and can best be accounted for in terms of neurophysiology, while others are more cogently explicated by using psychodynamic, learning, and sociocultural concepts and explanatory hypotheses. In the case of organic brain syndromes, the biologic substrate of man's symbolic processes is damaged or disturbed. In the case of reactive syndromes and deviant illness behavior, it is the *meaning* of illness-related information and distress for the particular individual and his attempts to cope with disability, symptoms, and so forth, that are the core determinants of psychopathology.[21] The latter is appropriately studied and explained by applying the methods and concepts of the behavioral sciences.

Psychiatric disorders have been traditionally classified into those caused by demonstrable brain damage and/or dysfunction and those in which evidence of cerebral pathology is either lacking or not considered to be a direct cause of the behavioral disorder. The former class of disorders constitutes the *organic brain syndromes*. Psychiatric syndromes belonging to the second category are referred to as *"functional."* This traditional dichotomy in psychiatric classification has a practical value, but it should not be viewed as sharp and immutable. Many gray areas exist that cannot be fitted readily into one or the other class of disorders. It suffices to mention depressive syndromes, which often accompany or follow viral infections, affective or schizophreniform psychoses arising in the course of Cushing's syndrome or systemic lupus erythematosus, and so on. Furthermore, it is generally acknowledged today that all disorders of behavior are *multidetermined*. There is yet heuristic value in distinguishing syndromes in which one or another class of etiologic factors, suggested by Zubin,[48] predominates. In the case of the organic brain syndromes, a pathologic process in the brain constitutes a necessary condition for their occurrence. In this limited sense, they have an etiologic implication. Limited, since their psychologic descriptive features allow only very tentative inferences about the nature and causes of the cerebral pathology and dysfunction. Psychologic symptoms provide only one set of relevant diagnostic criteria which must be supplemented by the use of neurologic, electroencephalographic, neuroradiologic, biochemical, and other nonpsychologic techniques for the identification of the type, location, and causation of the cerebral disorder. To diagnose an organic brain syndrome is practically important, however, since such a diagnosis draws attention to cerebral pathology whose nature and etiology must be identified as a basis for effective treatment, if such is currently available.

Organic brain syndromes may be defined as psychiatric syndromes resulting from cerebral damage (diffuse, focal, or both), and/or a temporary metabolic derangement involving the brain as a whole or some of its parts. "Cerebral damage" connotes destruction of neurons and is irreversible. All psychiatric syndromes represent clusters of specified psychologic impairments and abnormalities, or symptoms, that show a regular tendency to occur together. These syndromes, regardless of their etiology, are described in psychologic terms. This holds true also for the organic brain syndromes.

There is considerable confusion in the literature as to what criteria should be followed in the definition and diagnosis of organic brain syndromes. Clinical psychologists generally favor the concept of *"organicity,"* which connotes behavioral correlates of cerebral disease or damage. Some writers restrict the meaning of this concept to permanent or temporary impairment of so-called higher mental processes or highest integrative functions.[35] Chapman and Wolff[8] distinguish four categories of these functions:

1. The capacity for the expression of needs, appetites and drives
2. The capacity to employ effectively the mechanisms for goal achievement (learning, memory, perception, etc.)
3. The capacity to maintain appropriate thresholds and tolerance for frustration and anxiety and to recover rapidly from their effects
4. The capacity to maintain effective and well-modulated defense reactions

Reitan[31] asserts that it is misleading to consider "brain damage" as a meaningful diagnostic entity. He proposes that independent variables, such as whether the damage is diffuse, focal, focal and diffuse, or bilaterally focal; involvement of right or left cerebral hemisphere; lobular localization of areas of maximal involvement within each hemisphere; rate of onset and progression (if any) of the lesion; and category of the lesion in neuropathologic terms, that is, neoplastic, degenerative, vascular, traumatic, inflammatory, and so forth, are all relevant to psychologic effects. A major methodologic fallacy in neuropsychology has been to assume that brain lesions will produce a standard type of psychologic deficit, or at least cannot fail to cause psychologic defects. Neither of these assertions is supported by available evidence.[35]

Psychologic assessment of organicity includes mental status examination and the use of various batteries of psychologic tests designed to detect a range of "organic" signs. The level and type of performance on one or more psychologic tests, as compared with a normative standard, has commonly been used to identify organicity. Brain damage may produce in any individual three categories of psychologic signs: (1) a general deterioration in all aspects of functioning as compared to the subject's premorbid performance; (2) differential effects depending on the location, extent, and so forth, of the damage; and (3) highly specific effects if the damage occurs in a highly specialized area of the brain.[30] It follows that no single psychologic test is sufficient to identify both the presence and nature of organicity. For the purpose of diagnosis, organicity is assessed by tests of general intelligence, psychomotor functions, language and communicational skills, memory, learning, attention, aspects of perception and thinking. These psychologic abilities are impaired in various patterns and degrees of severity. It should be emphasized that the diagnosis of organicity depends heavily on the evidence of some degree of impairment of *cognitive functions*, that is, remembering, perceiving and thinking. More specifically, deficits of *abstraction, reasoning*, and *concept formation* are often considered as sensitive indicators of cerebral dysfunction. In general, detection of organicity has weighed strongly on signs of *impaired information processing*.

The approach of a clinician to the diagnosis and classification of psychopathologic effects of cerebral disorders differs from that of a neuropsychologist. Psychiatrists and neurologists are less concerned with defining and detecting "organicity" as the term is applied by psychologists. They are more likely to look for changes in a subject's *personality, affective state,* and *overall adaptive efficacy* as a source of diagnostic clues to an early detection of a cerebral disorder. Furthermore, clinicians tend to rely for their diagnostic inferences on observations made by the patient and/or other observers regarding the former's impaired performance and abnormal behavior in his everyday settings and tasks. Evidence of morbid *change* in subjective experience and objective performance provides an important diagnostic clue that may lead to formal psychologic and other special laboratory tests.

Organic brain syndromes, in contrast to organicity, are defined in terms of psychopathologic symptoms and signs elicited by history, mental status examination, and observations of patient's behavior in nonlaboratory settings. Furthermore, organic brain syndromes include those featuring aspects of mental functioning other than cognition, that is, motivation, affect, and impulse expression and control. In addition, an adequate classification of organic brain syndromes should reflect such variables as: (1) a relatively global versus selective psychologic impairment or abnormality; (2) rate of onset and duration of the syndrome; and (3) its degree of severity. These dimensions will be discussed in more detail after the following critique of the current "official" classification of organic brain syndromes.

The latest revision of the American Psychiatric Association's Diagnostic and Statistical Manual of Mental Disorders[11] revolves around a concept of *the* organic brain syndrome, which is defined as a "basic mental condition characteristically resulting from diffuse impairment of brain tissue function from whatever cause." This vague definition makes no allowance for the diversity of psychopathologic syndromes encountered in clinical practice that may result not only from diffuse, but also focal, or diffuse and focal, cerebral disease. The so-called "basic symptoms," according to the manual (p. 22), include:

1. impairment of orientation
2. impairment of memory
3. impairment of all intellectual functions, such as comprehension, calculation, knowledge, learning, etc.
4. impairment of judgment
5. lability and shallowness of affect

The above descriptive definition reflects an overly reductionistic conception of organic psychopathology. To speak of *the* organic brain syndrome is misleading, since it implies nonexistent homogeneity of psychiatric manifestations of cerebral disease and dysfunction. The adjective "basic" in this context is meaningless. In the majority of patients suffering from various types of cerebral tissue dysfunction, the impairment of the different mental capacities varies.[35] Relatively *uniform* impairment of a wide spectrum of psychologic functions corresponding to the "basic symptoms" does exist, but characterizes only *severe degrees* of widespread cerebral damage or metabolic derangement. Orientation, memory, judgment, and so forth, may be intact unless the brain disorder is relatively severe. The official definition makes no allowance for, say, frontal lobe syndrome, hallucinosis, and other incontrovertibly "organic" syndromes characterized by relatively circumscribed cognitive, motivational, and affective disorders. Lability and shallowness of affect are by no means a constant component of organic brain syndromes. Depression and anxiety are far more common, especially in the earlier stages and milder degrees of cerebral disorders. Anyone using the manual for diagnosis is liable to miss that which is practically most important: the early, the mild, the potentially reversible, the relatively selective and thus of localizing value, and the most eminently treatable psychologic impairment. There is an obvious need for a more differentiated and clinically useful classification of the syndromes designated "organic."

Two other features of the official classification call for comment. It propounds a division of the organic brain syndromes into *psychotic* and *nonpsychotic,* and *acute* and *chronic*. The former dichotomy imposes an ill-defined distinction of doubtful value in this area of psychopathology. "Acute" and "chronic," terms borrowed from medicine, have a connotation of rapid or gradual onset and of short or long duration, respectively. An *acute* brain syndrome is by official definition *reversible,* a *chronic* one, *irreversible*. This division is misleading. A reversible syndrome may set in gradually in the course of a chronic illness, like pernicious anemia or hypothyroidism, or follow a head injury and thus come on rapidly. An irreversible, "chronic," syndrome may come on acutely as a result of severe carbon monoxide poisoning or Wernicke's encephalopathy. Thus, the terms "acute" and "chronic," as they are used in the official classification, are ambiguous. It might be more logical to speak of reversible and irreversible syndromes. Reversibility, however, has disadvantages as a basis for classification. It is necessary to clarify whether reversibility refers to a cluster of psychopathologic symptoms or to the underlying cerebral disorder. For example, delirium is a reversible, "acute" brain syndrome par excellence. This implies that a set of symptoms that is called "delirium" never lasts permanently and always lifts within days or weeks, rarely months. This does not mean, however, that the patient's psychologic functioning will necessarily return to its premorbid level or that the integrity of the brain will be restored. In the majority of cases, delirium has a favorable outcome and is followed by restitution of the previous level of mental functioning. In some instances, however, it may be followed by coma and death, or by a different organic, such as the amnestic, syndrome, which may gradually clear up fully or only partially. Reversibility is not an all-or-none concept; it connotes *degrees* of restoration of the psychologic status quo. Its extent can often be established only retrospectively after a prolonged period of observation. Reversibility of psychologic impairment depends primarily on the nature of the underlying brain pathology and availability of specific treatment. In a strict sense, irreversibility should refer to *destruction of neurons* on the one hand, and the related *permanent psychologic deficits* on the other.

The classification of organic brain syndromes proposed herein combines traditional and novel features. It retains some of the ancient terms that many clinicians would like to see abolished. Yet, established terms, when clearly defined, are more useful than new ones, which tend to be ignored. The present classification is novel in that it distinguishes the relatively *global* (widespread) and *selective* (focal) organic brain syndromes. Further, within the global category, we distinguish three syndromes characterized by an *acute*, *subacute*, and *chronic* onset and/or course, respectively. These three syndromes—delirium, subacute amnestic–confusional state, and dementia —partly reflect the degree of reversibility of the psychopathology, although not necessarily of cerebral pathology. The global syndromes refer to those in which the core abnormality is a *relatively uniform impairment of cognitive or intellectual functions*. There are deficits in acquiring, evaluating, and retrieving information, and related impairment of learning ability, judgment, and capacity to use information for problem-solving and purposeful behavior. The term ''global'' does not imply that every patient displays equal impairment of every recognized higher mental function. The term connotes simultaneous or sequential impairment of cognitive functioning, but it does not gainsay the obvious fact that such impairment may vary in degree and need not be strictly uniform.

Relatively *selective* brain syndromes are labeled according to the predominant psychologic impairment or abnormality. The selective syndromes need formal recognition for several reasons. First, they are clearly distinct clinically from the more extensive global syndromes. Second, they point toward focal, rather than diffuse, cerebral pathology, and thus have a limited localizing diagnostic value. Third, they narrow the range of etiologic factors to look for. Fourth, they may require specific therapeutic measures designed to help the patient compensate for and cope with the given circumscribed defect.

The other novel feature of the classification is the proposed inclusion of syndromes that are usually classified as functional. These depressive, schizophreniform, paranoid, and manic syndromes may lack the features of "organicity," but they nevertheless appear to reflect specific derangement in some parts of the brain, such as the limbic system. They may be viewed as overlapping the organic and functional syndromes. To call these syndromes "toxic" or "infective–exhaustive" psychoses, as is often done in the literature, evades the issue of their pathogenesis. It can hardly be denied that they are caused partly by cerebral dysfunction and may clear up as the latter remits. These syndromes highlight the relativity of the organic–functional dichotomy in psychiatric classification.

The writer believes that this tentative modification of the classification of psychiatric disorders (Table 2-1) causally related to cerebral dysfunction reflects more faithfully observable facts and is clinically more useful than the current classification endorsed by the American Psychiatric Association.

Table 2-1
Classification of Organic Brain Syndromes

OBS with *global* cognitive impairment
  Delirium
  Subacute amnestic—confusional state
  Dementia
OBS with *selective* psychological deficit or abnormality
  Amnestic syndrome
  Hallucinosis
  Personality and behavior disorders
  Other circumscribed cognitive and psychomotor disorders
Symptomatic functional syndromes
  Schizophreniform
  Paranoid
  Depressive
  Manic

DEFINITIONS OF THE SYNDROMES

Bonhoeffer[5] recognized that somatic diseases can give rise to only a few psychiatric syndromes. He challenged the earlier views of Kraepelin and others who believed that every organic disease could lead to a distinct and diagnostically specific psychiatric disorder. Bonhoeffer distinguished five overlapping psychiatric syndromes occurring as a result of acute somatic illness: delirium, epileptiform excitement, twilight state, hallucinosis, and amentia. They were collectively designated as "exogenous psychic reaction types." The word "exogenous" in this context connoted the origin outside the brain. This was an erroneous view, since it is now generally acknowledged that both primarily cerebral diseases and systemic ones affecting the brain secondarily give rise to identical psychiatric syndromes[3] (See Chapter 3). The latter differ, however, in their clinical features, mode of onset, duration, and degree of reversibility.

The following are the descriptive definitions of the syndromes used in the classification proposed by the author.

Delirium is a transient psychiatric syndrome due to a widespread impairment of cerebral metabolism and consequent functional decompensation, and manifested clincially by a relatively global impairment of cognitive functioning. It represents one form of disordered (clouded) consciousness and is further defined by the following empirical criteria:

1. The onset is acute, generally a matter of hours or a few days.
2. The patient is awake and usually able to respond verbally.
3. There is evidence of impairment of attention, recent memory, thinking, and perception.
4. Cognitive impairment fluctuates in degree over time, but tends to be most severe at night.
5. There is impaired ability to process external and internal information inputs and relate them meaningfully to the patient's past experience and knowledge.
6. The patient manifests some degree of disorientation, that is, defective ability to orient himself in time and space, and a tendency to misidentify unfamiliar surroundings and persons for familiar ones.
7. There is in most cases a concomitant slowing, in some cases mixed with fact activity, of the background EEG frequencies which tends to vary pari passu with the level of awareness.
8. There is usually a disturbance of the normal sleep–wakefulness patterns, such as insomnia, daytime drowsiness, and, in some cases, intrusion of dreams into wakeful awareness.
9. Hallucinations and delusions may be present, but are not diagnostic.

The author uses the term delirium as synonymous with that of "acute confusional states" of other authors.[19] This syndrome is self-limited and rarely lasts more than several weeks. It typically accompanies an acute intracranial or systemic illness, but may, and often does, complicate chronic cerebral disease, especially in the elderly.

Two major clinical variants of delirium may be distinguished: *hyperac-*

tive and *hypoactive*. The former is characterized by marked psychomotor overactivity, excitability, a tendency to hallucinations and persecutory delusions, and a high degree of behavioral and autonomic arousal. This variant is typically seen in the withdrawal syndromes from alcohol and barbiturates, but is not confined to them. It may be associated with a lowered convulsive threshold and the appearance of mixed fast and slow EEG background frequencies. It is likely that this form of delirium is an expression of heightened cerebral cortical excitability and arousal associated with disorganization of cortical functions and corresponding clouding of consciousness. Normal sleep pattern is disrupted and intrusion of dream mentation in a wakeful state may occur (''oneiric'' delirium). The most extreme example of this variant is the so-called delirium acutum.[9]

The hypoactive variant of delirium features reduced psychomotor activity even to the point of stupor, apathy, somnolence during the day with or without nocturnal insomnia, reduced arousal and excitability, and generally slowed and impoverished thought processes. The patient is less likely to hallucinate than in the hyperactive state. The EEG background activity is predominantly or exclusively slowed. Wernicke's encephalopathy is a good example of this variant.

The two clinical variants of delirium may be regarded as two opposite poles of a continuum with common mixed forms in between. They likely reflect increased or decreased activity of the arousal system. Their unifying feature is the disorganization of cerebral cortical activity and the corresponding clouding of consciousness and global impairment of information processing. A necessary condition for the development of delirium is a widespread disturbance of cerebral metabolism.[19]

Subacute amnestic–confusional state (''reversible dementia'') designates an organic brain syndrome characterized by a potentially reversible global cognitive impairment, usually of insidious onset and/or protracted course. It consists of various constellations of cognitive deficits occurring in the absence, or with only a mild degree, of clouding of consciousness. This syndrome may follow an acute cerebral disorder, such as trauma or infection, or develop insidiously in the course of a chronic disorder: toxic, metabolic, neoplastic, and so forth. It may be viewed as an intermediate form between delirium and dementia.

An important practical reason for distinguishing this syndrome is to underscore the fact that slowly developed and/or protracted cognitive or intellectual impairment does not always signify irreversibility. Some authors refer to this syndrome as ''reversible dementia'' to stress its clinical similarity to the syndrome resulting from irreparable damage to the cerebral cortex. It is amenable to timely treatment[26] or resolves spontaneously over months or even a few years. This syndrome is most often seen after head injury, subarachnoid hemorrhage or encephalitis, or as a complication of pernicious anemia, chronic intoxication with barbiturates, bromides, or lead, a slow-growing, space-occupying, intracranial lesion, hypothyroidism, normal pressure hydrocephalus, hepatic or renal disease, and so forth.

Dementia is an organic brain syndrome due to cerebral cortical damage and characterized by a relatively global impairment of cognitive functions. It is further defined by the following criteria:

1. There is a decrement in the patient's intellectual functioning, as compared to his premorbid performance.
2. The cognitive deficits do not depend on a disorder of consciousness.
3. There is usually some degree of *personality change,* that is, either accentuation or alteration of the subject's characteristic personality style and traits.
4. The onset is sudden or insidious, course static or progressive, depending on the nature of the underlying brain pathology and its cause.
5. Not all cognitive functions are impaired to the same extent; some may be relatively intact, especially in the early stages of progressive dementia. Recent memory is usually the first cognitive function to be impaired.
6. There is evidence of cerebral damage, widespread or multifocal.
7. The EEG may be normal or show diffuse slowing of background activity and/or focal abnormalities (see Chapter 4). It is diagnostically less reliable than in cases of delirium.

It has been suggested that the term dementia is antiquated, ambiguous, and misleading.[37] There is no doubt that this word has acquired the narrow connotation of *severe* and *progressive* intellectual impairment associated with extensive cerebral cortical damage. The term may be retained, however, if it is generally agreed to use it in the sense proposed here. It must be emphasized that dementia, like any other syndrome, has *degrees of severity.* In its mild forms it may be relatively inconspicuous and manifest itself only in situations that are novel for the subject or demand a high level and speed of intellectual performance or information processing. Furthermore, the patient may effectively compensate for his deficits unless he is under stress and anxious or depressed. Functional decompensation may occur following bereavement or retirement, for example, and the patient may for a time manifest severe intellectual impairment that is still largely reversible. The concepts of *compensability* and *modifiability* of the cognitive deficits are useful in accounting for fluctuations in the patient's intellectual performance, which is to some extent independent of the severity of cerebral damage. The patient's premorbid level of adjustment and intelligence, his affective state, motivation, and access to environmental supports may help him compensate for even severe degrees of cerebral damage. These observations are relevant to diagnosis and management.

Amnestic syndrome designates an organic syndrome characterized by impairment of memory to a greater extent than that of any other cognitive function. The memory pathology is of two types: an impaired ability to recall information that had been acquired prior to the onset of illness *(retrograde amnesia)* and some degree of inability to form new memories *(anterograde amnesia)*. The extent of retrograde amnesia varies from patient to patient and often from one occasion to another. Older memories are less vulnerable than recent ones.[40] Anterograde amnesia implies a degree of incapacity for new learning. Amnestic syndrome may occur in the absence of any other cognitive impairment.[46] Many patients, however, display other symptoms, such as disorientation for time, defects in perception, impaired concept formation, lack of initiative and emotional blandness.[38] Confabulation may be present, but is neither an invariable nor a defining feature of the syndrome. There is often a striking lack of insight into the presence of memory deficit and a tendency to deny its existence. The patient is typically alert, responsive, has no clouding of consciousness or impairment of grasp of his surroundings and communications addressed to him. He is able to reason and solve problems within the limits of immediate attention.[38]

Amnestic syndrome may be reversible (transient) or irreversible. It must be stressed that any given patient may have potential for a partial or total recovery of his memory function. For example, a patient with Wernicke–Korsakoff encephalopathy, or one who has sustained head injury or suffered from encephalitis, may over a period of up to 2 years and occasionally longer show evidence of gradual recovery, partial or complete.[40]

Amnestic syndrome must be distinguished from memory pathology, which represents part of global cognitive impairment resulting from a widespread cerebral damage or metabolic derangement. The syndrome discussed here is selective in its psychologic manifestations and results from lesions of diencephalic–temporal structures, especially the medial dorsal nuclei of the thalamus, the mammillary bodies, and the hippocampal formations.[40]

Hallucinosis designates an organic brain syndrome in which hallucinations in one or more sensory modalities constitute the predominant, or only, psychologic abnormality. The additional diagnostic criteria are:

(1) lack of clouding of consciousness; (2) absence of a functional psychosis; and (3) recurrent or constant hallucinatory activity.

This syndrome, first defined by Wernicke in 1900, was included by Bonhoeffer among the so-called exogenous reaction types.[42] In the English literature, the term is most often used in regard to a variant of the alcohol withdrawal syndrome, the acute alcoholic hallucinosis. This, however, is not the only form of this syndrome. Hallucinosis may occur with intoxication from drugs, such as bromides, cocaine, or LSD. It can also be a manifestation of nontoxic conditions, including tumors compressing the optic nerves and chiasm, migraine, and diseases of the sense organs, such as bilateral cataracts or otosclerosis. In the last two conditions, concomitant cerebral disease appears to be needed for the hallucinosis to occur.[6]

The patient may display varying degrees of conviction that his hallucinations are real, that is, of external origin, or he may more or less firmly believe that they are internally derived. This aspect of hallucinosis determines whether the patient is considered psychotic or not. The more convinced he is about the veridical nature of his misperceptions and the more inclined to elaborate false beliefs regarding their source, the more delusional and psychotic he is deemed to be.

Personality and behavioral disorders are organic brain syndromes in which cognitive impairment is slight or absent, and pathology or affect, motivation, and/or behavior dominates the clinical picture.

The so-called frontal lobe syndrome provides a striking example of this type of brain syndrome. It combines mood changes (euphoria, irritability, apathy) with disorders of motivation and impulse control (impulsiveness, disinhibition, lack of initiative), as well as impaired appreciation of social norms and judgment. Thus, the syndrome comprises both deficient and excessive expression of affects and drives. Either may dominate the clinical picture or they may intermingle.

Bilateral thalamic lesions, induced by stereotaxic surgery for the treatment of tremor and rigidity in Parkinsonian patients, have resulted in reduced energy level, diminished responsiveness to environmental stimulation, and impaired emotional control.[33]

Lesions in the septal region, hypothalamus, and the medial temporal lobe may give rise to outbursts of rage and violent behavior.[28] Pathologic laughing and crying, with or without appropriate stimulation and corresponding affect, may accompany lesions of substantia nigra, cerebral peduncles, caudal hypothalamus, and ventral brain stem.[15]

Disorders of sexual behavior often accompany temporal lobe epilepsy.[4][39] A marked loss of libido, expressed by lack of desire for sexual intercourse and absence of erotic fantasies and dreams, has been reported in a large proportion of patients studied by Gastaut and Collomb.[12] Hypersexuality has been observed after bilateral rhinencephalic ablations. Transvestism[4] and exhibitionism[14] may be associated with temporal lobe epilepsy (see Chapter 10).

Ventromedial hypothalamic lesions may result in hyperphagia, outbursts of rage, and pathologic laughing and crying.[29]

Patholgic affects, such as fear, depression, or elation, may occur as ictal phenomena. Ictal depressions lasting from hours to weeks have been reported in patients suffering from uncinate fits. This type of depression could be due to subclinical hippocampal–amygdaloid–temporal lobe epilepsy.[43] Fear may be experienced with epileptic discharges from the anterior half of either temporal lobe.[45]

Thus, focal lesions in various areas of the brain—frontal, fronto-parietal, temporal, and parieto-occipital areas of the cortex, as well as in the corpus callosum, hypothalamus, and striathalamic region—may lead to conspicuous disorders of affect, mood, motivation, and to defective impulse control.[32] Such disorders may be accompanied by relatively little, if any, impairment of cognitive functions.

The psychopathologic manifestations discussed in this section have been accorded no place in the current "official" classification of the organic brain syndromes. This is illogical. It can hardly be denied that these syndromes result from cerebral lesions, usually focal ones, and that they are deviations from the normal. Thus, they fulfill the criteria for organically derived psychopathology, even though the intellectual capacity may be relatively or fully intact. These syndromes need to be included in the classification because of their diagnostic importance.

Other circumscribed cognitive, psychomotor, and/or perceptual disorders analogous to the amnestic syndrome, involve relatively selective psychologic impairment and/or abnormality in the absence of across-the-board intellectual deficits that are erroneously considered as the hallmark of organic mental disorders by the official classification.

Depersonalization syndrome, which implies a subjective sense of estrangement or unreality of one's environment, body, and/or self, may occur in inflammatory, neoplastic, toxic, and other cerebral disease.[1] It may be accompanied by other perceptual disturbances, including visual hallucinations, metamorphopsia (subjectively perceived alteration of the size of the objects—micropsia and macropsia), dysmorphopsia (alteration or distortion of shape), autoscopy (visual hallucination of the self), prosopagnosia (inability to recognize well-known faces), body image disturbances, and so forth. Parietal lobe disease and temporal lobe epilepsy may give rise to this syndrome.[10,17.]

Some patients may show relatively selective impairment of capacity for abstraction or of psychomotor performance, for example. Anyone looking for generalized intellectual deterioration or widespread derangement of information processing, which characterize the organic brain syndromes as officially defined, will be liable to overlook or ignore such subtle and relatively circumscribed deficits. Yet, the latter are no less "organic" than fully developed delirium or dementia. They have considerable diagnostic and practical significance for the physician and patient, respectively. The concept of the organic brain syndromes must be modified to accommodate various constellations or psychologic deficits and abnormalities.

Symptomatic functional syndromes refer to paranoid, schizophreniform, depressive, and manic psychoses, as well as depressive neuroses that are causally related to cerebral disorders. They may be accompanied by some constellation of cognitive deficits, but the latter may be absent.

The inclusion of these syndromes under the heading "organic" is controversial. Yet, they appear to have greater than chance association with some organic disorders. This does not gainsay the generally held belief that the majority of patients displaying one of these syndromes have no evidence of cerebral disease.

These syndromes are often vaguely called "toxic psychoses," since they may be caused by drugs, such as amphetamines, ephedrine, phenmetrazine, cortisone, ACTH, bromides, and so forth. Not only drugs can give rise to the symptomatic syndromes, however. They have been observed in infectious, neoplastic, metabolic, and endocrine disorders. It is sufficient to mention schizophreniform psychoses associated with limbic lesions; depressive syndromes often complicating Cushing's syndrome, viral infections, carcinoma of the body and tail of the pancreas, and Parkinson's disease; and paranoid psychoses due to quinacrine or amphetamines. Studies of these conditions may be expected to elucidate some of the metabolic pathways whereby cerebral functioning may be deranged to produce or facilitate an affective or personality disorder.

The question whether the above somatic disorders produce the various symptomatic syndromes or only trigger off a "preprogrammed" psychobiologic mechanism remains an open one. It is difficult to separate them from psychoses and neuroses that are best considered as reactive to the symbolic meanings of the given disease and its symptoms and consequences for the patient. These behavioral disorders span a wide spectrum of recognized psychiatric syndromes. It is plausible that at least some of the psychopathologic states having their onset in close temporal relationship to organic disease are manifestations of disordered cerebral metabolism or neurophysiologic dysfunction. The practical implication of this is that the clinician must always keep in mind the possibility that any given psychiatric disorder may be a manifestation of a somatic disease whose other symptoms it may overshadow and mask.

PATHOGENESIS OF THE ORGANIC BRAIN
SYNDROMES

Physical illness and injury constitute a major class of etiologic factors in disorders of mental function and behavior. Somatic disease of any type and origin may give rise to psychologic dysfunction through a variable constellation of the following potentially pathogenic and overlapping mechanisms[21]:

1. By causing irreversible damage to and/or temporary metabolic derangement in the brain.
2. By virtue of its disturbing subjective meaning, conscious and unconscious, for the individual and the resulting painful emotions and maladaptive modes of defending against them.
3. By impairing the patient's capacity to cope with his needs, conflicts, impulses, and affects, as well as with the demands of his social roles and tasks.
4. By altering the internal and/or external sensory inputs and feedback.
5. By changing the body image.
6. By disrupting the normal sleep–wakefulness pattern.

Any disease affecting the brain may also exert its effects on the individual's subjective experience and observable behavior through mechanisms 2 to 6 listed above. The extent to which these potentially psychopathogenic mechanisms are operating in a given subject, whether or not they give rise to a psychiatric disorder, and what form the latter takes will depend on the *complex interplay of multiple determinants inherent in the organic pathogenic factors, the patient, and his external environment.* The shared basis of the organic syndromes and the necessary condition for their occurrence is the presence of brain damage, cerebral metabolic derangement, or both. Psychobiologic and social factors influence the clinical manifestations, their severity and fluctuations, and thus the course and outcome of every brain syndrome. These factors tend to be most prominent when the cerebral disorder is mild or moderate and recede into the background as the mass of normally functioning cerebral cortical tissue diminishes.[8] The following summary of the relevant variables highlights the complexity of the determinants of the clinical picture in any given patient.

Characteristics of the Organic Factors

Absolute strength of the noxious agent. This refers to the quantitative aspects of the factors causing cerebral dysfunction. As a general rule, the higher the strength of the given noxious factor, the greater the probability that it will result in cerebral dysfunction. In turn, the greater the resulting deviation from homeostasis and normal cerebral functioning, the higher the incidence and severity of psychologic deficits and impairment of the subject's adaptive capacities. Examples are provided by the degree of hypoglycemia or hypoxia; degree of deviation from the normal blood pH and electrolytic concentration; amount of circulating toxin, such as ammonia or bromide; the force of impact of mechanical trauma to the head, and so forth.

Simultaneous presence of more than one pathologic factor. In many clinical conditions, a combination of pathogenic factors such as electrolytic imbalance, hypoxia, presence of toxins in the blood, and change in blood pH, potentiates their effectiveness in bringing about acute cerebral and functional decompensation. A common result is a global impairment of information processing exemplified by delirium. Instances include surgery,[25] infections,[41] or severe burns.[2]

Global or selective involvement or cerebral structures and functions. Metablic encephalopathies,[27] provide a good example of conditions that have a widespread effect on cerebral metabolism and usually bring about global impairment of higher mental functions. Delirium, subactue amnestic–confusional state, and/or dementia are the common consequences. Lesions involving the reticular formation of the brain stem are liable to result in a severe depression of consciousness, manifested as stupor, akinetic mutism, or coma. Certain drugs and viruses show specific affinity for certain cerebral structures, such as those composing the limbic system. Their psychologic effects appear to depend on the particular biochemical and pathophysiologic processes that they set in motion. LSD-25, for example, induces abnormal hypersynchrony (theta activity) in the hippocampus[18] and depresses the firing rate of the serotonergic raphé nuclei, which trigger show-wave sleep.[24] Similarly, thiamine deficiency is known to produce damage to diencephalic structures and a subsequent amnestic syndrome.

Rate of change in the physical–chemical milieu of the brain. The higher the rate of such change, the more likely is one to encounter an acute disturbance of consciousness, be it coma, epileptic seizure, akinetic mutism, or delirium. A rapidly rising intracranial pressure, sudden drop in blood glucose or serum calcium concentration, and other changes all favor a rapid onset of clouding of consciousness of varying degree of severity. A slow-growing brain tumor, chronic intoxication with barbiturates or carbon monoxide, gradually failing secretion of the thyroid gland, pernicious anemia—all these conditions tend to modify the natural history of the associated psychopathology in the direction of gradual onset and subacute or chronic course.

Duration of cerebral pathology. On the whole, the longer the pathologic process lasts, or the more often it recurs, the more likely is an irreversible and progressive psychopathologic syndrome to result. Examples are provided by prolonged nutritional deficiencies, chronic hypoxia, hypothyroidism, normal pressure hydrocephalus, repeated head trauma in boxers, recurrent severe hypoglycemic episodes, chronic subdural hematoma, and so forth.

Static versus progressive nature of pathology. Brain damage sustained as a result of severe head injury, acute carbon monoxide intoxication, or heart block is liable to result in some degree of *stationary* psychologic deficit, global and/or selective. Unless such a defect is both relatively global and profound, the patient has time to develop more or less effective compensatory functions or strategies that may allow him to attain a reasonable degree of adjustment and competence. Rapidly progressive pathology, such as an invasive malignant neoplasm, strains the patient's adaptive capacity to the breaking point and makes him prone to a breakdown of his coping and defense mechanisms and to related psychologic decompensation, resulting in delirium, functional psychosis, or both. In the acute stage of a diffuse cerebral pathology, as after severe head injury, or with a rapidly growing brain tumor, one is likely to see various patterns of gross denial of illness and disability.[44] Irregularly progressive cerebral pathology, as in cerebrovascular disease, introduces elements of uncertainty and unpredictability for the patient and, especially in the early stages, may give rise to severe depression and/or anxiety, sometimes with suicidal tendencies, and deployment of ego mechanisms of defense with resulting neurotic and/or psychotic symptoms.

Characteristics of the Host

Age. The same organic etiologic factor is liable to have different psychopathologic effects, depending on the age of the patient. Infection, intoxication, head trauma, or brain tumor in a child, adolescent, or young adult is most likely to result in delirium or amnestic–confusional state with somnolence and irritability. An irreversible brain damage of mild-to-moderate severity in this age group is liable to lead to behavioral disorders and circumscribed cognitive deficits, rather than to a typical dementia or amnestic syndrome.

In the age group of 40–60 years, there is an increasing tendency for chronic cerebral pathology to give rise to an *alteration of personality* with or without global or selective cognitive impairment. It is a good clinical rule to consider cerebral disease, primary or secondary, in anyone over 40 who presents with a ''personality change'' of any type and of recent onset.

In people 60 years old and over, there is a high incidence of some degree of cortical neuronal loss. Such brain damage may be well compensated and not apparent to the patient's environment, yet it predisposes him to cognitive decompensation in response to a wide range of noxious factors that would fail to have such consequences in a person with an intact brain. A mild respiratory or urinary infection, general anesthesia, dehydration, drugs, and so forth may precipitate delirium in the elderly. Cognitive disorganization in the aged may also follow psychologic stress, such as bereavement. Such acute decompensation may be readily reversed if appropriate management is promptly instituted, but there is an increased risk that a permanent intellectual deficit may be the aftermath of delirium in the elderly.

Differential vulnerability to a given pathogenic factor. It is a common clinical observation that individuals of the same age, and otherwise healthy, differ widely in their readiness to manifest cognitive and behavioral decompensation in response to the same type and dose of a drug, or to an equal degree of deviation from the normal of the concentration of various chemical constituents of the blood, such as oxygen, CO_2, glucose, or electrolytes. The determinants of such differential vulnerability are unknown, but are postulated to reflect genetic and/or acquired neurophysiologic and psychologic predisposition. An example of the acquired susceptibility is provided by a tendency of subjects with temporal lobe damage following head trauma to develop acute, pathologic alcoholic intoxication with violent behavior.[23]

Idiosyncrasy to specific drugs is another instance of selective vulnerability. Some people become delirious and may show various allergic symptoms in response to therapeutic doses of commonly used drugs, such as digoxin, antihistamines, tricyclic antidepressants, minor tranquilizers, or penicillin.

Addiction to alcohol, sedatives, and hypnotics predisposes to delirium and hallucinosis when blood levels of these agents drop rapidly following reduced intake or vomiting.

Personality factors. There is evidence that some individuals are more likely to respond with cognitive disorganization and/or a symptomatic functional psychosis to a wide variety of factors that impair normal cerebral functioning, be they chemical agents, fever, or sensory and sleep deprivation. This enduring psychologic predisposition is still poorly understood. It appears that the perceptual–cognitive style of field dependence may be one such predisposing factor.[7] Trait anxiety, reflecting relative inadequacy to employ ego mechanisms of defense, may be another. It is a common clinical observation that some people react with intense anxiety, thought disorder, body image disturbances, feelings of depersonalization, paranoid ideation, and/or hallucinations to any factor that causes even mild clouding of consciousness with impaired cognitive and perceptual functioning.

Sleep deprivation and/or fragmentation. These factors appear to facilitate the onset and increase the severity of delirium, especially in the elderly.[16] Sleep deprivation potentiates the deliriogenic effect of scopolamine and hallucinogenic properties of LSD.[34]

Presence of chronic systemic disease–renal, cardiovascular, autoimmune, hepatic, or pulmonary. These diseases may give rise to delirium, subacute amnestic–confusional state, or dementia, not only as a result of the specific metabolic derangement that they cause, but also because of impaired metabolism and detoxification of drugs, increased tendency to hypotension or hypertension and cerebral hypoxia, and greater susceptibility to infection.

Preexistent brain damage of any origin. Such brain damage predisposes to delirium.

Current emotional state. Not only enduring personality traits, but also the patient's current emotional state resulting from intense intrapsychic or interpersonal conflicts related to the symbolic meaning and other personal consequences of his illness, or to bereavement, or to other subjectively disturbing factors, may adversely affect his cognitive functioning, already impaired as a result of cerebral damage and/or metabolic derangement. Anxiety, depression, apathy, and euphoria may enhance cognitive disorganization and interfere with motivation, thus further impairing the subject's performance and capacity to compensate for psychologic deficits.

Characteristics of the Environment

Sensory input underload or overload. Either of these factors alone may cause some degree of cognitive impairment and abnormal behavior.[13,47] Susceptibility to the effects of these variables shows striking interindividual differences, as well as changes in the same person at different ages and in different situations. Elderly people are on the whole more vulnerable to the disorganizing effects of excessive or deficient sensory inputs. These factors may facilitate the onset and increase the severity of delirium, as well as enhance cognitive deficits in the brain—damaged.

Social isolation. This factor may have effects similar to those of sensory deprivation. It is of particular importance in the elderly and increases their cognitive deficits.

Unfamiliarity of the surroundings. It is a common clinical experience to observe acute cognitive decompensation when an elderly person is admitted to a hospital or moved to some unfamiliar environment. Widespread brain dysfunction, reversible or not, always impairs information processing to some extent. Such processing may be further compromised by information inputs that are novel, ambiguous, or discrepant. A common clinical example of this is provided by the intensive care units.

Quality of interpersonal relationships. Crises in interpersonal relations brought about by personally significant losses or conflicts are liable to elicit dysphoric affects, such as anger, grief, depression, and anxiety, and thus influence adversely an individual's ability to compensate for and cope with cognitive impairment of any origin.

Thus, multiple variables related to the causal organic factors, the spatial–temporal and other features of the resulting cerebral pathology, as well as those inherent in the patient and his environment, influence the form, clinical manifestations, severity, course, and prognosis of the organic brain syndromes. *All these factors have to be taken into account in planning diagnostic procedures and management of the patient.*

SUMMARY

The proposed classification of the organic brain syndromes embodies the following postulates:

1. It is practically useful to distinguish between syndromes due to demonstrable cerebral disease or dysfunction on the one hand, and those whose occurrence is more cogently explicated in terms of genetic, psychodynamic, sociocultural, developmental, and learning concepts and explanatory hypotheses, on the other. The criterion of "demonstrability" expresses no more than the limits of the present knowledge of cerebral processes and the methods for detecting their derangement.
2. The "organic" and the "functional" psychiatric syndromes depend on cerebral activity, are multidetermined, and represent a continuum, rather than a dichotomy. Their etiology is heterogeneous and includes varying contributions of a range of causal factors. The same syndrome may be the final common path for many etiologic factors, and the same factor may give rise to more than one syndrome.
3. The organic brain syndromes are viewed as a direct psychologic manifestation of brain damage, temporary cerebral metabolic derangement, or both. As such, they are distinguished from those psychiatric disorders that are more cogently accounted for by explanatory hypotheses using psychologic concepts. Admittedly, this distinction is a relative one, but it facilitates appropriate choice of diagnostic and therapeutic measures.

4. It is logical and clinically useful to distinguish between organic brain syndromes characterized by relatively global or by selective psychologic impairment, respectively.
5. Impairment of cognitive or intellectual functions is a common characteristic of organic brain syndromes, but it is not a necessary and invariable manifestation of cerebral dysfunction. Disorders of personality, motivation, and affect may be the only such manifestation in some cases.
6. Descriptive syndromes represent static and cross-sectional symptom clusters. The value of the descriptive classification is enhanced if *temporal* features of symptomatology are included. The *mode of onset* and *behavior over time* of the psychiatric disorder provide additional etiologic, diagnostic, and prognostic clues. Thus, every brain syndrome should be described not only in terms of its component sysmptoms, but also its mode of onset and course, which may be acute, subacute, or chronic. The syndrome is acute when its onset is sudden *and* its course short, that is, days or weeks; subacute, when the onset is insidious and/or the course protracted, that is, months or years; and chronic, when, regardless of the mode of onset, there is evidence that an irreversible cerebral pathology is present or, retrospectively, when the syndrome is judged to be irreversible on the basis of its course and lack of response to appropriate treatment.

REFERENCES

1. Ackner B: Depersonalization. I. Aetiology and phenomenology. J Ment Sci 100:838–853, 1954
2. Antoon AY, Volpe JJ, Crawford JD: Burn encephalopathy in children. Pediatrics 50:609–616, 1972
3. Bleuler M, Willi J, Bühler HR: Akute psychische Begleiterscheinungen Körperlicher Krankheiten. Stuttgart, Thieme, 1966
4. Blumer D, Walker AE: Sexual behavior in temporal lobe epilepsy. Arch Neurol 16:37–43, 1967
5. Bonhoeffer K: Die Psychosen im Gefolge von akuten Infektionen, Allgemeinerkrankangen und inneren Erkrankungen, in Aschaffenburg GL (ed): Handbuch der Psychiatrie, Spez. Teil 3. Leipzig, Deuticke, 1912, pp 1–60
6. Burgermeister JJ, Tissot R, De Ajuriaguerra J: Les hallucinations visuelles des ophtalmopathes. Neuropsychologia 3:9–38, 1965
7. Cartwright RD: Dream and drug-induced fantasy behavior. Arch Gen Psychiatry 15:7–15, 1966
8. Chapman LF, Wolff HG: Disease of the neopallium and impairment of the highest integrative functions. Med Clin North Am 677–689, 1958.
9. Chrisstoffels J, Thiel JH: Delirium acutum, a potentially fatal condition in the psychiatric hospital. Psychiatr Neurol Neurochir 73:177–187, 1970

10. Critchley M: The Parietal Lobes. London, Arnold, 1953
11. Diagnostic and Statistical Manual of Mental Disorders (ed 2). Washington, DC, American Psychiatric Association, 1968
12. Gastaut H, Collomb H: Etude du comportement sexuel chez les épileptiques psychomoteurs. Ann Med Psychol (Paris) 112:657–696, 1954
13. Gottschalk LA, Haer JL, Bates DE: Changes in social alienation, personal disorganization and cognitive-intellectual impairment produced by sensory overload. Arch Psychiatry 27:451–457, 1972
14. Hooshmand H, Brawley BW: Temporal lobe seizures and exhibitionism. Neurology 19:1119–1124, 1969
15. Ironside R: Disorders of laughter due to brain lesions. Brain 79:589–609, 1956
16. Johnson LC: Physiological and psychological changes following total sleep deprivation, in Kales A (ed): Sleep, Physiology and Pathology. Philadelphia, Lippincott, 1969
17. Kenna JC, Sedman, G: Depersonalization in temporal lobe epilepsy and the organic psychoses. Psychiatry 111:293–299, 1965
18. Killam KF Jr: Pharmacological aspects of limbic function, in Hocking CH (ed): Limbic System Mechanisms and Autonomic Function. Springfield, Ill, Thomas, 1972
19. Lipowski ZJ: Delirium, clouding of consciousness and confusion. J Nerv Ment Dis 145:227–255, 1967
20. Lipowski ZJ: Review of consultation psychiatry and psychosomatic medicine. II. Clinical aspects. Psychosom Med 29:201–224, 1967
21. Lipowski ZJ: The patient, his illness and environment. Psychosocial foundations of medicine, in Arieti S, (eds): American Handbook of Psychiatry (ed 2) Vol. 4, New York, Basic Books, (in press).
22. Lipowski ZJ, Kiriakos RZ: Borderlands between neurology and psychiatry: Observations in a neurological hospital. Psychiatry Med 3:131–147, 1972
23. Marinacci AA, von Hagen KO: Alcohol and temporal lobe dysfunction. Behav Neuropsychiatry 3:2–11, 1972
24. Morgane PJ, Stern WC: Relationship of sleep to neuroanatomical circuits, biochemistry, and behavior. Ann NY Acad Sci 193:95–111, 1972
25. Morse RM, Litin EM: Postoperative delirium: A study of etiologic factors. Am J Psychiatry 126:388–395, 1969
26. Nicol CF: Treatment of reversible dementia. NY State J Med 70:2432–2437, 1970
27. Plum F, Posner JB: The Diagnosis of Stupor and Coma. Philadelphia, Davis, 1966
28. Poeck, K: Pathophysiology of emotional disorders associated with brain damage, in Vinken PJ, Bruyn GW (eds): Handbook of Clinical Neurology, vol 3. Amsterdam, North-Holland, 1969
29. Reeves AG, Plum F: Hyperphagia, rage, and dementia accompanying a ventromedial hypothalamic neoplasm. Arch Neurol 20:616–624, 1969
30. Reitan RM: Psychological deficit. Ann Rev Psychol 13:415–444, 1962
31. Reitan RM: Psychological testing of neurological patients, in Youmans JR

(ed): Neurosurgery: A Comprehensive Reference Guide to the Diagnosis and Management of Neurosurgical Problems. Philadelphia, Saunders, 1973

32. Riggs HE, Rupp C: A clinico-anatomic study of personality and mood disturbances associated with gliomas of the cerebrum. J Neuropathol Exp Neurol 17:338–345, 1958

33. Riklan M, Levita E: Subcortical Correlates of Human Behavior. Baltimore, Williams & Wilkins, 1969

34. Safer DJ, Allen RP: The central effects of scopolamine in man. Biol Psychiatry 3:347–355, 1971

35. Smith A: Ambiguities in concepts and studies of "brain damage" and "organicity." J Nerv Ment Dis 135:311–326, 1962

36. Statistical Note 68: Department of Health, Education, and Welfare. Washington, DC, February 1973

37. Stengel E: Psychopathology of dementia. Proc Roy Soc Med 57:911–914, 1964

38. Talland GA: The psychopathology of the amnesic syndrome. Mod Probl Psychiatry Neurol 1:443–469, 1964

39. Taylor DC: Sexual behavior and temporal lobe epilepsy. Arch Neurol 21:510–516, 1969

40. Victor M: The amnesic syndrome and its anatomical basis. Can Med Assoc J 100:1115–1125, 1969

41. Wallace JF: Infectious delirium. Southwest Med 50:181–183, 1969

42. Walther-Büel H: Le syndrome de l'hallucinose. Psychiat Neurol 152:345–362, 1966

43. Weil AA: Ictal emotions occurring in temporal lobe dysfunction. Arch Neurol 1:87–97, 1959

44. Weinstein EA, Kahn RL: Denial of Illness. Springfield, Ill, Thomas, 1955

45. Williams D: The structure of emotions reflected in epileptic experiences. Brain 79:29–67, 1956

46. Zangwill OL: The amnesic syndrome, in Whitty CWM, Zangwill OL (eds): Amnesia. London, Butterworths, 1966

47. Zubek JP (ed): Sensory deprivation: Fifteen Years of Research. New York, Appleton-Century-Crofts, 1969

48. Zubin J: Classification of the behavior disorders. Ann Rev Psychol 18:373–406, 1967

Commentary

The teaching of acute (reversible) and chronic (irreversible) disorders has always been totally unsatisfactory. It was sheer nonsense to change a diagnostic label from chronic to acute when the patient's mental state cleared, particularly when such recovery may have occurred several months after the onset. The introduction of an intermediate state along with sharper guidelines between dementia and delirium is clearly a useful step.

All of the subheadings in this classification deserve further discussion, and many will be discussed in subsequent chapters. In particular, the editors believe that the personality and behavioral changes produced by focal organic lesions deserve much more attention than they usually receive. These problems will be discussed in part in Chapters 8, 9, and 10.

The reader is reminded that the classification presented by Dr. Lipowski is novel and has not been used by the other contributors to this volume. A certain confusion of terminology could not be avoided, but in truth, this semantic confusion quite accurately reflects the current state of the art.

Of all types of organic mental disorders, one of the least understood by present day psychiatrists concerns the acute organic mental syndromes. For detailed discussion of this problem, the editors have called upon Professor Manfred Bleuler. His presentation has already been published in German,[1] but has not appeared previously in English. It was considered of sufficient importance to merit translation for an English audience.

It should be noted that what Manfred Bleuler discusses under the title "Acute Exogenous Reaction Types" is referred to as "delirium," "the acute brain syndrome," and "the acute confusional state" in contemporary usage. Also, note the emphasis of the plural in the title: Acute Exogenous Reaction Types. Differentiation of the various types is essential for diagnosis, prognosis and treatment, and is discussed in the next chapter.

REFERENCES

1.   Bleuler M, Willi J, Bühler HR: Akute psychische Begleiterscheinungen körperlicher Krankheiten. Stuttgart, Thieme, 1966

Manfred Bleuler, M.D.

3
Acute Mental Concomitants of Physical Diseases

BONHOEFFER'S CONCEPT OF THE ACUTE EXOGENOUS REACTION TYPE

It is common knowledge that severe acute physical illness is frequently accompanied by mental disturbances; few escape painful experiences of this kind. Mental illness resulting from physical illness is observed by every physician as part of his daily routine, a fact documented in the scientific literature as far back as the history of medicine is recorded.

Until the late 1800s, the medical profession was totally alien to the idea that the mental concomitants of acute physical illness could be systematically sorted out and their symptoms separated from mental disturbances that have their roots elsewhere. For decades after the development of psychiatry as a discipline in its own right—way beyond the middle of the nineteenth century—no relationship between psychopathologic manifestations and acute physical disorder was detected. Among the causes of psychiatric illness, the most diverse physical diseases were mentioned in the same breath as overwork, ill-fated love affairs, sudden reverses of fortune, modern haste and stress (there were complaints of modern haste and stress as long as a century ago), unbearable working conditions in factories, and "hereditary taint." The opinion prevailed that these and many other circumstances would lead to identical mental derangement. It was still unknown whether, and to what extent, these causes or clusters of causes would result in *specific* psychopathologic syndromes, and it was even less possible to establish a causal therapy from the existing psychopathologic symptomatology. Accordingly, the concept of a "unitary psychosis" was widely accepted; it was believed that any traumata affecting the psyche could result in any of the psychopathologic syndromes. This idea was developed by, among others, Morel (1809–1873) in Paris. According to him, mental disturbances of all types indicated "deterioration" or "degeneration," caused by the most diversified acquired as well as inherited traumata.

By the end of the last century, the view was first established that, on the contrary, each specific insult would lead to a specific clinical picture, that is, each individual physical illness would result in a particular mental disturbance. This conviction was enhanced by the brilliant progress of bacteriology which ascribed a specific pathologic syndrome to a specific pathogenic species of microbe. Small wonder, therefore, that the Linnean system once more became, semiconsciously, the idol of psychopathology. The designation of illnesses with Latin generic names (for example, chorea minor, typhus abdominalis), like plants and animals, stood in high repute.

The German psychiatrist Emil Kraepelin[7] (1855–1926) sought with particular earnestness and devotion to further this new concept scientifically. He attempted to ascribe a specific psychic disturbance to each type of physical insult, especially to each exogenous or endogenous poison. How profoundly he was fascinated by this aim is apparent from such statements as "It is with particular satisfaction that I consider the fact that, according to the results of our experiments, each individual substance discussed here corresponds to a fully characteristic effect on our psychic life" (from Kraepelin's book *On the Influence of Certain Medicaments on Simple Mental Processes,* 1892; the medicaments investigated for their influence on the psyche were alcohol, tea, paraldehyde, morphine, chloral hydrate, ether, and others).

Attempts were also made to ascribe a specific mental disturbance not only to each poisonous substance, but to each metabolic disorder and each infectious disease. Psychic concomitants of infections were not only differentiated according to the pathogen, but in terms of other variables: If they arose during an episode of fever, they were ascribed to the fever; if they occurred prior to the increase in temperature, they were ascribed to the toxin of the specific pathogen; if they became evident after termination of the illness, they were considered phenomena of exhaustion. It was expected that the psychoses resulting from fever, infection, and exhaustion could be symptomatologically differentiated.

But this turned out not to be the case, as did many other hypotheses based on the assumption that each specific physical illness was associated with its own specific psychosis.

It was left to Karl Bonhoeffer[3] (1868–1948), at that time a resident of Breslau, to recognize the essence of the relationship between physical illness and acute mental disturbance. First, he determined that the majority of acute mental disturbances caused by physical illness display a clinical picture that differs widely from the numerous psychoses that arise without physical illness (that is, from the ''endogenous'' psychoses—dementia praecox and manic–depressive illness—and also from psychoreactive disturbances). According to Bonhoeffer, the psychoses accompanying acute physical illness run their course as symptomatologically specific ''exogenous psychic reaction types.'' They were subsequently given the comprehensive designation, in the singular, of ''acute exogenous reaction type of Bonhoeffer.'' Next, Bonhoeffer noted that within the overall framework of the acute exogenous reaction type, the symptomatology of a psychic disturbance is by no means primarily dependent on the type of physical illness causing it. Accordingly, the psychopathologic syndrome arising from physical illness must be determined by circumstances other than the nature of the physical disease. Entirely different physical illnesses can lead to identical psychopathologic syndromes.

This teaching, for which we are indebted to Bonhoeffer, occupies a middle ground between the two earlier views: the one assuming that physical disabilities (as all other traumata affecting the psyche could lead to any given psychosis, and the other postulating a single specific psychopathologic syndrome for each individual physical illness. Time has proved that Bonhoeffer's teaching most closely represents the facts.

This can be formulated simply: *All acute mental concomitants of physical diseases can be fitted in the overall framework of the acute exogenous reaction type*. This reaction type is fundamentally different from psychic disturbances that occur independently of physical illness. However, within the framework of the acute exogenous reaction type, no specific connections between the type of physical illness and the mental syndrome can be established. The circumstances determining more precisely the symptomatology within the framework of the acute exogenous reaction type remained to be investigated following Bonhoeffer's fundamental work.

The term ''exogenous'' derives from the ancient concept that the body is an entity separate from the brain and in particular from what was originally conceived as the ''psyche.'' An exogenous insult, then, signifies anything that penetrates from the extracerebral sphere into the brain and mind and there wreaks damage. Without this semantic insight, it could be easily assumed that psychologic reactions to a shattering experience (such as a reactive depression or the paralysis from fear) are exogenous. In common usage, however, this is not so. Exogenous disturbances may be defined as those that derive from the *body* and lead to mental disturbances.

Singular or plural? The acute exogenous reaction type or the acute exogenous reaction types? Bonhoeffer employed the plural. Gradually and imperceptibly, the singular has also taken hold. I prefer the singular. We are dealing pathogenetically with a single type of mental illness—that which manifests a mental disturbance as a result of physical illness. If the "type" refers not to the pathogenesis but to the clinical picture, then it is admittedly arbitrary whether the singular or the plural is used. The use of the singular can also be justified because the syndromes alternate and, for the most part, are mixed with each other. Perfectly pure syndromes, independent of one another, are rarely seen. In addition, if the plural were used, the temptation would be great to use the term "exogenous" in the sense that a psychic trauma had come to the patient from sources outside the body.

Bonhoeffer's theory has grown slowly but steadily, and has become increasingly significant for psychiatric thinking. To be sure, in the textbooks and handbooks published in the meantime, the concept was dealt with only brieflly, and hardly in accordance with its significance. Conrad does discuss it extensively in *Psychiatrie der Gegenwart*[4] but he concerns himself primarily with the "Gestalt change" of psychic experience. He examines how the individual psychopathologic symptoms are the manifestation of changes in the totality of psychic life, but worries little whether these changes are palpably rooted in the body. A large number of short contributions, and scattered remarks in publications on other subjects, have added significantly to the development of Bonhoeffer's concept. Above all, many clinicians have adopted the concept into their psychiatric thinking, and it has thus been broadened and kept alive in dialogues between psychiatrists.

Surprisingly, even though he remained active for 36 years after offering the concept of the acute exogenous reaction type, Bonhoeffer himself did not participate in its further development. It is an open question why he avoided doing so. Perhaps it was due to the fact that he had carried out his investigations as an empiricist and observer, and because of natural modesty could not propose his concept as a basic principle of psychiatric thinking.

The most significant extensions of Bonhoeffer's concept are the following:

1. Whereas Bonhoeffer addressed only a limited number of physical illnesses as causes of mental disturbances of the acute exogenous type, it now appears that *every* severe physical disturbance that affects the mind leads to acute disturbances within the framework of this reaction type.
2. The symptomatologic frame drawn by Bonhoeffer has had to be widened.
3. It is now possible to differentiate more simply, more clearly, and more naturally among the clinical syndromes within the overgrown framework of the acute exogenous reaction type by grouping them into three series of syndromes.
4. For each of these three series, characteristic relations to pathogenesis, diagnosis, prognosis, and therapy can be established.

The three series of syndromes will be discussed in the following sections.

However, it should first be noted that investigators concerned with the relationship between physical causes and psychopathologic syndromes followed divergent paths and arrived at different conclusions in France, England, and the United States.

The leading French schools were primarily concerned with classifying the acute psychic disturbances according to gradations in the *dissolution de la conscience,* with the term *conscience* used in a somewhat different sense than the German *Bewusstsein. Conscience* refers not only to clarity and light in mental life, but also to an active principle that creates clarity and order. Following the neurologic theories of Hughlings Jackson, investigations sought the order in which mental processes dissolved under the influence of the most diversified acute insults. This line of inquiry was most fruitfully pursued by Henri Ey.[6] He classified acute mental disorders, quite independent of cause, by the degree and type of breakdown of rational behavior, internal coherence, and inner clarity. This produced superb insights into the structure of psychic life, but by virtually disregarding the problem of causal damage, excluded causal prophylaxis and therapy from the clinical picture.

At about the same time as Bonhoeffer, Adolf Meyer (1866–1950) worked out his theory of "reaction types" in the United States. One of his significant contributions, "The Problems of Mental Reaction-Types, Mental Causes and Diseases,"[8] appeared in 1908, 4 years before Bonhoeffer's principal publication. Meyer developed the concept of "ergasia" for orderly and rational activity, by which he meant something resembling the term *conscience* used by many French investigators. The reaction type designated by him as "dysergasia" includes most of the psychopathologic syndromes that Bonhoeffer described within the framework of the acute exogenous reaction types. In addition, however, Meyer also included deliriumlike conditions without physical causes. On the other hand, some of Meyer's other reaction types embrace clinical pictures that result from acute physical illnesses; his "anergasia" corresponds to the amnestic psychosyndrome, and his "thymergasia" covers mood changes of widely divergent origins, including physical causation. Meyer searched for physical, environmental, and constitutional causes in each of his reaction types.

Important schools of thought in the Anglo-American region were also not inclined to differentiate between physically determined mental disturbances and those otherwise determined. Rather, they attempted to elucidate the psychologic significance of each mental disturbance, including those of physical origin. The psychiatrist of this school devotes himself primarily to the analytically oriented investigation of psychodynamics and leaves the clarification of physical causes to the internist and the neurologist. He often relies on the psychologist for evidence of the physical origin of a psychopathologic picture, rather than on his own clinical findings. Accordingly, many Anglo-American schools, including the leading ones, scarcely concerned themselves with the development of Bonhoeffer's concept of the acute exogenous reaction type. Instead, the psychoanalytic investigation of the physically ill was promoted, neurologic diagnostics were extended, and a vast, statistically oriented investigation of the reactions of the physically ill in a variety of test situations was carried out, all in very loose connection with one another.

Clinical psychopathologic research—and not just test-oriented psychopathology or psychodynamics—is in need of continuation and must include the further development of the *clinical* concept of the acute exogenous reaction type based on *clinical* experiences and genetic investigations.

Bonhoeffer's Contribution

The acute mental concomitants of all physical disturbances fit into the framework of the acute exogenous reaction type. By 1912 Bonhoeffer had investigated a considerable number of physical illnesses for their psychiatric concomitants. His definition of acute exogenous reactions at that time was based on his experiences with infectious diseases, cachectic and anemic states, polycythemia, heart diseases, uremia, eclampsia, diabetes, gout, hyperthyroidism, tetany, myxedema, Addison's disease, and gastrointestinal conditions. On the basis of his studies, he felt justified in assuming that the acute mental disorders accompanying all illnesses termed at the time as "general and internal" could be included in the concept of the acute exogenous reaction type. On the other hand, Bonhoeffer almost completely excluded intrinsic brain diseases, the toxic effects of external poisons, and the epilepsies from his considerations. Nevertheless, he indicated that their mental complications lead to the same clinical syndromes as did those of the "general and internal" illnesses.

One of the most important further developments of the theory of the acute exogenous reaction type lies in the discovery that acute brain diseases, acute exogenous intoxications, and acute states of genuine epilepsy result in the same psychopathologic phenomena as "infections, general and internal diseases."

Why was this not specifically determined by Bonhoeffer himself? No doubt an entirely extraneous reason played a role: For his contribution to Aschaffenburg's *Handbuch*, he was simply assigned "the psychoses associated with acute infections, general and internal diseases." The description of toxic psychoses, brain diseases, and of the epilepsies was reserved for other clinicians and Bonhoeffer had no desire to encroach on their spheres of work. Furthermore, it was in line with the tendency of the period to organize pathology according to the organs, so that psychoses associated with brain diseases and those with "general diseases" were not likely to be considered together.

Today it is obvious that psychoses associated with *exogenous intoxications* fit very well into the syndromatic framework of those associated with infectious, metabolic, and circulatory diseases. This is true, for example, for acute alcohol psychoses, for amphetamine psychoses, for withdrawal psychoses of chronic abuse of hypnotics, and for the "experimental" psychoses induced by mescaline, LSD, and other so-called hallucinogens.

Cerebral diseases had been included by Bonhoeffer among the causes of psychoses of the acute exogenous reaction type, although with some hesitation and almost as an aside. Among others, he ranks the manic excitement of fever or hyperthyroidism as similar to that of general paresis, cerebral trauma, or apoplectic cerebral insult. He fully admits the psychoses associated with chorea minor—unquestionably related to brain disease—into the area of his studies. Today we recognize that *all* acute brain disease affecting the psyche acutely leads to mental disturbances within the framework of the acute exogenous reaction type. This includes such diverse disorders as infections, trauma, circulatory disorders and even acute phases of senile dementia and hereditary degeneration (such as Huntington's and Pick's diseases).

Furthermore, we clearly recognize today what some decades ago could only be surmised or suspected: that general physical disorders affect the mind via the brain. This has been demonstrated by both pathologic–anatomic and electroencephalographic investigations. What has emerged particularly clearly and unambiguously is that functional changes of the peripheral endocrine glands affect the psyche through the brain and not, as formerly supposed, through some other, unexplainable manner. The functions of the extracerebral endocrine organs originally exert their influence on specifically attuned cerebral systems, through humoral and neural paths. At first these influences are merely functional, but with severe disturbances they become structural and extend into large portions of the brain. Once it was established that the noxious effects of extracerebral disease affect the psyche via the brain, it became clear that the effects of acute generalized brain disease are identical with those of acute extracerebral illness. Today, any attempt to differentiate the psychopathologic pictures of cerebral and of general illness lacks all rational basis.

It is true that Ewald[5] raises a justifiable objection against including acute cerebral diseases with the other illnesses that lead to "exogenous" reaction types. He points out that the term "exogenous" is no longer suitable for a concept that includes cerebral illness; originally it described those diseases that penetrate from the extracerebral region into the brain and thereby to the psyche. He writes:

Even if one still speaks of exogenous damage from . . . extracerebral physical illness in which something alien to the body or to the brain (Kleist) may develop . . . one can hardly refer to exogenous damage when speaking of brain tumor or cerebral sclerosis, and definitely not when speaking of senile dementia and its variants (Alzheimer and Pick). And yet these disorders resemble, in their symptomatic picture, so accurately the chronic final states due to exogenous damage and are so frequently accompanied by more acute delirious phases that the need exists to include them, *as far as the syndrome is concerned*, with the exogenous rather than with the endogenous or psychogenic illnesses. Thus the concept of the organic psychosis appears to be the more comprehensive and more accurate one.

This now raises the question whether, after the inclusion of brain diseases among the causal factors of the reation type in question, the label "exogenous" reaction type should be dropped. With the modern extension of the concept, the term "acute organic psychosyndrome" presents itself as a logical and tempting substitute for "acute exogenous reaction type." I personally prefer the older term, even though in a literal sense it is a paradox; it has secured a place for itself in psychiatric language usage. Replacement of well-established terms for pedantic reasons tends to produce confusion. It is also my belief that we owe it to the great scientist Bonhoeffer to adhere to the term coined by him. The expression "organic psychosyndrome" comes from Eugen Bleuler and was reserved for the chronic psychopathologic states associated with widespread brain disease. To use Bleuler's term for a concept for which we are entirely indebted to Bonhoeffer would be offensive. And finally, in science, we are accustomed to adhering to labels that have an historic basis, even when, with modern knowledge, they would be phrased differently.

As Bonhoeffer has repeatedly stated, acute *epileptic disorders*—epileptic dysphoric and twilight states—are symptomatologically identical to the mental disorders originally included among the acute exogenous mental disorders. In fact, Bonhoeffer has emphasized the "epileptiform excitements" as one of the principal syndromes among these disorders. Today it is obvious that epileptic phenomena are based on cerebral processes. Thus, acute epileptic psychoses belong among the group of acute cerebral psychoses. The fact that they were not originally included in the acute exogenous reaction type was due to ideas that today are obsolete and that used to lead to a paradoxical terminology: Until quite recently the epilepsies (or at least the idiopathic epilepsies) were considered among the "endogenous" psychoses. If this were justified, it would be ridiculous to include the "endogenous" disease epilepsy among "exogenous" psychoses. This contradiction is resolved as soon as epilepsy is taken out of the category of "endogenous" psychoses, such as schizophrenia and manic–depressive states. Aside from the fact that in many cases of epilepsy heredity plays a role, epileptic phenomena have been proved to be most closely associated with cerebral phenomena, whereas schizophrenic and manic–depressive states are not, at least insofar as our current state of knowledge indicates. Accordingly, the manifestations of epileptic psychoses can be included with the organic psychoses; this, however, is not the case for schizophrenic and manic–depressive conditions. The close relationship of the epilepsies to the diseases of the acute exogenous reaction type is demonstrated by the fact that identical physical diseases often lead to both psychoses and epileptic seizures.

The Extension of the Symptomatology of the Older Acute Exogenous Reaction Type

In the closing chapter of Bonhoeffer's principal work,[3] he summarizes the different forms of the exogenous reaction type as follows:

These reaction types are deliria, epileptoid agitations, twilight states, hallucinoses, forms of amentia—at times hallucinatory, at times of a catatonic or an incoherent character. These syndromes are indicative of specific types of courses: critical or lytic development, the appearance of emotional–hyperesthetic fatigue states, amnestic phases of the Korsakov type, intensification to acute delirium and to meningism. I believe that this lists the principally occurring states and courses, but it is certain that this does not exhaust the totality of the syndromes that can occur. I call attention, for example, to the occurrence of manic states . . . .

Among the reaction types listed, the deliria, twilight states, hallucinoses, and emotional–hyperesthetic fatigue states are well-defined syndromes that are still diagnosed today almost exactly as they were 50 years ago. The same is true of acute delirium.

Delirium is characterized by disorderly and incoherent thinking, disturbed orientation, difficulty in comprehension, illusions, and hallucinations (partly of a dreamlike-scenic, partly of an elementary type), delusional thoughts, anxiety, and other moods, with abrupt changes of these symptoms from hour to hour, and even from minute to minute. The patients are still concerned with their environment, even though they respond to it with difficulty, in an illusional and confused manner. In *twilight states* the patients are completely absorbed in a dreamlike hallucinatory–delusional inner life and are scarcely accessible to their environment. In *acute delirium* all coherent expression is suspended, there exists only senseless agitation (wriggling, rolling, striking, grimacing, screaming, and moaning); only a few words are repeated in a stereotyped fashion. *Hallucinoses* are characterized by hallucinations; all other symptoms of delirium are pushed into the background or else are not discernible at all. The *emotional–hyperesthetic fatigue state* consists of discomfort, weakness, and hypersensitivity to sensory stimuli. To these are added difficulty of perception and lability of mood, which particularly expresses itself in plaintiveness and irritability. The dream life assumes exaggerated importance during sleep and even during semiconsciousness and greatly agitates the patient; the limits between the dream life and the waking experience become blurred. The more they are blurred, the more readily the fatigue state can turn into one of delirium or twilight.

Clinical experiences since 1912 now force us to extend not only the etiologic, but also the old symptomatologic, limits of the acute exogenous reaction type significantly.

1. The term *amentia* is no longer valid and must be extended, perhaps to that of "confused state."
2. The term *epileptic excitement* can be enlarged to the "state of excitement."
3. Unconsciousness, coma, and their precursors must be included in the acute exogenous reaction type.
4. The term *emotional–hyperesthetic fatigue state* must be extended.
5. *Amnestic phases of the Korsakov type* must be fully integrated into the acute exogenous reaction type and can no longer be mentioned marginally as "developmental phases." Furthermore, their symptomatology must be broadened.
6. The view that the clinical pictures of the acute exogenous reaction type are invariably identical with "disorders of consciousness" must be opposed. It also includes states with maintained consciousness.

Amentia.   Even the most brilliant psychiatric authors have never succeeded in defining an "amentia" syndrome convincingly, let alone segregating it from the syndrome of "delirious states." For this reason, the majority of modern writers avoid this term assiduously. All attempts to differentiate between delirium and amentia need to be exaggerated only slightly to arrive at a satire: Amentia is characterized by incoherence accompanied by an obtunded state, and delirium by an obtunded state accompanied by incoherence. In delirium there is an obtunded state; in amentia "a certain degree of obtunded state." In delirium, one can find "occupational delirium and jactation; in amentia the motor manifestations go beyond these" (but where to?). Amentia differs from delirium because of "deliriumlike hallucinations." And so on.

   And yet the concept once had a certain justification and one is loath to drop it. Perhaps that which the majority of authors have preferentially understood by it can be circumscribed, in retrospect, as follows: There are conditions that display an incoherence in the thought processes resembling a delirium and that occasionally manifest all the other individual symptoms of delirium, but in which one gets the impression, upon first contact, of awareness, of the ability to communicate, and even of circumspection. It is only upon more extensive conversation that one is surprised at how far removed from reality and from true contact the patients are. Many assertions concerning amentia can be understood in this light. The degree of the obtunded state is difficult to establish because it is concealed by alertness; the motor restlessness is not manifested as purposeless individual motions or as mere "occupational delirium" but on the surface appears at first rational. Thus the patient with amentia would be a delirious person who on superficial contact appears to be a healthy one. Accordingly, amentia runs a course that is less acute and less stormy than that of delirium. (It is true that some other authors, on the contrary, considered amentia as a particularly severe form of delirium, so that their "amentia" closely resembles "acute delirium.")

To me this circumscription fails to justify a defense of the old concept of "amentia." Common usage has abandoned it; it would be hopeless to oppose the trend.

The vacancy left by the abandoned term must be filled, however. There are in fact conditions arising from physical illness that fall outside the common concept of delirium and yet closely resemble a delirium; for these a term must be found. In my opinion the term "amentia" is successfully replaced when the syndrome of "simple confusional state" or merely "confusional state" is added to the syndrome of delirium. Such a designation is self-explanatory; it aptly describes conditions where incoherent thinking is in the foreground without an immediately apparent disorder of consciousness and without the appearance of gross symptoms, such as illusions or hallucinations. Most of the clinical pictures formerly designated in the literature as amentia can be readily classified as belonging either to the deliria or the the confusional states.

Epileptic excitement. Like the term "amentia," the term "epileptiform excitement" has fallen into disuse. Bonhoeffer characterized it as "severe, usually anxious agitation." As in the epileptic twilight state, "fantastic fearful ideas, impulsive urges to get away, loss of orientation in space and in time" appear acutely. However, in acute physical illness we have observed agitations of *all* kinds, not just of the type mentioned. Therefore, it will be necessary to include an unqualified "state of excitement" among the syndromes of the acute exogenous reaction type. What was formerly designated as "epileptiform agitation states" may now be divided into "twilight states" and mere "excitements."

Unconsciousness, coma, and their precursors. Bonhoeffer emphasized that acute exogenous reaction types are usually encountered in general hospitals and far less frequently in psychiatric institutions. For this reason, the exogenous syndromes of delirium, twilight state, and so on, easily escaped the notice of the psychiatrist.

Unconsciousness, or coma, is a particularly frequent side effect of severe physical disease and of agony. Coma, precoma, and their preceding stages, as routinely observed by the internist and the surgeon, belong to the acute exogenous reaction type. They have been excluded from psychiatric considerations for the simple reason that in general they fall within the working sphere of the internist, the surgeon, and the neurosurgeon; the psychiatrist has little contact with them. With today's broadening of psychiatry beyond the walls of the old psychiatric institution, their inclusion into psychiatric considerations has become imperative, just as the inclusion of organic deliria and twilight states was in Bonhoeffer's days.

Even if unconsciousness was not, "the obtunded state" was included among the exogenous reaction types at an early date. Insofar as it concerns simply a relative suspension of psychic activity, with difficulty of perception and with apathy, it must be considered a preliminary step toward coma. "Acute delirium" can constitute a passing stage between delirium and coma.

Emotional—hyperesthetic fatigue state. The concept of "hyperesthetic–emotional fatigue state" by no means encompasses all the mild forms of the acute exogenous reaction type. The ones most frequently encountered are simple moodiness with irritability, anxiousness or whining, but also with exalted moods of short duration; the excitability is either aggravated or diminished (the patients are "excited" or "apathetic"); individual elementary urges are often reduced when compared to their normal strength but, suddenly, may become evident (change from lack of appetite and aversion to drink to overwhelming hunger or thirst, from the need to move about to the need to rest, from the more common extinction of sexual needs to the sudden, strong need for sexual gratification or for tenderness, and so on).

Amnestic phases. According to Bonhoeffer's formulation, the "amenstic psychosyndrome of the Korsakov type" is an after effect of acute exogenous disorders rather than one of their number. This interpretation is justified to the extent that the more acute exogenous disorders frequently change over into an amestic syndrome. Disorders are now observed, however, in which an amnestic syndrome appears acutely, sometimes following an episode of unconsciousness. This happens most frequently, of course, after cerebral concussion or contusion, but also after brain surgery, carbon monoxide poisoning, chronic alcoholism, or a cerebral vascular accident. Often the amnestic syndrome is but of short duration and clears after a few hours or a few days—for example, after concussion or slight cerebral insult. Therefore, it is also useful to include acute amnestic syndromes (acute Korsakov psychoses, when the milder forms have intensified to the social significance of a psychosis) among the *acute* exogenous reactions and not merely under the chronic syndromes.

Furthermore, the concept of the amnestic syndrome requires amplification. According to the classic descriptions, it involves above all memory and orientation, and in addition a tendency toward confabulation and perseveration. It has long been known that in chronic cases an increasing paucity and simplification of the thought processes and of the entire intellectual capability, as well as an emotional dedifferentiation, are added to these symptoms, with the result that the patients become indifferent and apathetic, although when they do comprehend something they react in an elementary and emotionally uninhibited fashion. In some cases the amnestic symptoms, in others the intellectual disorder, and in still others the emotional disturbances are in the foreground. For this reason, Eugen Bleuler used the term "amnestic psychosyndrome" in a purely symptomatologic sense for disorders dominated by the amnestic symptoms. For chronic sequelae to widespread cerebral (and especially cortical) damage he introduced the term "organic psychosyndrome." In general, insufficient note is made of the fact that both impoverishment of thought and emotional disturbance are part of the "amnestic syndrome," in both acute and chronic brain disorders. Sometimes the amnestic disturbances are overshadowed by the intellectual and emotional disturbances. When acute, they should be included in the acute exogenous reaction type. So long as no comprehensive name is generally accpeted for them, one can refer to them as "Korsakov syndrome" in a more general sense when one wishes to classify the cases exhibiting the typical intellectual or emotional disturbances (with only mild amnestic disturbances) together with the amnestic syndrome. (In a narrower sense, the Korsakov syndrome would then be a purely amnestic syndrome.)

Disorders of consciousness. It is true that, by Bonhoeffer's formulation, "disorders of consciousness" constitute the principal forms of the acute exogenous reaction types. In his view deliria, twilight states, forms of amentia, and epileptiform excitements unequivocally represent disorders of consciousness. It is a misconception of his views, however, to claim that any acute exogenous reaction type must *invariably* have a disorder of consciousness. Mere moodiness, which Bonhoeffer numbers among the syndromes of the acute exogenous reaction type, is not a disorder of consciousness, at least not if the concept of "consciousness" is used in its customary meaning. (Moodiness belongs to the disorders of consciousness only when the term *Bewusstsein*—consciousness—is given far broader meaning than in German language usage. Henri Ey includes moodiness among the disorders of the *conscience* in the French sense.) Also, the amnestic syndrome, the emotional–hyperesthetic fatigue states, and most exogenous initial symptoms are not disorders of consciousness.

On the other hand, there are classical disorders of consciousness without any organic basis: hysterical twilight states, alternating personalities, and acute schizophrenic disorders of consciousness.

The equalization of disorder of consciousness and acute exogenous reaction type has often resulted in confusion—for example, when the argument was advanced that the hallucinoses resulting from LSD were not an acute exogenous reaction type but schizophrenic, because they were not disorders of consciousness.

Natural Order of the Various Syndromes of the Acute Exogenous Reaction Type

With extension, the framework of the acute exogenous reaction type became so broad that the concept is beyond the grasp of the novice and loses its significance. The entire multilevel symptomatology of the acute exogenous reaction type can, however, be made readily accessible by first eliminating the noncharacteristic initial symptoms and then sorting the essential and characteristic syndromes into three series. Such a classification becomes readily understandable, even for the student; deductions concerning causation, prognosis, and therapy can now be drawn from the totality of the symptoms.

In very mild cases and those with a subacute course during onset or convalescence, the mental concomitants of physical diseases are not characteristic. They are so routine that everyone recognizes them from his own experience: fluctuations of mood, excitement or apathy, and unpredictable fluctuations of the ordinary instinctive needs. At the outset, the mood is often exalted. On the eve of an innocuous infection one may experience a sensation of elation, during which the accomplishment of daily tasks appears more interesting, easier, and more satisfying—only to be doubly affected when the physical illness makes active life impossible. Instead of this euphoria, other moods (whiny, irritable, hostile, anxious, and so on) may appear and alternate with each other in unpredictable sequences. General agitation can alternate with apathy and inertia. Thirst, hunger, the need to rest or move about, sexual urges, somnolence, reactions to heat or cold—all these manifest themselves in a manner that is temporally more irregular and unpredictable than usual. Identical phenomena can be triggered through purely psychic shock. They can be the initial symptoms of a schizophrenic or manic–depressive breakdown.

At times the moodiness, excitement and apathy may increase, beyond what is common with mild physical illnesses, to a state that in effect approaches a psychosis. For the most part, however, the symptoms of the characteristic exogenous disorders (listed below) are associated with them. Still, there may exist, as concomitants of physical diseases, purely manic or depressive mood changes and pure excitements of severe degree whose psychopathologic profile is indistinguishable from classic disorders such as manic–depressive psychoses. Such symptoms usually disappear promptly or increase to the more characteristic syndromes of the acute exogenous reaction type.

Leaving aside these uncharacteristic initial conditions, *the bulk of the symptoms of the acute exogenous reaction type can be assigned to three following series:*

1. States of Reduced Consciousness. Clinical pictures that are characterized by a *dampened or fading mental life:* The extreme case is unconsciousness, coma.

   When onset is gradual, this state increases from a simple obtunded state to torpor and semicoma, which changes into coma.

2. States of Altered Consciousness. Here the mental life is not dampened but *has fallen into disorder.* Confused thinking (particularly in the form of incoherent thinking) is in the foreground. The sense of perception can likewise fall into disorder by no longer communicating that which is essential and comprehensive. Much that ought to be noticed remains unnoticed, and what ought to remain unnoticed moves into the foreground. The interpretation of sensations gets mixed up with the sensations themselves; this leads to illusions. Ideation and perception are no longer differentiated; this leads to dreamlike hallucinations. Disorganized irritative phenomena in the central nervous system lead to elementary hallucinations. Attention is split.

   The emotional life is just as disordered as the intellectual processes; the most diversified moods and urges keep alternating. The most typical syndromes of this series are: delirium, acute delirium, simple confused state, twilight state, and hallucinosis. In delerium, the disorder affects the entire mental life—thinking, orientation, perception, and sensation—but the patient remains receptive to simple impressions from his environment (but in a confused fashion). In acute delirium, the confusion is combined with extreme agitation and reaches a degree that makes all communication between the patient and others impossible. In twilight states, the patient is preoccupied with his dreamlike, confused inner life, so that he is more shut off from his environment than a delirious person. In the confusional state, the confused thinking and, in the hallucinosis, the confusion of all perception are entirely predominant.

3. States of Mental Life Organized on a Simplified Level. The *Korsakov syndrome* belongs here, but also included are those forms characterized less as amnestic psychosyndromes than as organic disorders of thought or affect.

   An orderliness of mental life is preserved; thus we are not dealing with an alteration of consciousness. Neither can we speak of a mere dampening or diminution of the entire mental activity. Rather, mental life continues actively, albeit on a simplified level. The simplification is characterized by impoverishment of memory and ideation, and above all by impoverishment of creative thinking. This is associated with dedifferentiation of feeling to the point of maximum dullness, and gross, boundless excitement upon coarse impression.

If desired, a differentiation can be made, depending on whether the memory is most severely affected (amnestic psychosyndrome or Korsakov syndrome in its narrowest sense), whether the capacity for thinking and judgment are most impaired, or whether the severest effects are on emotionality (for the last two there are no familiar terms; they have to be labeled by phrases such as "acute Korsakov Syndrome with greater involvement of thought processes than of memory," as "acute state resembling an organic dementia," as "Korsakov Syndrome with predominant emotional disorder," or as "acute organic emotional change with mild amnestic disorder," and so on).

It must be emphasized that the symptoms of the different series can be mixed—in fact, careful observation frequently demonstrates such a mixture. In particular, the amnestic disorders are often associated with delirium.

Epileptic seizures can occur with any disorder of the acute exogenous reaction type. The pathogenesis appears related to that of the acute organic psychoses. Motor awkwardness, fidgetiness, dysarthric speech, and tremors are frequent accompaniments. Other neurologic and general physical symptoms depend upon the underlying disease. The underlying physical disease can often be determined by physical findings, whereas the psychopathologic findings at best suggest that some physical illness forms the basis for the psychosis.

It is not difficult to demonstrate the character of these three series of syndromes to the beginner, but one may be guilty of oversimplification. An example of a grossly simplified demonstration would be the following: A severely affected sufferer from a physical ailment becomes increasingly difficult to communicate with and finally stops speaking altogether (reduced-consciousness series); or he talks incoherently, "crazily" (altered-consciousness series); or he talks in simplistic manner (series of mental life organized on a simplified level).

An interpretation of the dynamics of events may be approached by the analogy of the life of a patient and the activity of a platoon of soldiers. It fades when each man loses his capacity for action; it becomes disordered, aimless, and ineffective when the commander is eliminated and each group or individual acts according to his own judgment; it is orderly but spiritless and awkward when, after the loss of a capable commander, another steps into his place whose capacity to command is limited. This kind of analogy approaches the concepts of Jackson, as transmitted by Henri Ey and others into modern psychiatry. It is possible to conceive that with reduced consciousness, cerebral function is affected in its totality; in altered consciousness, on the other hand, those differentiated connections could be perturbed without which mental life cannot proceed in an orderly and homogeneous fashion. With organization on a simplified level, a primitive order and organization based on reduced potentials for making connections would have become reestablished. Are these plausible similes or do they contain elements of neuropathologic facts? We do not know.

The Concept of the Acute Exogenous Reaction Type and the Knowledge of Pharmacologic and Endocrinologic Psychiatry

If the extended version of the concept of the acute exogenous reaction type is correct, then the effects of drugs and endocrine disorders on the mind must fit into the framework. They do.

The drugs commonly used in psychiatry today influence, above all, the moods and the degree of general excitement. Their effects correspond to the initial symptoms of the acute exogenous reaction type. Each syndrome of "reduced consciousness" and "altered consciousness" can be produced with some dosage of some drug. A Korsakov syndrome is produced when, after poisoning with a sedative or a narcotic, or as a result of prolonged use of certain drugs, an extended loss of consciousness has occurred. It can also be set off by drug-induced epileptic seizures.

It is a basic precept of psychopharmacology that sleep and anaesthesia can always be induced by means of certain drugs, but that the effects of stimulants do not always agree with expectations; delirious, twilight, hallucinatory, and confusional syndromes can appear after administration of many drugs, but these effects are extraordinarily unpredictable (except for the hallucinogenic effect of a few drugs); the effects on mood are the most unpredictable.

The mental disorders in physical diseases are analogous. Many disorders lead to reduced consciousness (increased intracranial pressure, severe traumata, severe cerebrovascular accidents, diabetic coma, and so on). On the other hand, the incidence with physical diseases of excitement and particularly of mood changes cannot be predicted. States of altered consciousness may be either present or absent with identical illnesses.

When endocrine diseases or iatrogenic endocrine changes have an acute onset and acute sequelae, they fit squarely within the framework of the acute exogenous reaction type. The general drive is either lessened or enhanced, the mood is changed in the most varied manner, and prompt changes of the sex drive may take place (for example, the sexual needs of males disappear within a few hours after administration of massive doses of estrogen). If there are any acute psychoses, there are either dileria, twilight states, hallucinoses, or confusional states, just as with other physical diseases (for example, with cortisone or after radical removal of the thyroid or parathyroid gland).

The Relationship of the Three Series of
Syndromes of the Acute Exogenous Reaction
Type to Course, Prognosis, Diagnosis,
Pathogenesis, and Therapy

With respect to the *final outcome* of mental disorders from the acute exogenous reaction type, three possibilities usually present themselves:

1. Final outcome is death.
2. Final outcome is a chronic organic psychosyndrome, that is, either a chronic Korsakov psychosis or an organic dementia.
3. Final outcome is recovery.

Death is generally due to the underlying illness. In the case of irreversible coma resulting from severe brain damage, the complications of coma will eventually terminate life, even with the best of care. In states of disordered consciousness, a number of life-threatening situations arise: injuries, exhaustion, neglect, or resistance in the treatment of the basic illness.

Outcome in a chronic organic psychosyndrome instead of recovery probably occurs whenever coma has lasted more than a few weeks or when a Korsakov psychosis with acute onset shows no tendency toward recovery for a period of more than a few months. (So long as a Korsakov psychosis shows any sign of improvement, further improvement may be anticipated even if the psychosis has already been of very long duration.)

An altered consciousness in itself does not generally lead to chronic organic psychosyndrome. Some danger in this respect, however, arises when the state of altered consciousness was associated with coma or when its symptoms have become mixed with those of the Korsakov syndrome (as is often the case in delirium tremens, for example).

The chronic organic psychosyndrome is by far the most common disorder whenever a syndrome of the acute exogenous reaction type turns chronic. But *states of disordered consciousness may also become chronic*. This is particularly true of hallucinoses and simple confusional states. The following examples may be listed: chronic alcoholic hallucinosis, the "paranoid state associated with malaria," and chronic hallucinoses and confusional states following acute epileptic states.*

The magnificent tendency toward recovery, innate to human nature,

---

*The following fact is extremely difficult to interpret: in rare cases, syndromes of altered consciousness (especially hallucinoses and confusional states) gradually develop into psychoses that are either schizophrenic or at least cannot be distinguished from schizophrenias. The problems presented by these cases have been studied by many but have never been solved completely and unequivocally. I will not discuss them at this point. Recently, Eliot Slater et al[9] have investigated them thoroughly with respect to schizophrenialike psychoses in epilepsy. In Zurich, they have been studied by G. Bennedetti[2] with respect to alcohol hallucinoses.

consistently surprises the inexperienced. Everyone realizes that recovery from coma may be complete. However, an inexperienced observer will have doubts when a delirium is prolonged. It must be pointed out to him that an acute or subacute Korsakov psychosis may still heal, unless there has been no improvement over several months. I have often observed that the prognosis for patients with alcoholic or posttraumatic Korsakov syndromes was made too unfavorable.

As far as the course is concerned, with acute severe insult, coma results; but coma also develops with slowly increasing damage.

By comparison, the "acute" Korsakov psychosis follows a rather subacute course, occurring most frequently as an aftermath of a severe reduction of consciousness or of an unconsciousness. It can develop without these, but then usually in a subacute form.

Alterations of consciousness may appear and fade without any of the symptoms of the other two series. They may precede a state of reduced consciousness or else intervene between unconsciousness and Korsakov syndrome in the course of return to a normal state.

The most common courses are: (1) very severe acute trauma → unconsciousness → possible alteration of consciousness → acute Korsakov syndrome → chronic organic psychosyndrome or recovery. (2) reduced consciousness → alteration of consciousness → recovery. (3) reduced consciousness → possible alteration of consciousness → unconsciousness death. Many other courses are frequently observed.

The consideration of these courses leads to a certain confirmation of the presumed dynamic bases: reduction of all brain function most commonly results from the most acute and most severe traumata; disturbances of connections, and thus of organization, occur with somewhat less acute and less severe traumata; organization on a simplified level does not occur acutely.

The significance of the three series of syndromes for diagnosis varies. The following rule of thumb can be established: Distinct symptoms of reduced consciousness (that is, torpor and coma) and distinct symptoms of simplification of mental life (that is, Korsakov syndrome in the broad sense of the term) constitute *proof* of an underlying physical illness. Once these symptoms are detected, there can be no let-up or pause until the physical ailment is discovered. On the other hand, states of altered consciousness cannot be unequivocally diagnosed as an indication of physical conditions because they may also result from endogenous or psychogenic disorders.

This rule of thumb requires some elucidation:

1. A slight reduction of consciousness, a mildly obtunded state, cannot be established as being physically rooted solely by psychodiagnostic methods. There is a considerable risk of confusing this state with mild depression (in which retardation is in the foreground), with emotional stupor, and even

with incipient "association-poor" schizophrenia. This type of mildly obtunded state may be considered exogenous without hesitation only when a close temporal relationship with a physical insult is known. However, we are certain of the exogenous causation when the obtunded state changes to torpor, precoma, and coma. In any event, nature rarely allows formulations of absolute certainty, and emotional fainting spells, among others, could be cited in contradiction of the above formulation.

2. It is easy to diagnose the Korsakov syndrome in severe cases. Once this diagnosis is confirmed, the presence of an underlying disease is assured. Milder and less characteristic cases may be confused with retarded depression and with hysterical pseudodementia.

3. With altered consciousness the situation is different: Deliria, twilight states, confusional states, and hallucinoses of a very similar or apparently identical type can be observed on other than organic bases. For example, hallucinoses can also occur in late-onset schizophrenia and in prison psychosis. There exist not only exogenous but also hysterical and schizoprenic twilight states. The simple confusional states of certain physical diseases and of the simple type of schizophrenia can be similar. As everywhere in medicine, it becomes necessary to compare the total clinical picture and the entire course of the condition. The presumption that a state of altered consciousness is of organic etiology must be confirmed by establishing the underlying physical disease and the temporal relationship between physical and mental disorder. (This relationship can admittedly be loose.) There is, nevertheless, some significant psychopathologic evidence: Above all, it is essential to know whether symptoms of reduced consciousness or of the Korsakov syndrome are associated with a delirium, a twilight state, and so on. If such symptoms are in evidence, an organic state is confirmed. Of further importance, the utterances of a patient with organic disorders of consciousness generally provide an immediate impression of his inner situation. We note whether he is sad, irritable, anxious, preoccupied, perplexed, confused, or lucid; we are not faced, as is so often the case with acute schizophrenics, with the sinister impression of the false, the eccentric, the artificial, the incomprehensible. Elementary irritative hallucinations are common with organically ill patients but otherwise rare. Dreamlike hallucinations may occur in both. A number of other differential diagnostic investigations could be considered, but are extremely delicate (for example, the differential diagnosis between "brain-confused," incoherent thinking and "schizophrenic-confused," scattered thinking). On the other hand, it has been correctly emphasized for decades that catatonic symptoms can occur both in organic and schizophrenic alterations of consciousness. They cannot be employed in the differential diagnosis discussed here.

Today, hypotheses concerning the basic cerebral processes in the acute exogenous reaction type are beginning to take shape. To be sure, they remain uncertain. With increasing extinction of the mental life, the electrical activity of the brain is at first synchronized, the alpha waves disappear, slow and irregular waves take their place, and ultimately all electrical activity ceases. The oxygen consumption decreases despite normal or increased cerebral circulation. The extinction of mental life corresponds to that of cerebral electrical activity and metabolism. With states of altered consciousness the situation is different: A significant but diversified change of the electrical activity occurs. There are electrical arousal responses, for example, in the excitation stage preceding anesthesia; dreaming occurs with the electrical pattern of light sleep; in other cases "forced normalization" (Landolt) of a previously abnormal electrical activity is observed. There is reason to believe that the oxygen consumption in twilight and delirious states is as little reduced as during sleeping or dreaming. With simplification of mental life, no electroencephalographic changes take place, or else they are mild, uncharacteristic, and diffuse. So far as can be concluded from the few investigations made to date, the oxygen consumption in the brain is reduced.

Very little is known about the relationships between the various forms of the acute exogenous reaction type and well-localized brain damage. It is certain that pressure or hemorrhage affecting the midbrain lead to coma (often with dilated, fixed pupils and extensor spasms). Most likely unconsciousness can also result from other brain lesions. Excited confusional states and deliria following cranial trauma do not indicate cerebral compression with midbrain damage, as do simple reduction of consciousness and unconsciousness. Rather, it may be presumed that cortical damage causes them. In cases of Korsakov syndrome, damage has been found both in the cortex and in the brain stem. There is evidence that impairment of recent memory (and to a lesser extent impairment of remote memory) are due to changes in the limbic system. In a recent comprehensive report, Akert and Hess[1] have pointed out that the hypothalamus, because of its marked vascularization and particular permeability of the blood–brain barrier in the ventral gray matter of the third ventricle, is markedly vulnerable to chemical, microbial, and toxic damage coming from the bloodstream, just as it is also a preferential site for mechanical microtraumata. The same authors further note that it is possible in animal experiments to activate some behavior patterns from the hypothalamus that appear identical to those in deliria and twilight states (excitement, adynamia, unprovoked aggression). Also acetylcholine and the catecholamines are concentrated in the diencephalon, and toxic effects upon them can lead to deliria. The best-known example is atropine delirium. Important central nervous systems that mediate relations between endocrine system, brain, and instincts, between excitement and phasic nature of psychic events reside in the hypothalamus and epithalamus. However, so far no differentiation by cerebral localization has been established for the various forms of the acute exogenous reaction type.

The most important *therapy* of mental disorder due to acute physical diseases is the somatic therapy of the underlying disease. Over and above this, however, the classification of these disorders into three series yields three significant, specific therapeutic indications:

1. The *therapy of unconsciousness*, properly developed only in the last two decades, has proven so overwhelmingly successful that it is now universally recognized. Its essence lies in the notion that, in addition to artificial food and fluid intake and to avoiding decubitus and pressure damage to peripheral nerves, respiration must be kept free at all costs. Formerly, unconsciousness of long duration was fatal, because of respiratory complications; with today's care, fatalities occur virtually only because of exacerbation of the primary disease.

2. The *alterations of consciousness* are amenable to psychiatric therapy. It cannot be overemphasized that the optimal and least dangerous form of tranquilization for excitement or confusion due to physical cause—even in the most severe deliria—is a most simple, but patient and painstaking psychotherapy. When nurses and relatives are constantly in attendance, and when frequent visits by the physician convey a sense of security and confidence, these efforts not only have a soothing, solacing, and calming effect but often exert a healing effect on the mind. Psychotherapy, however, should not consist only of comforting talk, consolation, and intimate chats; rather, the patients should be encouraged to regain strength by carrying out tasks as soon as their physical condition permits and, as soon as possible, they should resume familiar responsibilities. For example, a housewife—as soon as accessible—should be asked what instructions she has for cooking meals or how the children are to be occupied. Occupational therapy is not indicated for chronic mental patients alone, nor is schizophrenia its only indication; in exogenous acute confusional and excitatory states it can accomplish a great deal. If a patient with impaired consciousness is treated for his physical ailment only, if he is regarded with astonishment or veiled dread and disgust, if one does not communicate or have compassion for him, and if he is isolated or even put between side rails, the effect may be deleterious. What these patients need most, to be sure, is now in short supply: time and more time, on the part of physicians, relatives, and nurses. Tranquilizing medication seems simpler and more time-saving. We are all the more conscious of this as more and more tranquilizers have appeared on the market (with increasingly obtrusive advertising pitches). Without question, tranquilizers are often indicated for agitated patients with disordered consciousness. But their dangers must be

kept in mind. In physically caused mental disorders they have, more often than in other conditions, paradoxical effects, for example, they are exciting instead of calming, and aggravate confusions. Moreover when, in excitatory and confusional states, a tendency toward progression into precoma and unconsciousness exists, the tranquilizers often aggravate the clinical picture. In addition, there are numerous physical dangers and contraindications (risk of hypotension, liver damage, agranulocytosis, precipitation of seizures, and many others). Untoward side effects appear less pronounced with the newer tranquilizers that are not primarily hypnotics. Nevertheless, with their use, a patient in a delirious or twilight state may become completely inaccessible and fall into torpor and subcoma. Paradoxical effects, with aggravation of excitement, confusion, hallucinations, and delusional thinking occur with all of the neuroleptic drugs. Thioridazine (Mellaril), among others, is a mild and often effective phenothiazine preparation. At times an intravenous dose of Librium has a prompt calming effect. In some cases, though, the agitation can be controlled better with hypnotics than with neuroleptics. But the hypnotics carry an even greater risk of reinforcing the tendency toward torpor and coma, and they too can augment confusion and hallucinatory tendencies, and can, paradoxically, excite instead of promote sleep.

3. The *Korsakov psychoses* also demand (aside from the etiologic therapy) full consideration of psychiatric indications, particularly when they persist over extended periods of time. The key words here are: occupational therapy, organization of leisure time, careful balance of adding or taking away responsibility, and general precaution and care. To this may be added special problems, such as evaluation of judgment in business matters, competence in legal matters, and so on.

CONCLUSION

Is there still any sense and significance today in surveying and classifying the mental disturbances due to physical illness, and to delimit them against other mental disorders? Or has the extension of the framework of their clinical pictures rendered this endeavor absurd?

There is no lack of weighty opinions to the effect that it has indeed led to absurdities. Conrad[4] eyes the pursuit to delimit the exogenous reaction types with a certain amount of skepticism. He bases his attitude on the premise that "there is practically no psychotic syndrome that cannot be found with physically based psychoses as well." This statement is correct, but it requires an immediate amplification: But there exist psychotic syndromes that can be found exclusively with physically based psychoses (the states of reduced consciousness and the Korsakov syndrome in the broader sense of the term). If one were to postulate Conrad's statement without qualifying it, then it would indeed be futile to lose any more words about the acute exogenous reaction type, and Bonhoeffer's concept could well be consigned to oblivion. We would be justified in renouncing all further attempts to establish the causes of disease from psychopathologic syndromes and could again be satisfied with the old image of the "unitary psychosis." The qualification, however, implies an obligation: to make use, for prevention and treatment, of the diagnostic clues provided by nature. This is an essential truth that would be irresponsible to ignore, even with our psychiatric philosophy and our psychiatric research orientation.

The statement that "there is practically no psychotic syndrome that cannot be found in physically based psychoses as well" requires critical scrutiny in other respects as well: It ignores all distinction between what is frequent and what is rare. There are a great many common psychotic syndromes that can be found only rarely in connection with physically based psychoses. Certainly it can happen, for example, that acute schizophrenias arise that, for a limited period of time, are indistinguishable from physically rooted states of confusion (such as the one that used to be designated as amentia). But how rare are such cases! Certainly, there are occasions when a hysterical twilight state temporarily cannot be distinguished from an epileptic one—but how much more frequently they are easily differentiated!

In principle, and in the overwhelming majority of cases, the psychopathologic symptoms of physically caused psychoses are readily differentiated from those that arise without demonstrable physical disorders. This claim can be made for the acute psychoses. The symptoms of chronic psychoses associated with physical illnesses are, in an even more overwhelming majority, clearly distinguishable from those of the chronic psychoses of physically healthy individuals.

The basic feasibility of distinguishing mental disorders that are physically rooted from others signifies not only a decisive element concerning their diagnosis, prophylaxis, and therapy but also concerning the planning of further research on the organic psychoses. Far more, the inferences of this concept radiate into all areas of psychiatry, including the theory of schizophrenia. With the schizophrenic clinical pictures, we can define disorders that, in the vast majority of cases, differ from the psychoses associated with physical disorders—and yet despite all efforts we find no sign of physical disorders in these schizophrenic clinical pictures (at least none to which under scientific scrutiny causal significance can be ascribed). Certainly, it does not serve the cause of schizophrenia research to pass over in silence these two results, which complement each other so impressively. How to utilize these results is not the object of our discussion. What we may say for certain is the following: if and insofar as schizophrenias are physically based, then they are so in an entirely different way than those psychoses that according to today's knowledge have an obvious and intimate connection with physical disorders.

REFERENCES

1. Akert K, Hess WR: Über die neurobiologischen Grundlagen akuter affektiver Erregungszustände. Schweiz Med Wochenschr 92:1524–1530, 1962
2. Benedetti G: Die Alkoholhalluzinosen. Stuttgart, Thieme, 1952
3. Bonhoeffer K: Die Psychosen im Gefolge von akuten Infektionen, Allgemeinerkrankungen und inneren Erkrankungen, in Aschaffenburg G (ed): Handbuch der Psychiatrie. Leipzig und Wien, Deuticke, 1912, p 106
4. Conrad K: Die symptomatischen Psychosen, in Gruhle HW, Jung R, Mayer-Gross W, Muller M, (eds): Psychiatrie der Gegenwart, vol 2. Berlin, Springer, 1960
5. Ewald G: Psychosen bei akuten Infektionen, bei Allgemeinleiden und bei Erkrankung innerer Organe, in Bumke O (ed): Handbuch der Geisteskrankheiten, Ergänzungsband, 1. Teil. Berlin, Springer, 1939
6. Ey H: Etudes psychiatriques. Structure des psychoses aigües et déstructuration de la conscience. Paris, Desclée de Brouwer & Cie, 1954
7. Kraepelin E: Über die Beeinflussung einfacher psychischer Vorgänge durch einige Arzneimittel. Jena, Gustav Fischer, 1892
8. Meyer A: The Problems of Mental Reaction-Types, Mental Causes and Diseases. Psychol Bull 5:245, 1908
9. Slater E, Beard AW, Glithero E: The schizophrenia-like psychoses of epilepsy. Br J Psychiaty 109:95–150, 1963

Commentary

Obviously, the disorders discussed under the term exogenous reaction types by Professor Bleuler are of importance to all physicians. In actual practice, most patients with these disorders are treated by internists, surgeons, neurologists, neurosurgeons, and other practitioners and are not routinely seen by psychiatrists. The psychiatric aspects of the acute mental reactions, however, are poorly understood by the physicians who care for these patients, and the help of enlightened specialists would be of value for both the patient and the attending physicians.

The next two chapters discuss the dementias, a disparate group of disorders that have evoked little interest for the past few decades. Recent discoveries have reawakened interest in dementia and our next two chapters will explore a number of recognized dementing disorders, emphasizing the treatable forms and the means of diagnosing them.

Richard N. Harner, M.D.

4
EEG Evaluation of the Patient With Dementia

Patients with intellectual deterioration comprise 10 percent of the admissions to the neurology service at the Graduate Hospital of the University of Pennsylvania. Intellectual deterioration represents the third most common cause for admission to the hospital among all patients with a suspected neurologic disorder.

Definition of the term may vary according to one's specialty. Many psychiatrists consider dementia to be an untreatable degenerative disorder of the nervous system associated with mental and social deterioration. The neuropathologist views dementia as a disorder of neuronal metabolism that sometimes shows characteristic histologic alterations at postmortem examination or brain biopsy. The neurologist usually considers dementia to be a symptom characterized primarily by intellectual deterioration that might be due to a variety of underlying causes including infection, tumors, metabolic disorders, subdural hematoma, or neuronal degenerative disease,[6,17,35] with emphasis on those causes of dementia that may respond to treatment. The prognostic evaluation of those disorders that are not presently treatable is an important secondary consideration.[28] The usefulness of the electroencephalogram as a diagnostic adjunct is in exactly two areas. Most treatable causes of dementia are associated with prominent EEG abnormalities, while the "degenerative" disorders, which for the most part are untreatable, show few EEG abnormalities in the early stages of development unless the rate of progression is rapid.

EFFECTS OF AGING

In the aging process, sporadic opportunities for serial EEGs, as well as planned investigations, reveal a decrease in group mean alpha frequency, which begins in the seventh decade[5,9,14,21,23–25,30] but does not affect all individuals (Fig. 4-1). When present, a change in alpha frequency is ordinarily not accompanied by prominent focal abnormalities, signs of cortical irritation, or voltage depression, which might suggest other types of pathologic process. Signs of intellectual deterioration, increased reaction time, or loss of recent memory may occur in elderly patients, but reported correlations with slowing of alpha activity have been good only in (more severely involved) hospitalized subjects.[26]

Another finding seen in populations of individuals aged 50 years and older is that of intermittent delta and theta activity occurring predominantly in temporal regions, more in the left hemisphere,[3] as shown in Figure 4-2. Intermittent temporal slowing occurs with increasing frequency in the seventh decade, and beyond and has been viewed as a normal finding because of poor correlation with signs of intellectual deterioration. Many clinical electroencephalographers believe tht intermittent temporal slowing is related to diminution in cerebral blood flow[2,7] but technical difficulties have prevented accurate measurement of blood flow in the temporal region.

We have examined our recent experience at the Graduate Hospital of the University of Pennsylvania, where more than one third of the patients are 65 years of age or older. In the 13-month period beginning January 1, 1973, 661 of 1797 electroencephalograms were recorded on patients 60 years of age or older. Routinely, semiquantitative evaluations of the frequency, amplitude, amount, and distribution of EEG waveforms and a statement of the degree of EEG abnormality are performed prior to any knowledge or correlation with clinical symptoms and these data form the basis for this retrospective study.

Table 4:1 shows the distribution of EEGs according to age and presenting symptom or reason for referral. Patients with MIN (minimal) symptoms included those with head and neck pain, leg weakness, minor antecedent trauma, and so forth. Those in the DIZ group had the isolated complaint of dizziness without other neurologic signs or symptoms. The TIA (transient ischemic attack) group had recurrent, transient neurologic deficit, including syncope. DEM (dementia) patients had the primary symptom of chronic intellectual impairment or memory loss, unaccompanied by a history of cerebrovascular disease, acute neurologic deficit, or obvious etiology. CVA ("cerebrovascular accident") patients had acute stroke syndromes, presumably of vascular etiology in the majority; SEIZ patients had seizures as a predominant symptom; CONF patients were acutely confused and dis-

Table 4-1
Reasons for EEG Referral of Patients Aged 60–90 years

| Symptom | Number of EEGs | | | |
	60–69 Years	*70–79 Years*	*80–90 Years*	*60–90 Years*
MIN	38	20	0	58
DIZ	37	27	4	68
TIA	36	38	13	87
DEM	25	5	2	32
CVA	36	39	22	97
SEIZ	36	14	10	60
CONF	17	28	10	55
COMA	21	21	15	57
Miscellaneous	56	71	20	147
Totals	302	263	96	661

oriented; COMA patients were stuporous or unresponsive; and MISC patients were those who could not be classified. The distribution of patients according to symptoms is quite even, except for the lack of MIN patients in the 80–90 group and the (surprising) lack of DEM patients in the 80–90 group.

The distribution of normal, mildly abnormal (grade 1), and more abnormal (grades 2–5) EEG according to symptoms is shown in Table 4:2. Note that the criteria utilized allow a great majority (87 percent) of the MIN group to be interpreted as normal while the reverse is true of CVA, SEIZ, CONF, and COMA groups. Occasional (10%–20% of recording time) low-to-medium voltage (20–40 mV) 4–5/sec activity was present in the majority of EEGs interpreted as normal, increasing in incidence from the seventh decade (40%) to the ninth decade (87%) but was not correlated with any symptom group.

Table 4:3 shows the incidence of more than mild EEG abnormalities in our study. There are clear trends of increasing abnormality in association with increasing age and with increasing severity of symptoms. In the DEM group, the amount of major abnormality is similar to that seen in the TIA group but less than that in the CONF, CVA, and SEIZ groups.

In patients with minor or less severe symptoms, a significantly higher incidence of abnormalities of all types occurs in TIA and DEM groups compared to MIN and DIZ groups (Tables 4:2 and 4:3). Of special interest are the mild abnormalities that occur with significantly greater frequency ($p <$

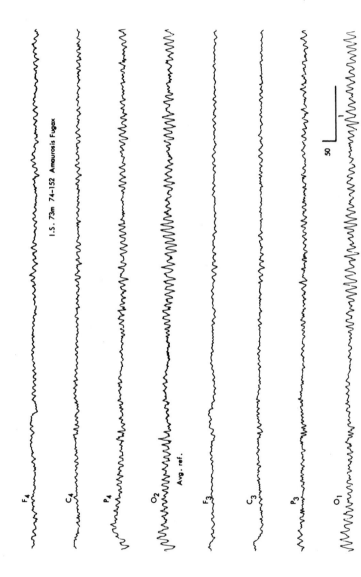

Fig. 4-1.   Normal EEG in a 73-year-old man with recent transient loss of vision in one eye. Alpha frequency is 9 cps. Electrode positions in this and subsequent figures according to international 10–20 system.

Table 4-2
Distribution of EEG Abnormalities According to Symptoms in Patients Aged 60–90
Years

Symptoms		EEG		
	N	Percent Normal	Percent Mild Abnormality	Percent > Mild Abnormality
MIN	58	83	14	3
DIZ	68	71	12	18
TIA	81	32	25	43
DEM	32	25	34	41
CVA	97	13	8	78
SEIZ	60	7	17	77
CONF	55	4	7	89
COMA	57	0	0	100
Miscellaneous	147	15	17	68

Table 4-3
EEG-Abnormality According to Age and Reason for Referral in 661 EEGs from
Patients Aged 60–90 years.

Symptom	Percent of EEGs with more than mild abnormality.			
	60–69 Years	70–79 Years	80–90 Years	60–90 Years
MIN	0	10	—	3
DIZ	14	19	50	18
TIA	33	50	46	43
DEM	44	20	50	41
CVA	69	79	91	78
SEIZ	78	64	90	77
CONF	83	93	90	89
COMA	100	100	100	100
Miscellaneous	58	75	70	68
All	49%	63%	79%	59%

0.01) in TIA and DEM groups than in any other group. The abnormalities
were two types: (1) an alpha frequency less than 8.0 cps in the DEM group
and (2) a moderate amount (20%–40% time) of medium voltage (40–80 mV
1–3.5 cps activity, maximal in temporal regions.

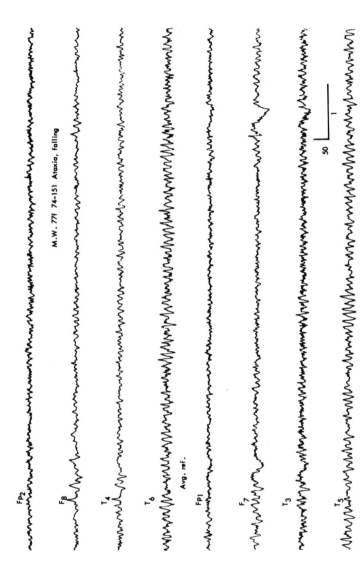

Fig. 4-2. Intermittent bitemporal 2/sec medium voltage activity, more on the left (F7,T3). Recent onset of ataxia and falling.

Further quantitative information concerning alpha frequency in DEM patients was obtained by including the EEGs that were interpreted as normal. Table 4:4 shows the mean alpha frequency in normal and mildly abnormal EEGs from MIN, DIZ, TIA, and DEM patients in each age group. Decrease in alpha frequency is seen with advancing age and in DEM patients. In the MIN group, only four had an alpha frequency of 9.0 cps, while the majority of EEG's for the DEM group had a mean alpha frequency of 8.5 or less (Fig. 4-3). On the other hand, DEM group EEGs overlapped the MIN group EEGs in 11 cases, indicating lack of exact correspondence between symptoms of intellectual impairment and alpha frequency, in spite of a highly significant statistical difference. Practically, a mean alpha frequency of less than 8.0 cps can be regarded as abnormal, an alpha frequency of less than 8.5 cps should be suspect in patients under the age of 80 years.

Slowing of mean alpha frequency and the presence of a moderate amount of intermittent delta activity, especially in temporal regions, have been regarded by some as obligatory effects of the ''normal aging process.'' Our results confirm the correlation of such findings with advancing age in the seventh decade and beyond. In addition, however, these same findings occur with significantly higher frequency in patients with intellectual impairment and transient ischemic attacks and, therefore, cannot be regarded as normal. Studies of regional cerebral blood flow will be important in establishing the possible relationship between EEG abnormalities, clinical symptoms, and cerebral ischemia.[11,16,27]

PRIMARY CEREBRAL DEGENERATION

The *onset* of presenile dementia (Alzheimer's disease), Huntington's chorea, or senile dementia is usually not associated with striking EEG abnormalities, although there may be a slight slowing of alpha frequency or a slight excess of delta activity. Over the course of 1 or more years, progressive diffuse slowing and loss of fast activity occur[19,20,34] but lag behind clinical symptoms[31] until the last stages. Then paroxysmal or ''triphasic'' activity can even be seen.[22] Occasionally, the availability of serial EEGs of a patient with dementia may be helpful when slowing of alpha occurs rapidly, rather than gradually, as expected in the uncomplicated aging process (Fig. 4-4).

The usefulness of EEG evaluation in patients with dementia is dependent on the stage of development of symptoms. In the early stages, a normal EEG constitutes good evidence against metabolic, toxic, focal, or infectious causes (see below). In the later stages, the presence of diffuse slowing helps in the distinction between organic causes of dementia and psychotic reactions of functional origin.[8,25,28]

Table 4-4

Relationships of Age and Symptoms to Alpha Frequency in 179 Normal or Mildly Abnormal EEGs From Patients Aged 60–90 Years

Alpha	60–69 Years	70–79 Years	80–90 Years	60–90 Years
Symptoms	Frequency ± SC (n)	Frequency ± SE (n)	Frequency ± SE (n)	Frequency ± SE (n)
MIN	9.8 ± 0.1 (38)	9.4 ± 0.2 (18)	—	9.7 ± 0.1 (56)
DIZ	9.6 ± 0.2 (31)	9.1 ± 0.2 (22)	8.8 ± 0.8 (2)	9.4 ± 0.1 (55)
TIA	9.7 ± 0.2 (23)	9.4 ± 0.3 (19)	8.8 ± 0.4 (7)	9.4 ± 0.1 (49)
DEM	8.9 ± 0.3 (14)	8.6 ± 0.7 (4)	7.0 (1)	8.7 ± 0.3 (19)
All	9.6 ± 0.1 (106)	9.3 ± 0.1 (63)	8.6 ± 0.3 (10)	9.1 ± 0.1 (179)

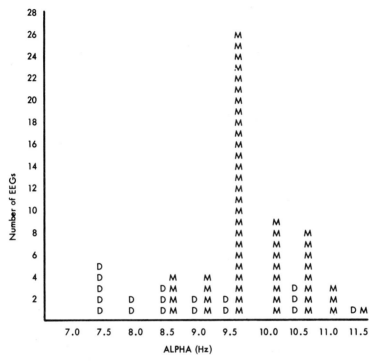

Fig. 4-3. Mean alpha frequency in EEGs from DEM and MIN patients, aged 60-79 years.

Confusion can arise when clinical symptoms such as language disturbance, focal weakness, or seizures occur in the course of a degenerative
disorder. These clinical findings may be mirrored in the EEG as focal slow
waves or focal irritative activity (sharp waves, spikes). The recognition that
such focal features can occur in as many as 10 percent of patients with
degenerative diseases does not eliminate the need to look for other types of
focal process that may be treated.

TREATABLE DEMENTIAS

If the incidence of EEG abnormalities in the early stages of intellectual
impairment due to primary metabolic or "degenerative" cerebral disorders is
low, then the exact reverse is true of secondary metabolic encephalopathies
with few exceptions.[12] Hyponatremia, hypothyroidism, hypercalcemia, pernicious anemia, uremia, hepatic encephalopathy, and pulmonary

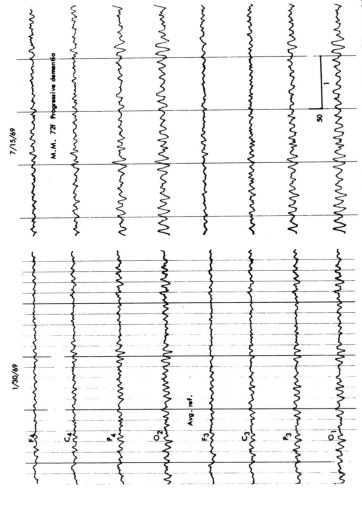

Fig. 4-4. Reduction in occipital alpha frequencies from 9 cps after 6 months of progressive dementia in a 72-year-old woman.

72

insufficiency are characterized by diffuse slow activity, which usually ante-dates the onset of mental symptoms and correlates with the degree of mental impairment. In addition, *irritative features* are common in anoxia and disorders of electrolytic metabolism; *triphasic waves* (Fig. 4-5) appear in 20 percent of patients with uremic and hepatic encephalopathy;[13] and *focal slow activity* may occur, apparently resulting from preexisting areas of decreased resistance in the brain. Since dementia represents a late stage of metabolic encephalopathy that develops on a chronic basis, the EEG is abnormal in almost every case and, therefore, is a very useful screening procedure.

A particular point of confusion can arise in relation to hypothermia, hypothyroidism,[36] and vitamin B_{12} deficiency,[33] each of which can produce gradual slowing of alpha activity indistinguishable from the slowing that can occur as part of the aging process or in the early stages of primary degenerative disorders of the brain, such as Alzheimer's disease (Fig. 4-6). Biochemical screening tests are essential in these cases.

In a similar fashion, the EEG is an excellent screening procedure for the detection of localized brain lesions,[31] even more so for those that have grown sufficiently large to produce symptoms of dementia. Rapidly growing primary brain tumors and metastatic lesions are most easily detected, but even parasagittal and basal meningiomas are usually evident in the electroencephalogram by the time they have become large enough to produce dementia.

One of the most difficult lesions to detect by EEG, and yet eminently treatable, is *subdural hematoma*. In the majority of cases, unilateral or bilateral slow activity is present in patients with subdural hematoma. However, it is the depression of the rhythmic fast and medium frequencies that gives the best clue as to the location of the largest subdural collection (Fig. 4-5). In some cases, voltage asymmetry at medium and high frequencies may be the only finding. In such situations, meticulous technique and thoughtful interpretation are required to make the diagnosis.

In part because of these cases, we routinely utilize sonoencephalography (SEG) to determine the midline location in patients hospitalized for suspected brain lesions.[29] The combined information obtained from consideration of *brain function* (EEG) and *brain mass* (SEG) is especially helpful in eliminating false positives in diagnosis of subdural hematoma (Fig. 4-7). Voltage depression due to hemispheric cerebral atrophy or a recent cerebral infarction are common and may be distinguished from subdural hematoma by lack of midline displacement or even midline displacement toward the side of voltage depression in the presence of atrophy. In our experience, the electroencephalogram shows some abnormality in 90 percent of cases of subdural hematoma and is lateralizing in perhaps 80 percent. The use of sonoencephalograph has markedly reduced the false positives and has served to in-

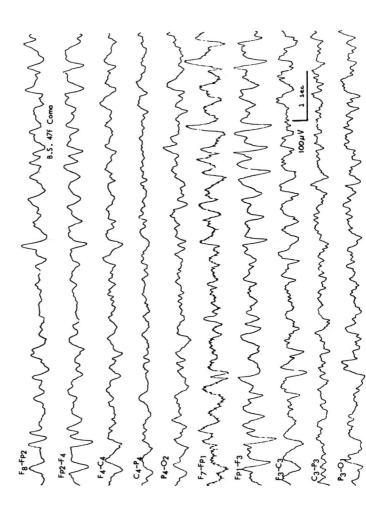

Fig. 4-5. Prominent bifrontal triphastic waves, more on the left, in a 47-year-old patient with known hepatic failure who became comatose. Reduction of fast activity over the entire right hemisphere (upper five channels) lead to the evacuation of a large, coexistent

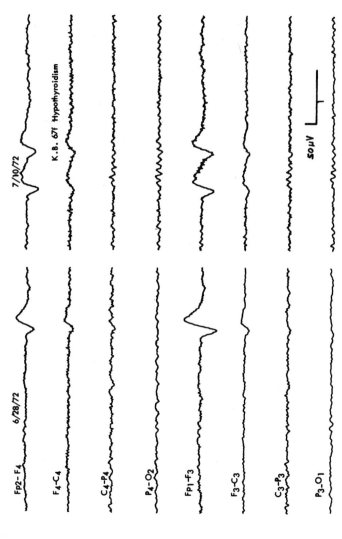

Fig. 4-6. Hypothyroidism, before and after treatment. Low voltage rhythmic 4-6/sec activity was associated with wakefulness on June 28, 1972 (no eye blink artifact in channels one and five). Twelve days later, there was striking improvement, but alpha frequency was still only 7.5 cps.

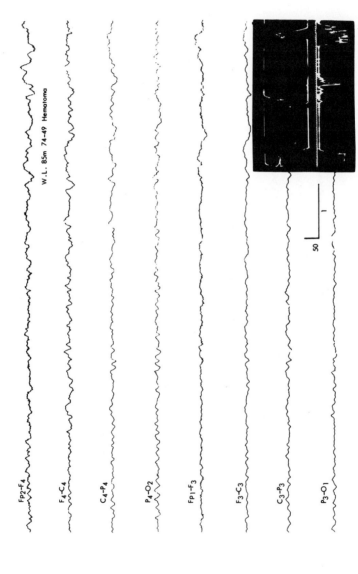

Fp2-F4

W.L. 85m 74-49 Hematoma

F4-C4

C4-P4

P4-O2

Fp1-F3

F3-C3

C3-P3

P3-O1

50

Fig. 4-7. Persistent confusion and impaired level of consciousness associated with 7.5 cps alpha rhythm on the right and depression of rhythmic activity over the entire left hemisphere (Channels 4 to 8). Insert shows sonoencephalogram with 10-mm displacement of the midline echo toward the right. The combined findings indicated a large left hemisphere mass. A hematoma was evacuated.

crease the clinician's attention when we mention the possibility of a subdural hematoma.

EEG findings in patients with *increased intracranial pressure* have long been controversial. It is apparent that mere increase in intracranial pressure may not be associated with EEG abnormality. For example, in patients with "benign" intracranial hypertension and small lateral ventricles, EEG abnormalities are rare. However, distension of the ventricular system, due to obstruction of cerebrospinal fluid flow, is associated with slowing of EEG activity, which appears as intermittent rhythmic bursts of slow activity usually reaching a maximum in the anterior regions of the head.[4]

In "normal pressure hydrocephalus," Brown and Goldensohn[1] reported only mild abnormalities in 5 of 11 cases, aged 62–80 years. As described, these findings are similar to those in our patients with minor symptoms, TIAs, or dementia. More data are needed in this important area, but it is true that bursts of slow activity in a patient with dementia should raise the possibility of increased intracranial pressure, which is reflected in ventricular dilatation.

Cerebral infections in the ordinary sense are not usually associated with dementia. A brain abscess may be viewed as a tumor, and the expectation would be localized slow activity that is indistinguishable from that seen in primary or secondary tumors. However, chronic meningeal infection, tuberculosis, for example, often produces striking EEG changes, particularly when the base of the brain is involved.[32] These changes may revert after appropriate treatment (Fig. 4-8). High voltage bursts of slow activity seen in tuberculous meningitis or cryptococcal meningitis may mimic the findings of intraventricular hypertension.

Jakob-Creutzfeldt disease is a rapidly progressive "degenerative" disorder of the brain that has now been transmitted to chimpanzees and probably represents a viral infection.[10] The EEG pattern is characteristic in later stages and consists of periodic bursts of spike and slow wave activity occurring at regular intervals. Similar patterns may be observed in childhood lipidoses, anoxic encephalopathy,[18] and in subacute sclerosing panencephalitis. However, in a patient over 40 years of age with progressive dementia, such periodic complexes constitute extremely good evidence of Jakob-Creutzfeldt disease.

The presence of characteristic abnormality in the EEG does not eliminate the possibility of other types of pathologic process. In one patient, sagittal sinus thrombosis coexisted with Jakob-Creutzfeldt disease and accounted for an accelerated clinical course that was reflected in EEGs obtained over the course of several weeks (Fig. 4-9).

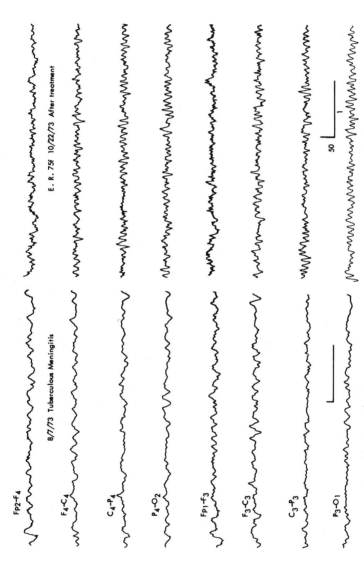

Fig. 4-8. Tuberculous meningitis before and after treatment in a 75-year-old woman. Amplification on August 7, 1973 was reduced by one half.

78

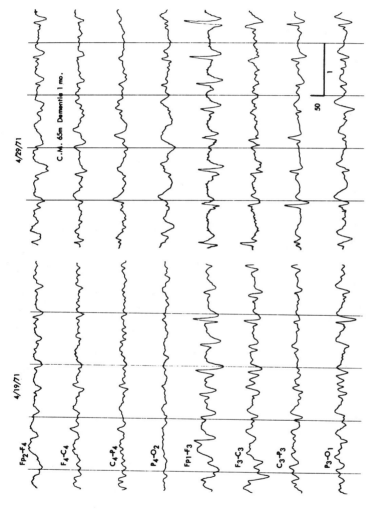

Fig. 4-9. Rapidly progressive intellectual impairment associated with periodic spike discharge maximal over the left hemisphere (April 19, 1971). An EEG 2 weeks earlier was normal. Ten days later (April 29, 1971) spike activity was persistent, but medium voltage 1–2/sec slow activity appeared more on the right. Cerebral angiography demonstrated nonfilling of the sagittal sinus. On autopsy, thrombosis of the sagittal sinus was present, and characteristic microscopic findings of Jakob–Creutzfeld disease were found.

SUMMARY

Dementia should be viewed as a symptom that may be due to a variety of causes. One of the most common causes is primary metabolic or "degenerative" disease of the brain, in which the EEG is usually normal or shows only a slight degree of slow activity in the early stages. Diffuse slowing, focal slow and irritative activity, voltage depression, and specific wave forms occur frequently in the treatable dementias. Thus, the EEG performs a useful screening function for the physician and may also point the way toward general diagnostic categories that aid in the evaluation of treatable dementias.

REFERENCES

1. Brown DG, Goldensohn ES: The electroencephalogram in normal pressure hydrocephalus. Arch Neurol 29:70–71, 1973
    phalus. Arch Neurol 29:70–71, 1973
2. Bruens JH, Gastaut H, Giove C: Electroencephalographic study of the signs of chronic vascular insufficiency of the Sylvian region in aged people. Electroencephalogr Clin Neurophysiol 12:283–295, 1960
3. Busse EW, Barnes, RH, Friedman EL, Kelty EJ: Psychological functioning of aged individuals with normal and abnormal electroencephalograms. J. Nerv Ment Dis 124:135–141, 1956
4. Daly DD, Whelan, JL, Bickford RG, MacCarty CS: The electroencephalogram in cases of tumors of the posterior fossa and third ventricle. Electroencephalogr Clin Neurophysiol 5:293–216, 1953
5. Davis PA: The electroencephalogram in old age. Dis Nerv Syst 2:77, 1941
6. Drachman DA: The senile patient. Gen Pract 36:78–87, 1967
7. Frantzen E, Lennox-Buchthal M: Correlation of clinical electroencephalographic and arteriographic findings in patients with cerebral vascular accident. Acta Psychiatr Scand 36 (Suppl 150):133–134, 1961
8. Frey TS, Sjögren H: The electroencephalogram in elderly persons suffering from neuropsychiatric disorders. Acta Psychiatr Scand 34:438–450, 1959
9. Friedlander WJ: Electroencephalographic alpha rate in adults as a function of age. Geriatrics 13:29–31, 1958
10. Gibbs CL Jr, Gajdusek DC, Asher DM, Alpers MP, Beck E, Daniel PM, et al.: Creutzfeldt–Jakob disease (spongioform encephalopathy): Transmission to the chimpanzee. Science 161:388, 1968
11. Gustafson L, Risberg J, Hagberg B, Hougaard K, Nilsson L, Ingvar DH: Cerebral blood flow, EEG and psychometric variables related to clinical findings in presenile dementia. Acta Neurol Scand 48 (Suppl 51):439–440, 1972
12. Harner RN, Katz RI: Electroencephalography in metabolic coma, in Naquet R, Harner R (eds): Handbook of Electroencephalography, vol 10(in press)

13. Harner RN, Simsarian JP: Triphasic waves in metabolic encephalopathy. Electroencephalogr Clin Neurophysiol 36:222, 1974
14. Harvald B: EEG in old age. Acta Psychiatr Scand 33:193–196, 1958
15. Ingvar DH: Cerebral blood flow and metabolism in complete apallic synfunctions. Acta Anaesthesiol Scand, 45 (Suppl):110–114, 1971
16. Ingvar DH: Cerebral blood flow and metabolism in complete apallic syndromes, in states of severe dementia and in akinetic mutism. Acta Neurol Scand 49:233–244, 1973
17. Karp HR: Dementia in systemic diseases. Postgrad Med 202–208, Sept., 1971
18. Lesse S, Hoefer PFA, Austin JH: The electroencephalogram in diffuse encephalopathies. Arch Neurol Psychiatry 79:359–375, 1958
19. Letemendia F, Pampiglione G: Clinical and electroencephalographic observations in Alzheimer's disease. J Neurol Neurosurg Psychiatry 21:167-172, 1958
20. Liddell DW: Investigations of EEG findings in presenile dementia. J Neurol Neurosurg Psychiatry 21:173–176, 1958
21. Mankovsky NB, Belonog RP: Aging of the human nervous system in the electroencephalographic aspect. Geriatrics 26:100–116, 1971
22. Müller HF, Kral VA: The electroencephalogram in advanced senile dementia. J Am Geriat Soc 15:415–426, 1967
23. Mundy-Castle AC, Hurst LA, Beerstecher DM, Prinsloo T: The electroencephalogram in the senile psychoses. Electroencephalogr Clin Neurophysiol 6:245–252, 1954
24. Obrist WD: The electroencephalogram of normal aged adults. Electroencephalogr Clin Neurophysiol, 6:235–244, 1954
25. Obrist WD, Busse EW: The electroencephalogram in old age, in Wilson WP (ed): Applications of Electroencephalography in Psychiatry. Durham, NC, Duke Univ Pr, 1965, pp 185–205
26. Obrist WD, Busse EW, Eisdofer C, Kleemeier RW: Relation of the electroencephalogram to intellectual function in senescence. J Gerontol 17:197–206, 1962
27. Obrist WD, Chivian E, Cronqvist S, Ingvar DH: Regional cerebral blood flow in senile and presenile dementia. Neurology 20:315–322, 1970
28. Obrist WD, Henry CE: Electroencephalographic frequency analysis of aged psychiatric patients. Electroencephalogr Clin Neurophysiol 10:621–632, 1958
29. Sandok BA, Reiher J, Whisnant JP: Combined electroencephalography and sonoencephalography. Mayo Clin Proc 43:628–634, 1968
30. Short MJ, Musella L, Wilson WP: Correlation of affect and EEG in senile psychoses. J. Gerontol 23:324–327, 1968
31. Short M, Wilson P: The EEG in dementia, in Wells CE (ed): Dementia. Philadelphia, Davis, 1971, p 81
32. Turrel SW, Schmidt RP, Levy LL, Roseman E: Electroencephalographic studies of the encephalopathies. Serial studies in tuberculous meningitis. Electroencephalogr Clin Neurophysiol 5:53–63, 1953
33. Walton JN, Flynn RE, Sullivan JF: The electroencephalogram in pernicious anemia and subacute combined degeneration of the cord. Electroenceph Clin Neurophysiol 6:45–64, 1954

34. Weiner H, Schuster DB: The electroencephalogram in dementia. Some preliminary observations and correlations. Electroencephalogr Clin Neurophysiol 8:479–488, 1956
35. Wells CE (ed): Dementia. Philadelphia, Davis, 1971
36. Wilson WP: The electroencephalogram in endocrine disorders, in Wilson WP (ed): Applications of Electroencephalography in Psychiatry. Durham, NC, Duke Univ Pr, 1965, pp 102–122

Commentary

From this review it is obvious that dementia is neither a single nor a specific disorder and that among the causes of dementing changes are a number of treatable disorders. The use of the EEG to define the treatable conditions producing dementia may appear elementary but actually represents a major step; almost without exception the dementing disorders that are amenable to treatment produce distinctly abnormal EEG patterns. In contrast, the presently untreatable dementing disorders (particularly the presenile and senile dementias) maintain relatively normal EEG patterns until late in their course. The following chapter also deals with disorders causing dementia, but these are the more serious disorders that produce change in anatomic structure—dementia accompanied by hydrocephalus. This group of disorders has consistently been considered irreversible but it is now clear that a number of these disorders, if correctly diagnosed, can be treated successfully.

D. Frank Benson, M.D.

5
The Hydrocephalic Dementias

Not many years ago, an individual suffering a chronic/progressive disorder of cognitive ability faced an uncompromisingly dismal future. If seen by a psychiatrist, he was likely to be considered an example of "chronic brain syndrome," a wastebasket diagnosis supposedly manifested by one or more of five major symptoms (but more truly characterized by a lack of response to psychotherapy). The diagnosis alone precluded psychiatric treatment other than appropriate custodial management. If seen by other practitioners, the same patient was likely to be called demented. Dementia was considered almost universally to be an irreversible disorder, again obviating treatment. Under either nomenclature, the predicted course was one of progressive deterioration unaltered by therapy. Such a situation is unacceptable and, fortunately, also untrue. Recent discoveries, combined with the resurrection of older knowledge, offers most individuals with chronic/progressive disorders of cognition an accurate diagnosis, and many of the disorders so diagnosed are amenable to therapy. For some, this means actual cure; for many more, amelioration of the symptomatology is achieved. Comparatively few dementing disorders cannot be helped in some way.

The preceding chapter has already indicated that many causes of dementia are treatable. Most disorders discussed there, however, were caused by disturbances of brain function in the absence of structural changes. When disorders produce changes in mentation without causing death of cerebral neurons their reversibility following corrective measures does not seem surprising. What of those dementias associated with hydrocephalus and presumed cell death? They have consistently been considered incurable, and the

83

term "irreversible" specifically referred to the hydrocephalic dementias. This irreversibility has been disproved by Hakim and colleagues,[1,10] who demonstrated that the condition known as normal-pressure hydrocephalus (NPH) could be corrected. Dementia, often severe, and massive ventricular enlargement are consistently seen in this disorder. Appropriate treatment (shunting of cerebrospinal fluid) returns many individuals with NPH to an essentially normal mental state. Most disorders producing hydrocephalus and dementia do not respond to treatment so dramatically; nevertheless, many available treatments relieve to some extent, the dementing disorders associated with hydrocephalus. It will be the purpose of this presentation to discuss the differentiation, management, and prognosis of the hydrocephalic dementias.

DIFFERENTIATION

Until recently there has been little benefit obtained by differentiating the disorders that produced both dementia and hydrocephalus. This unfortunate truth was so firmly established that most early series of shunts performed for NPH included cases with suspected degenerative brain disease, specifically selected to see if shunting relieved all individuals with hydrocephalus.[17] Several serious investigations have denied any important differences in types of hydrocephalus except for magnitude and have advocated shunting all cases with sufficiently large ventricles.[2,19] Experience, however, suggests that shunting alleviates only certain types of hydrocephalus. Therefore, a number of diagnostic techniques have been devised to select cases most likely to benefit from shunting. While far from being totally effective in guiding selection, these techniques do offer information for differentiating varieties of hydrocephalic dementia. Table 5-1 presents a classification of hydrocephalic dementia based, at least in part, on recent findings.

An initial step in the process of differentiation is the establishment of what should be called dementia (see Chapter 2). While most clinicians use this term, a precise definition is difficult and many different processes are included under this term. For present purposes, we will characterize dementia as a deterioration of intellectual functions (including some or all of the following: cognition, memory, personality, constructional skills, and word finding) caused by brain disease. This definition is indefinite but directs attention to many different disorders, some of which may be relieved by present therapy techniques. To demonstrate hydrocephalus some variety of contrast study is necessary. When both hydrocephalus and dementia are present, an extensive work-up is indicated in searching for a remediable etiology. Full work-up includes careful clinical examination (history, general physical, neurologic, and psychiatric condition, including detailed mental status exams) and an EEG (see Chapter 4). Depending on the results of these examinations, the

Table 5-1
Hydrocephalic Dementias

Nonobstructive
  Degenerative
    Alzheimer's, Pick's, Senile, etc.
  Destructive
    Arteriosclerotic, traumatic
Obstructive
  Noncommunicating
    Ventricular obstruction
  Communicating
    Normal-pressure hydrocephalus
Other
  Cerebral cyst
  Ectatic basilar artery

---

condition of the patient, and the availability of facilities, additional study should include one or more of the following: pneumoencephalography, cerebral angiography, radioisotope cisternography, and/or spinal infusion pressure studies.* By correlating the information obtained from these tests, a differentiation and often a specific diagnosis can be made, which in turn allows more reliable therapeutic measures. Differentiating features of the principal varieties of hydrocephalic dementia will be outlined, followed by remarks about treatment and prognosis.

VARIETIES OF HYDROCEPHALIC DEMENTIA

Table 5-1 shows that hydrocephalic dementia can be divided into obstructive and nonobstructive groups. Obstructive hydrocephalus can be subdivided into communicating and noncommunicating, while the nonobstructive varieties of hydrocephalus can be subdivided into degenerative and destructive. In addition, several abnormalities such as cerebral cysts and the ectatic basilar artery syndrome remain unsettled and could be considered under either subcategory.

Degenerative Disorders

The classic examples of "dementia" have always been the degenerative disorders producing cerebral atrophy, the best-known of which are

---

*Since the writing of this chapter computerized axial tomography has been introduced and promises to be a valuable tool for the evaluation of dementia.

Alzheimer's disease and/or senile dementia. Whether these two entities are separable as suggested[16] or are the same disorder presenting with slightly different clinical pictures based on difference in the age of onset[11] is not important for the present discussion. Other degenerative disorders producing hydrocephalus include Pick's disease, Jakob–Creutzfeldt disease (actually a slow-virus encephalopathy), and possibly some of the so-called subcortical dementias (Huntington's chorea, Parkinson's disease,[13] the Steele-Richardson syndrome,[21] some of the spinal–cerebellar degenerations,[8] the "subcortical gliosis of Neumann"[15] and so forth).

There is considerable variation in the clinical picture of these entities, but they all share one diagnostically useful characteristic: their natural courses are relentlessly progressive. Although they begin and continue without dramatic or specific incident and the course is rapid in some and insidious and slow in others, the progressive and relentless downhill course is constant.

Table 5-2 outlines significant features of diagnostic studies in the degenerative disorders. Of prime importance is the relative normality of the EEG in the face of serious clinical disability (see Chapter 4). Angiography and spinal infusion studies are normal. Cisternography is also comparatively normal, although a demonstrable slowing of cerebrospinal fluid circulation is often noted. Pneumoencephalography shows a mild-to-moderate degree of ventricular enlargement, most specifically a widening of the third ventricle[22] and, when properly performed, demonstrates widening of the cortical sulci, producing an appearance of both central and peripheral atrophy. In more advanced cases, the callosal angle of Lemay[3,12] *becomes increasingly obstuse* (from 130° to 140°).

The characteristic history, the lack or late onset of elementary neurological findings (paralysis, visual field disturbance, sensory loss), the presence of severe dementia and the distinctive features of the laboratory studies usually allow a positive diagnosis of degenerative brain disease. The exact etiologic variety, however, may be difficult to ascertain and is primarily dependent on concomitant findings. Thus, the differentiation between Alzheimer's disease and Pick's disease rests on the early clinical state. Alzheimer's disease almost invariably begins with biparietal and bitemporal degeneration, producing memory loss, visual–spatial disturbance, word-finding disability, and problems in judgment and manipulation of knowledge. In contrast, Pick's disease involves the frontal and temporal lobes, initially producing memory problems along with severe personality changes. In Alzheimer's disease, the personality is usually preserved while "intelligence" suffers, whereas in Pick's disease, intellectual functions are comparatively well maintained in the face of severe personality alterations. Diagnosis of other varieties depends on the presence of characteristic neurologic findings, such as the movement disorders of Parkinson's disease, the Steele-Richardson syndrome, and

Table 5-2
Degenerative Disorders

Isotope cisternogram
  Some concetration of isotope in ventricles but variable in intensity and duration
  Slow (delayed) isotope flow
  Good sagittal concentration by 48 hr
Pneumoencephalogram
  Moderate enlargement of lateral and third ventricle and occasionally of fourth
    ventricle
  Frontal horns usually less than 300 mm in height
  Callosal angle (LeMay) obtuse, 130°-150°
  Air over cortical surface (but may not be present)
Arteriography
  Usually normal
Electroencephalography
  Normal in early stages
  Diffuse and fairly symmetrical slow activity in advanced stages

---

Huntington's chorea. Sometimes the clinician must await the pathologist's report to know the exact type of degeneration.

Arteriolosclerotic Disorders

There is considerable controversy surrounding the legitimacy of the term arteriolosclerotic or athrosclerotic dementia. Most of this controversy is a legitimate reaction to the tendency of many clinicians to use the label "arteriolosclerotic dementia" for any elderly patient with dementia. The postulation that vascular insufficiency produces a decrease in cerebral blood flow that in turn produces a dementing process[9] appears valid but lacks proof; in most individuals with dimentia, evidence of vascular insufficiency cannot be demonstrated at autopsy. However, the opposing belief that no one becomes demented on the basis of vascular disease is certainly untrue. Individuals who have suffered multiple strokes (large or small), particularly when both hemispheres are involved, may well become demented along with developing other problems. The natural course differs from that seen in the degenerative disorders. While the course is downhill and usually progressive, it is stepwise; a number of separate incidents combine to produce the final picture of dementia. Usually some of these steps are recognized as true strokes, but often "little strokes" are called "flu," "virus," "nervous exhaustion," and so forth. In contrast to Alzheimer's disease, multiple cerebral vascular accidents usually produce elementary neurologic dysfunction and are most often asym-

Table 5-3
Arteriosclerotic Dementia

Isotope cisternogram
  Ventricular filling inconstant
  Good sagittal concentration
  Cortical infarcts may appear as "hot spots"
Pneumoencephalogram
  Variable amount of ventricular enlargement, often asymmetrical
  Callosal angle (LeMay) obtuse, but if asymmetry is great, may be acute
Arteriography
  Often demonstrates significant extra–or intracranial vascular disease
Electroencephalography
  Usually abnormal, focal slowing and/or seizure activity; may show multiple foci

---

metrical. Thus, in most instances, the alert practitioner readily differentiates vascular and degenerative dementia on the basis of clinical findings alone.

Table 5-3 gives some of the diagnostic criteria from the various studies. In this situation, the EEG almost invariably shows significant abnormality, usually asymmetrical and often showing several destructive foci. The spinal infusion study is usually normal, but both the cisternogram and the pneumoencephalogram show evidence of ventricular enlargement. The cisternogram usually demonstrates a slower circulation of CSF and often shows areas of concentrated isotope uptake, the so-called "hot spots." Asymmetrical ventricular enlargement is frequently present on PEG (if the asymmetry is pronounced the callosal angle becomes acute). Angiography often demonstrates vascular stenosis or occlusion and may demonstrate other diagnostic features, such as luxury perfusion.

Obstruction of Ventricular Outflow

The problems produced by obstruction to the ventricular outflow channels are well recognized. Acute obstruction produces rapid increase in ventricular size, accompanied by nausea, vomiting, obtundation, papilledema, and, if not corrected quickly, tentorial or tonsilar herniation and death. If the obstruction of ventricular outflow is incomplete or develops slowly, an enormous dilatation of the ventricles occurs, accompanied by few basic symptoms. Change in intellectual function is always present, but, unfortunately, the clinical history is often vague. Personality changes often appear first, with problems of judgment, intellect, and memory appearing simultaneously or shortly after. The clinical picture produced by the partial obstruction often resembles that seen in degenerative disease, and differentiation may be necessary.

Demonstration of obstruction can be accomplished by appropriate laboratory studies. The EEG will almost always be abnormal in obstructive hydrocephalus; whether the abnormality is focal or widespread depends on the location of the pathology. Spinal infusion study is usually not helpful and may be dangerous. Cisternography from the lumbar approach often fails and cannot be considered diagnostic. Similarly, air studies using the lumbar approach may fail to fill the ventricular system and, in addition, are potentially life-threatening. Introduction of air into the ventricles (ventriculography) may be necessary and is usually diagnostic, not only demonstrating hydrocephalus but also the location of the obstruction. Arteriography may be helpful in delineating the location and type of pathology but may fail to give useful information.

Normal-Pressure Hydrocephalus (NPH)

The demonstration by Hakim and colleagues[1-10] of a massive degree of hydrocephalus despite free communication between the ventircular system and the lumbar subarachnoid space and a normal CSF pressure produced great interest. Of particular significance was the demonstration that appropriate therapy (shunting) could produce a dramatic clinical improvement. The criteria for diagnosing NPH, however, have not been clear, leading to both inappropriate selection of cases and failure of shunting.

The clinical picture of NPH is usually given as a triad of dementia, gait disturbance, and incontinence.[3] It is readily admitted, however, that all three are quite variable, and one or more may be absent in any given case. Some degree of dementia is usually present but may vary from a mild memory disorder or alteration in personality to a totally vegetative state. Similarly, the gait disturbance varies from almost undetectable to total incapacity. Incontinence is frequently, but not invariably, present. Most cases of NPH have a comparatively dramatic starting point, such as subarachnoid hemorrhage, other acute vascular incident, trauma, meningitis, and so on. Some cases have been reported, however, in which no specific etiology is known. While occult neoplasms have eventually been demonstrated in some of these, others have remained "idiopathic." The degree of clinical disability varies considerably in NPH, but dementia is usually a prominent feature.

Table 5-4 presents the diagnostic laboratory findings in NPH. Despite recent suggestion that the EEG may be fully normal,[4] our experience suggests that widespread slowing is usual. The diagnostic features of the laboratory

Table 5-4
Normal-Pressure Hydrocephalus

Isotope cisternogram
  Ventricular filling—persists 48–72 hr
  Ventricles large
  No isotope collection in sagittal area
Pneumoencephalogram
  Ventricles large
  Frontal horns over 32 mm in height
  Callosal angle (LeMay) is less than 120°
  Little or no air over cortex
Arteriography
  Bowing of anterior cerebral artery
  Lateral displacement of sylvian vessels
  Displacement of thalamo-striate veins
Electroencephalography
  Usually diffusely slow but often with focal slowing

---

studies are not completely reliable,[3] but with multiple studies NPH can usually be diagnosed with confidence. The spinal infusion study is positive in NPH.[14] However, both false-positive and false-negative results can occur.[25] Arteriography will usually show enlarged ventricles (bowing of anterior cerebral arteries, lateral displacement of the Sylvian mantle and the thalamo-striate veins). Cisternography gives a characteristic picture. There is immediate isotope concentration in the ventricles (ventricular reflux) where it may remain for many days. There is little or no movement of isotope into the cortical subarchnoid space and to the sagittal region. Pneumoencephalography also gives a characteristic picture with massive enlargement of the ventricles, a distinct decrease in the callosal angle (often less than 100°) and uneven ventricular enlargement with the frontal horns increasing in size more than the other portions of the lateral ventricles. Unfortunately, false findings can occur in either cisternography or air contrast studies, but when the features of several diagnostic studies are combined with the clinical information, a confident diagnosis can be made in most cases.

Cerebral Cysts

Porencephalic cyst is a pathological diagnosis denoting a developmental arrest that allows development of a cystic cavity with connection to the ventricle. Damage to the cerebral hemisphere, however, can also produce a cyst that communicates with either the ventricle or the subarachnoid space.

Table 5-5
Cerebral Cyst

Isotope cisternogram
  Isotope concentrates in cyst
  Cyst often demonstrable for many days
Pneumoencephalogram
  Some degree of ventricular enlargement
  Cyst often fails to fill with air—however, often demonstrable in 24-hr film
Arteriography
  No diagnostic findings—but may well be abnormal and reveal etiology

---

Cystic cavities may result from absorption of an intracerebral hematoma, a large infarction or tissue destruction by trauma, or surgical decompression. These cysts have also been called porencephalic cysts.[20] They can become enlarged and, at times, act like mass lesions. Isotope cisternography demonstrates many more apparent cerebral cysts than had previously been suspected. It has been suggested that the cyst wall, lacking an ependymal lining, absorbs and holds the isotope and thus produces an area that remains ''hot'' for many days.

There is no consistent clinical picture suggesting the presence of cerebral cysts except for the characteristic etiologic background noted above. Table 5-5 gives our present impression of findings that suggest the presence of cerebral cysts. It seems probable (although not definitely proven) that symptom-producing cerebral cysts develop only when there is abnormality of CSF circulation (essentially NPH). If this is true, shunting should produce improvement in the clinical picture, and some individuals with cerebral cysts are reported to have had clinical improvement after shunting.

Ectatic Basilar Artery

The possibility that a heavily arteriolosclerotic, high-riding, ectatic basilar artery could encroach on the floor of the third ventricle causing a partial obstruction of CSF outflow, hydrocephalus, and mental changes was first suggested by Swedish physicians.[5,6] They reported that shunting improved the mental state of these patients. Ectatic basilar artery can exist, however, without producing either hydrocephalus or dementia. In our practice, in fact, individuals with ectatic basilar artery, hydrocephalus, and dementia have always had a disturbance of CSF circulation of the type seen in NPH. Of patients with demonstrable ectatic basilar artery only those who also have the findings of NPH appear to benefit from a shunt procedure.

Table 5-6
Ectatic Basilar Artery

Isotope cisternography
  May be normal or abnormal
Pneumoencephalography
  Identation of floor of third ventricle by highly placed basilar artery
  Ventricles may be mildly or markedly enlarged
Arteriography
  Basilar artery protrudes above tentorium
Electroencephalography
  No diagnostic finding—will be diffusely slow if there is marked hydrocephalus

---

There are no specific clinical findings indicative of ectatic basilar artery except the advanced age of the patients, but, if suspected, the diagnosis can be made by appropriate studies. Table 5-6 presents the diagnostic features. Note that the EEG, the spinal infusion study, the pneumoencephalogram, and RISA cisternogram are all likely to be abnormal and similar to normal pressure hydrocephalus. The ectatic basilar artery itself can be illustrated best by angiography, but its presence can also be detected from an indentation of the floor of the third ventricle in a pneumoencephalogram. Demonstration of an ectatic basilar artery, however, does not prove that it is the cause of a dementia.

TREATMENT

Until recently, there was little reason to think that individuals with sufficient brain disease to produce both hydrocephalus and dementia were amenable to treatment. On rare occasions, a slow-growing tumor such as a colloid cyst of the third ventricle or a tentorial mengioma was discovered, and the symptoms, including dementia, were corrected by appropriate neurosurgical procedures. Most patients with dementia and hydrocephalus, however, were considered untreatable, a therapeutic nihilism that has been abandoned in the past decade. Some of the current methods of treatment will be reviewed here.

Degenerative Disorders

Degenerative diseases have proved to be the least amenable to therapy. At present, none can be cured, and even the ameliorative value of treatment is limited. For instance, Huntington's chorea responds to treatment, but only in a limited manner. Thus, a disabling chorea may be improved considerably with appropriate drugs; the improved motor status allows freer response on mental tasks with apparent improvement in mentation but does not truly improve the dementia. In fact, the sedative side effects may increase problems of mentation. In a similar way, patients with Parkinson's disease may show improved motor function with treatment. In many instances, patients with severe Parkinsonism who were considered demented improved greatly after treatment loosed the shackles of the movement disorder. Unfortunately, others remain severely demented despite greatly reduced rigidity. It appears unlikely that present therapy for Parkinsonism alters the state of mentation.

Jakob–Creutzfeldt disease, usually classified among the degenerative disorders, produces cerebral wasting, secondary hydrocephalus, and a severe dementia. In recent years, a viral etiology has been demonstrated.[18] A number of treatments are currently available for treatment of virus disorders, but none have been effective in changing the course of Jakob–Creutzfeldt disease. This does not mean, however, that the appropriate therapy will not be found in the future. Whether control of the virus would allow return of mental facility would be yet another question, one that only the future can answer. Nonetheless, Jakob-Creutzfeldt disease is a variety of hydrocephalic dementia in which treatment of sorts is available and with hope of improved therapeutic measures for the future.

The major varieties of degenerative hydrocephalic dementia, Alzheimer's disease, senile dementia, and the less common Pick's disease, do not respond to therapy at the present time. Management remains custodial. It is well known that patients with this disorder fare best when left in a familiar environment, since their condition deteriorates severely if they are removed to strange surroundings. This deterioration may be reversible as the patient comes to know his surroundings, but not infrequently mental function remains below previous levels. At present, considerable research is being performed in the field of the degenerative disorders, and it seems possible that in the future specific treatment will be available. At present, however, we must consider these disorders untreatable.

Arteriosclerotic Dementia

Fisher[7] suggested vascular insufficiency as a possible explanation for senile dementia, and the possibility that treatment to improve cerebral vascular circulation would be of use in this disorder has followed. Walsh, a major proponent of this idea,[23,24] demonstrated distinct improvement in mentation in a small series of patients with recent cerebral vascular accidents by using anticoagulant therapy. Unfortunately, he provided no control group, and how much of the demonstrated improvement would have occurred spontaneously can only be conjectured. Nonetheless, it is possible that anticoagulant therapy can improve cerebral blood flow and, if cerebral oxidation is increased, improved mentation could result. This premise lacks proof, and it must be emphasized that anticoagulant therapy carries a considerable risk for this group of patients.

In a similar vein, surgeons have suggested that correction of major extracerebral vascular disorders might improve cerebral circulation and hence improve mentation. Correction of great-vessel stenosis or occlusion potentially increases the amount of blood circulating in the head. Individual cases have been cited in which rather severe disability including obtundation, mental confusion, aphasia, and poor cognition have improved significantly following surgical correction of involved extracranial vessels. While these studies also lack control and remain anecdotal, surgical therapy may be considered in an individual with dementia and a suspicion of extracranial cerebrovascular disease.

Ventricular Obstruction

In the past, this variety of hydrocephalic dementia has been treated with the most success. Treatment is dependent on diagnosis of both the location and the cause of obstruction. When possible, removal of an obstructing mass should be carried out early. Thus, colloid cyst of the third ventricle, tentorial mengioma, papilloma of the fourth ventricle, cerebellar hematoma, and others can often be treated by direct surgery. Frequently, however, the problem is not truly correctable by surgery (that is, metastases, gliomas, intracerebral hematomas, and so on, can be treated but rarely cured by surgical decompression). At times, the location of the disorder makes removal impossible or very dangerous. In this situation a shunt is often helpful. For many years, the Torkildsen shunt, a tube connecting the lateral ventricle to the cisterna magna, has been used successfully. In more recent years, ventricular–atrial shunting has also been used with success. Obstruction to the ventricular outflow almost always deserves correction, and, if dementia is one of the symptoms, it is often improved.

Normal-Pressure Hydrocephalus (NPH)

When NPH was first recognized as a separate disorder, a rational treatment was also presented. This was shunting of CSF through a tube running from the ventricular region through the jugular vein into the atrium of the heart, the so-called ventricular–atrial shunt. Dramatic improvement has been recorded with this procedure. Individuals who were amnesic, incontinent, bedfast, apathetic, and unable to computate or perform any simple cognitive tasks have been returned to their previous mental state.

Unfortunately, not all cases of suspected NPH have responded to shunting. In fact, in most series, only a small percentage of treated individuals (from 20 to 40%) have made the dramatic improvement outlined above. Others show some improvement but have considerable residual deficit. At least some of the failures of shunting are based on inappropriate selection of patients. With improved diagnostic acumen, a better percent of good results can be anticipated. Even so, a sizable number of individuals with appropriate findings for the diagnosis of NPH do not obtain significant improvement with shunting and other causes of failure must be considered. These include:

1. The time from onset until treatment. It seems probable that prolonged delay of treatment reduces the chance of a full recovery.
2. The presence of structural brain damage other than that produced by NPH. Thus, NPH secondary to trauma often responds only partially to shunting because of extensive underlying brain damage.
3. Incorrect pressure. In the ventricular–atrial shunt the possibility of an inappropriate opening pressure of the valve must be considered. Cases have been recorded in which use of a medium-pressure valve produced no change; replacement with a low-pressure valve produced return to normal mentation.
4. Complications of shunting. The most serious complication is formation of a subdural hematoma, but meningitis and embolism have also been reported.
5. Plugging of the shunt. Shunts originating in the ventricle are often occluded, partially or completely, either by retraction into the periventricular tissues or by entanglement in processes from the choroid plexus.

At least some of the problems associated with ventricular–atrial shunting can be obviated by the use of a lumbar–peritoneal (theco–peritoneal) shunt. This shunt can operate without a valve, there is less chance for obstruction, and, if complications occur, the shunt is at a distance from the brain. Experience with lumbar–peritoneal shunts is still limited, but so far they appear satisfactory. Even so, the present means of treating NPH are crude, and improved methods should be sought.

Cerebral Cysts

As noted earlier, many cerebral cysts may be artifacts of the testing procedures. Nonetheless, when large cysts are demonstrated by both isotope and pneumoencephalographic techniques, an obstruction of CSF flow is often present. One would anticipate that shunting would decrease the size of the cyst by correcting the abnormality of CSF flow. In our experience, however, the improvement following shunting has not been impressive. Many neurosurgeons believe that direct surgical opening of these cysts is indicated, but, again, encouraging results are scanty. Nonetheless, the presence of a large cerebral cyst in a patient with hydrocephalic dementia warrants treatment.

Ectatic Basilar Artery

As already noted, in our experience an abnormality of CSF circulation has been present in all individuals with ectatic basilar arteries whose dementia improved after shunting. Whether the disorder of CSF circulation is produced by the abnormal situation of the basilar artery or is the result of some other factor is unknown at present. It is sufficient to note that some demented elderly individuals who show a highly placed arteriosclerotic basilar artery and evidence of disordered CSF circulation on appropriate testing can enjoy considerable recovery of mental function with shunting. Both ventricular-atrial and lumbar–peritoneal shunts have produced gratifying results in the author's practice. Shunting, of course, does not benefit every patient with ectatic basilar artery; selection of candidates based on the positive diagnostic criteria mentioned earlier will offer a reasonable chance for success.

SUMMARY

This chapter has emphasized two points: first, that dementia is *not* irreversible and, second, that differentiation of hydrocephalic dementia is important because treatment is at least somewhat specific for a given variety. We have described several categories, outlined some criteria for diagnosis, and reviewed some of the therapeutic maneuvers available at the present time. It is recognized that some of the disease categories, some of the criteria for diagnosis, and many of the treatment methods will be altered in the future. Nonetheless, we believe that the clinician who recognizes dementia may profitably use the guidelines suggested here in providing care for his patient.

REFERENCES

1. Adams RD, Fisher CM, Hakim S, Ojemann R, Sweet W: Symptomatic occult hydrocephalus with "normal" cerebrospinal fluid pressure: A treatable syndrome. N Engl J Med 273:117–126, 1965
2. Appenzeller O, Salmon JH: Treatment of parenchymatous degeneration of the brain by ventriculo–atrial shunting of the cerebrospinal fluid. J. Neurosurg 26:478–482, 1967
3. Benson DF, LeMay M, Patten DH, Rubens AB: Diagnosis of normal-pressure hydrocephalus. N Engl J Med 283:609–615, 1970

4. Brown DG, Goldensohn ES: The electoencephalogram in normal-pressure hydrocephalus. Arch Neurol 29:70–71, 1973
5. Ekbom K, Greitz T, Kalmer M, Lopez J, Ottosson S: Cerebrospinal fluid pulsations in occult hydrocephalus due to ectasia of basilar artery. Acta Neurochir 20:1–8, 1969
6. Ekbom K, Greitz T, Kugelberg E: Hydrocephalus due to ectasia of the basilar artery. J Neurol Sci 8:465–477, 1969
7. Fisher CM: Senile dementia—a new explanation of its causation. Can Med Assoc J 65:1–7, 1951
8. Greenfield JG: The Spino-cerebellar Degenerations. Springfield, Ill, Thomas, 1954
9. Greitz T: Effect of brain distension on cerebral circulation. Lancet 1:863–865, 1969
10. Hakim S, Adams RD: The special clinical problem of symptomatic hydrocephalus with normal cerebrospinal fluid pressure—observations on cerebrospinal fluid hydrodynamics. J Neurol Sci 2:307–327, 1965
11. Lauter H, Meyer JE: Clinical and nosological concepts of senile dementia, in Müller CH, Ciampi L (eds): Senile Dementia. Bern, Hans Haber, 1968
12. LeMay M, New PFJ: Radiological diagnosis of occult normal pressure hydrocephalus. Radiology 96(2):347–358, 1970
13. Loranger AN, Goodell H, McDowell F, Lee J, Sweet RD: Intellectual impairment in Parkinson's syndrome. Brain 95:405–412, 1972
14. Nelson JR, Goodman SJ: An evaluation of the cerebrospinal fluid infusion test for hydrocephalus. Neurology 21: 1037–1053, 1971
15. Neumann MA, Cohn R: Progressive subcortical gliosis—a rare form of presenile dementia. Brain 90:405–418, 1967
16. Noyes AP: Modern Clinical Psychiatry. Philadelphia, Saunders, 1953
17. Ojemann RG, Fisher CM, Adams RD, Sweet WH, New PFJ: Further experience with the syndrome of "normal" pressure hydrocephalus. J Neurosurg 31:279–294, 1969
18. Roos R, Gajdersek DC, Gibbs CJ Jr.: The clinical characteristics of transmissable Creutzfeldt-Jakob disease. Brain 96:1–21, 1973
19. Shenkin HA, Greenberg J, Borizarth WF, Gutterman P, Morales JO: Ventricular shunting for relief of senile symptoms. JAMA 225:1486–1489, 1973
20. Silverberg GD, Castellino RA, Goodwin DA: Porencephalic cysts demonstrated by encephalography with radioiodinated serum albumin. N Engl J Med 280:315–316, 1969
21. Steele JC: Progressive supranuclear palsy. Brain 95:693–704, 1972
22. Tavaras JM, Wood EH: Diagnostic Radiology. Baltimore, Williams & Wilkins, 1964
23. Walsh AC: Senile dementia—a report on the anticoagulant treatment of thirteen patients. Pa Med 71:65–72, 1968
24. Walsh AC: Arterial insufficiency of the brain: Progression prevented by long-term anticoagulant therapy in eleven patients. J Am Geriatr Soc 17:93–104, 1969
25. Wolinsky JS, Barnes BD, Margolis MT: Diagnostic tests in normal-pressure hydrocephalus. Neurology 23:706–713, 1973

Commentary

The previous two chapters have strongly emphasized that the presence of dementia does not indicate an irreversible, untreatable situation with grave prognosis. Rather than dismissing this disorder with a label of ''chronic brain syndrome'' and a generally hopeless prognosis, dementia deserves as much diagnostic work and treatment as any other disorder in medicine.

Theoretically, depression and dementia appear quite dissimilar, but, for practical purposes, differentiation may be extremely difficult. In both disorders, psychomotor retardation is a cardinal sign, and, as noted earlier, misdiagnosis is common; dementia and depression represent one of the major interfaces of neurology and psychiatry. With the ability to treat both disorders constantly improving, appropriate diagnosis is imperative. The following chapter will discuss this problem in full.

Felix Post, M.D., F.R.C.P., F.R.C. (Psych.)

6
Dementia, Depression, and Pseudodementia

The clinical differentiation between dementia and depression in elderly people is discussed. Differentiation may prove impossible at first contact with suddenly and severely disordered patients, but it can be effected in the great majority of cases, provided assessment is carried out competently. Only a few patients will continue to present the phenomena of depressive pseudodementia, which is shown to be of no therapeutic importance or prognostic significance. However, observations related to depressive pseudodementia have led to investigations indicating the importance of cerebral aging in the etiology of affective illnesses occurring late in life, and on some of the mechanisms operating in the depressive illnesses of all ages.

DEFINITIONS AND SYMPTOMATOLOGY

The relationship between dementia and depression presents problems mainly in middle and late life, and since the psychiatry of late life is not a very well-taught subject, an introductory discussion of some elementary matters seems unavoidable.

First, it should be pointed out that at any age both dementia and depression are characterized by impairment of psychologic functioning. The term dementia is applied differently by neurologists, psychiatrists, and geriatricians. Neurologists tend to use it as a synonym for cognitive impairment.[16,27] Depending on the underlying causative condition, the dementia as defined by a neurologist may or may not be recoverable. By contrast, many psychiatrists reserve the use of the term for patients whose cognitive impairment has been demonstrated to be due to irreversible or progressive structural brain damage of a diffuse and widespread type: In the elderly, this is most commonly associated with cerebrovascular disease, either characterized by the cerebral changes first described by Alzheimer or by those associated with the rarer types of presenile dementia. Geriatricians dislike the term dementia altogether, since it seems to imply hopelessness and therapeutic inactivity. They prefer to speak of persistent confusion. They tend to encounter patients with long-standing physical disease and socially deprived lives, whose mental impairment can be lessened by medical treatment and social rehabilitation. There are also national differences: The American terminology speaks of acute and chronic brain syndromes; the British use the terms acute and chronic confusional states to differentiate brief and transitional from persistent and irreversible conditions. The term "delirious reaction" is used synonymously with acute confusion. To escape this terminologic jungle, we shall try to avoid all these terms in this discussion and shall refer to all organic psychosyndromes very simply in terms of different instances of cerebral failure.

By contrast, the term depression is much more uniformly applied by physicians (including geriatricians), neurologists, and psychiatrists. Thus, there is no need to define the disorder or (for present purposes) to discuss whether or not differentiations such as those between biologic–endogenous –psychotic and psychogenic–reactive–neurotic depressions are useful. More important than this is the need to recognize the various disguises by which a depressive illness can emerge. The disorder can start abruptly and cause a sudden and profound disruption of all personality functions, very much like what occurs in sudden cerebral failure. Those depressives whose symptoms develop gradually, however, may initially appear to be suffering from slowly occurring cerebral failure. Finally, but by no means always, a severe state of cognitive and psychomotor disruption may occur in severe melancholia and in depressive stupor, and this disruption may also bear striking resemblances to that seen in severe cerebral failure.

Tables 6-1 and 6-2 attempt to portray the extent to which symptoms and signs of cerebral failure and of affective illnesses may overlap, and they illustrate how similarities in the development of these conditions can give rise to diagnostic difficulties. Table 6-1 indicates the rapid, almost simultaneous, appearance of clinical phenomena associated with these conditions with the divergence becoming evident only in the course of time. Table 6-2 shows the gradual development of the two conditions. Obviously, not all features named will occur in every patient or in the depicted sequence. It will be seen that the early signs of cerebral failure down to the appearance of mild memory defects may also occur in neurotic and self-limited anxious—hypochondriacal

Table 6-1
Rapid Onset of Disorder

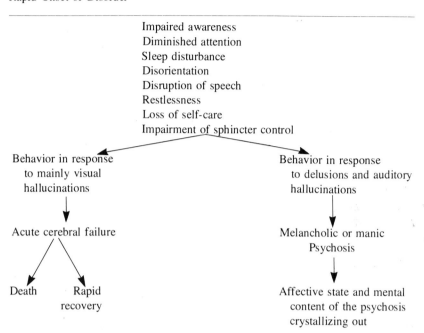

Impaired awareness
Diminished attention
Sleep disturbance
Disorientation
Disruption of speech
Restlessness
Loss of self-care
Impairment of sphincter control

Behavior in response
to mainly visual
hallucinations

Behavior in response
to delusions and auditory
hallucinations

Acute cerebral failure

Melancholic or manic
Psychosis

Death   Rapid
recovery

Affective state and mental
content of the psychosis
crystallizing out

–depressive conditions, while severe affective psychoses can share with organic mental disorders fleeting delusional ideas and suicidal propensities, as well as some more clear-cut cognitive defects. Impaired verbal communication may cause considerable difficulties in eliciting abnormal thought content characteristic of a manic or melancholic state. How then should we set about to unscramble these combinations of clinical phenomena in order to arrive at correct diagnoses, and even more important, at correct decisions concerning management?

DIFFERENTIATION OF ILLNESSES OF ABRUPT ONSET

Even the most experienced clinician may be unable to decide whether he is dealing with a cerebral or an emotional disorder when first seeing a patient exhibiting the array of symptoms shown in Table 6-1. The patient is likely to be in a state of panic, he may be aggressive, and he will be completely or almost completely inaccessible. Paradoxically, the need to make the precise

Table 6-2
Gradual Onset of Disorder

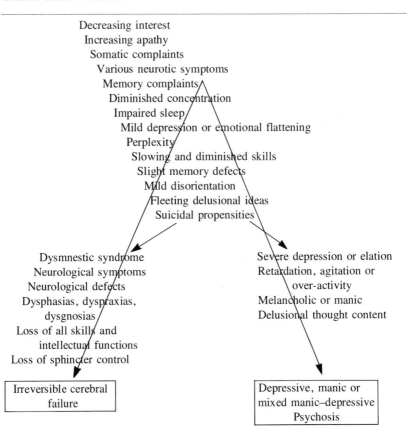

Decreasing interest
Increasing apathy
Somatic complaints
Various neurotic symptoms
Memory complaints
Diminished concentration
Impaired sleep
Mild depression or emotional flattening
Perplexity
Slowing and diminished skills
Slight memory defects
Mild disorientation
Fleeting delusional ideas
Suicidal propensities

Dysmnestic syndrome
Neurological symptoms
Neurological defects
Dysphasias, dyspraxias,
dysgnosias
Loss of all skills and
intellectual functions
Loss of sphincter control

Severe depression or elation
Retardation, agitation or
over-activity
Melancholic or manic
Delusional thought content

Irreversible cerebral failure

Depressive, manic or mixed manic–depressive Psychosis

and final diagnosis immediately is least imperative in these most urgent situations. Of foremost importance is the elimination of acute cerebral failure, since this may prove fatal if left untreated. Admission to hospital is indicated. As complete a physical examination as the patient will permit should be carried out, which may give the physician leads as to other tests that may be needed. To facilitate these, or to observe the patient further in those areas where physical examination had been negative, it will be necessary by means of medication to render him less disturbed and less likely to exhaust himself. Substances likely to impair his level of awareness even further (for example, barbiturates or paraldehyde) or to induce neurologic symptoms (for example, haloperidol) should be avoided as much as possible. Repeated doses of chlormethiazole by mouth or of tranquilizers like promazine by intramuscular injection should be the first choice. Skilled nurses, who can utilize lucid intervals in the patient's awareness to improve contact with him, should obviate the need for heavy medication, thus rendering the patient more accessible.

In the vast majority of patients with acute or subacute cerebral failure, the causal pathology will be speedily elicited. Where all findings have been negative during the first few days of observation, the clinical picture of a functional psychosis will have begun to emerge: In the present context, this might be a mixed manic–depressive state, a manic, or a severe melancholic condition, either agitated or stuporose in type. Obviously, a schizophrenic or a so-called psychogenic reaction, although much rarer in elderly subjects, will have to be considered as well. However, decisions on management can as a rule be made at an early stage, where external informants have been available from the start. A history should be taken from these informants with three broad possibilities in mind: (1) a functional psychosis of sudden onset; (2) acute cerebral failure; and (3) acute cerebral failure complicating chronic cerebral failure (that is, an acute brain syndrome in a patient with a long-standing chronic brain syndrome, a delirious reaction occurring in the course of the dementing process). A summary of some useful differentiating features follows.

Functional psychoses hardly ever truly arise abruptly. When time is taken to obtain a thorough history, evidence of milder, prodromal symptoms is usually forthcoming. Restricting our discussion to affective illnesses, there may have been over the preceding weeks changes like loss of interest, appetite, and sleep, possibly after a bereavement or other kinds of "loss." Mild elation might have preceded severe depression, or mild depression may have turned suddenly into a severe mixed manic–depressive or manic state. The patient himself and his home surroundings are likely to look well cared for. In most patients with acute cerebral failure, this will also usually be the case. There may, however, be a history of physical illness, and too often in these times evidence suggesting injudicious use of medications where the patient looks dishevelled or is discovered in dirty surroundings, the possibility of alcohol or drug abuse must be considered. Finally, a history of failing memory and mental ability and of failing physical health will always be obtained (provided it is sought) where acute cerebral failure has occurred as a complication of a dementing illness. In the case of an elderly person living alone, the neglected state of his person and of his home will strongly point to this possibility. Another observation may be helpful: Patients with acute cerebral failure will show variations in their level of awareness. During lucid intervals, they may demonstrate adequate recall of events immediately preceding the acute breakdown, confirming that until very recently their mental functioning had been intact. Demented patients whose condition is compounded by acute confusion may also become more accessible in relation to fluctuations of consciousness but will have a poor grasp of recent events, and they will betray ignorance of matters with which a healthy person of their age and educational status should be conversant.

In summary immediate differentiation between depression and ''dementia'' may not be possible in the absence of an independent history in cases of severe illnesses of sudden onset. Exclusion of any treatable physical disease and its management should be one's main concern, since the correct diagnosis will emerge on observation. Certain features of the mental state, and above all an independent account of the development of the disorder, will remove diagnostic difficulties at a much earlier stage.

DIFFERENTIATION OF ILLNESSES OF GRADUAL ONSET

While the nature of rapidly developing conditions will become apparent in the light of further information, observation, and response to treatment, well-established disorders will require full diagnostic assessment in order to avoid instituting unsuitable therapies and management of the cases based on faulty prognostications. In patients not regarded as ''old'' (a judgment that tends to change with the psychiatrist's own age!), the appearance of anxiety, depression, or elation together with related disorders of mental content and behavior will immediately suggest an affective illness. The possibility that affective symptoms may be part of a cerebral disorder is often not considered for a long time, especially when the patient has suffered earlier attacks of an affective illness. The discovery of intracranial neoplastic, inflammatory, or degenerative conditions (for example, presenile dementia) or of a general disorder (for example, myxedema) is often considerably delayed. By contrast, the appearance of any kind of psychologic symptom in older persons immediately gives rise to a suspicion of cerebral impairment due to normal or pathologic aging. The frequency with which the depressions of late life were misdiagnosed in the past as dementia has been exaggerated. I have made this point in the past,[29] and as long ago as 1951 I had been able to show in a follow-up of case records prepared by other psychiatrists that a differentiation between functional and organic mental disorders had been made correctly in the great majority of patients briefly evaluated during their passage through a mental observation unit. After a study of elderly patients in a mental hospital, Roth and Morrissey[39] recommended a diagnostic classification based on differences of prognosis as well as of symptomatology, which has been widely accepted and used. Since then, several long-term follow-up studies[18,19,30,34,37] of elderly depressives seen in widely differing settings have demonstrated that signs and symptoms of cerebral failure do not appear in them subsequently any more frequently than in the general elderly population: The occurrence of depressive symptoms in the elderly only occasionally foreshadows the onset of one of the dementias of late life.

While both in the past and in the present well-trained psychiatrists have been able to distinguish easily and correctly between depression and dementia, it would be unrealistic to suggest that problems of differential diagnosis did not occasionally arise. We noted (Table 6-2) that both during the development and at the height of affective illnesses there may be a considerable overlap of clinical phenomena with those of cerebral failure. As the incidence of cerebral deterioration begins to increase after the age of 40, gaining considerable momentum after 65, a careful assessment of neurologic and cognitive functioning becomes especially necessary in elderly persons presenting with affective disorders. Such evaluation will demonstrate in the great majority of patients that there are neither physical signs nor psychologic defects pointing to cerebral disease or deterioration. In a few elderly depressives, clear and incontrovertible evidence will be obtained for the presence of some type of cerebral pathology. Finally, there will be some depressed patients exhibiting some cognitive impairment and also perhaps some neurologic abnormalities. In this last group alone, difficulties will be experienced by the knowledgable clinician.

SCREENING AFFECTIVELY ILL ELDERLY PATIENTS FOR THE PRESENCE OF CEREBRAL FAILURE

It has been pointed out repeatedly (Table 6-2) that personality and character changes associated with early cerebral failure may for some time remain indistinguishable from those seen in mild depression or hypomania and also that cognitive malfunction may be very striking in severe affective psychoses. A careful assessment of the patient's cognitive and neurologic status has, therefore, been recommended in the preceding section. Before discussing this further, it cannot be overstressed that the examination for cognitive defects of an emotionally distressed patient may (from a diagnostic point of veiw) be much less useful than a history taken from an observant friend or relative. This is the case because there are important differences in the course of the development of purely affective illnesses in comparison with those occurring in a setting of progressive cerebral failure. As a general rule, depressions start with loss of interest, confidence, and drive, but objective failure at work or a memory disorder will become a problem only by the time the depression has become well established. However, these failures rather than the preceding mood disorder may have led to referral. In contrast, symptoms that might be attributed to an affective illness usually appear in the course of cerebral failure after cognitive deterioration had been progressing for some time: Advice may have been sought primarily for anxiety, hypochondriacal complaints, depression, euphoria, or paranoid behavior, but on specific inquiry it will emerge that these symptoms had been foreshadowed by many months of failure at work, episodes of disorientation (especially during a stay in unaccustomed surroundings), lapses of memory, repetitive talk, and so forth.

Turning to the examination of the patient, certain screeening procedures have been devised for use by busy clinicians. The slowly developing cerebral deteriorations of late life show themselves with few exceptions (such as Pick's disease) initially through impairment of memory functioning, especially of new learning, and secondary to this, of orientation. Tests of these abilities are easily devised and administered. This makes them useful screening procedures, which will help to exclude the presence of cerebral failure. Very brief questionnaires[13,15] have been found reliable and valid in situations where it seems desirable (for example, in geriatric practice) to quantify serious cognitive defects. When incipient cerebral failure, however, is suspected in emotionally disturbed patients, several aspects of memory function and orientation need be examined and compared. Above all, allowance has to be made for impairment due to age alone, and many time-honored tasks of the so-called sensorium examination have been found to be too difficult for the majority of elderly psychiatric subjects;[31,43] these include the recall after some minutes of a name or address, the retelling of a simple story, the serial subtraction of sevens starting from 100, and so on. In the writer's department, a number of questionnaires[31] have been developed that can be completely and correctly answered by a well-preserved person in his 80s. The first questionnaire assesses orientation, the second covers events in the patient's past life, the third tests his recall of recent events in his life, for example, concerning his admission to the hospital, and the fourth questionnaire refers to recent national and international events, as well as to names of Prime Ministers, Presidents of the U.S., and the British Royal Family. With a total possible score of 42 points, patients scoring more than 35 points only rarely prove to be suffering from cerebral failure. A lower score indicates that further assessment should be carried out, unless the patient's work and educational record suggests a low level of original intelligence. Most patients will cooperate in brief vocabulary tests, which will allow a rough estimate of their original I.Q. Thus, poor performance on the questionnaire concerning recent political events and names can be ignored in a patient of low intellectual background, but would raise suspicions of deterioration in a person of higher status. In fact, the actual scores obtained form the least important results of these simple clinical tests. For this reason, any clinician may design his own questionnaires, provided they tap orientation and various kinds of information, and thus allow patchiness of performance to be demonstrated. It is well recognized, for instance, that excellent recall of past life events but poor recall of recent events is highly suggestive of cerebral failure. This may also be indicated by great variability in the knowledge of recent historical and political matters, by telescoping (transposing order) of the sequence of events, by perseveration and confabulation. By and large "near miss" answers are suggestive of cerebral deficits, while "don't know" answers are more typical of the unwilling and possibly depressed patient.

Even in the absence of demonstrable defects of memory and orientation or of neurologic signs, the patient should be examined for the presence of focal signs of cerebral dysfunction, whenever the history is suggestive of early cerebral failure. It is usually possible to obtain the cooperation of anxious and agitated patients in a brief assessment of their abilities to name objects, write, read, use numbers, copy simple designs, and in right–left orientation. Finally, emotional lability and affective incontinence are sometimes mistaken for depression by the inexperienced. These disorders (so characteristic of some elderly demented patients) can often be elicited through making the patient laugh or cry, almost to order, by suggesting sad or cheerful themes. Truly depressive affect is little influenced by these maneuvers: at best a social smile may be evoked.

In summary, the presence of cerebral failure will thus be made evident in affectively ill patients on the basis of a history of diminishing memory and other cognitive functions that were noticed some time before the onset of depression, and as a result of an examination demonstrating patchy defects of orientation and recent memory. Even in the absence of unmistakable neurological defects, cerebral failure will be indicated by the presence of dysphasia, apraxia, or agnosia. Defects of this kind, as well as the presence of frequent perseverations and of near-miss or confabulatory answers, should not be ignored even in a severely depressed patient, and should lead to a double diagnosis: cerebral disorder plus affective illness.

ASSOCIATION BETWEEN DEPRESSIVE ILLNESS AND CEREBRAL DISEASE

The association of severe depression with Parkinsonism is well known. What is less often recognized is that depressive illnesses occur more commonly in relation to cerebrovascular disease than can be explained in terms of chance association.[30] These patients have a frequency of family histories of affective illnesses similar to elderly depressives without cerebral changes and tend to have suffered from depressions earlier in life, before there could possibly have been any cerebral process at work. Thus, it is important to recognize the presence of depression in elderly people who have a history of epileptiform convulsions or strokes, since they may be as severe a suicidal risk as cerebrally intact depressives.

The association between senile dementia and severe depression seems to be much less frequent, but whatever the cause of cerebral failure any associated depression should be vigorously treated in its own right, except where cerebral impairment is of recent origin and (as in some cases of myxedema) is expected to yield to medical or surgical treatment fairly rapidly.

Just as in depressions associated with Parkinsonism, those occurring in patients with cerebrovascular disease tend to make good remissions with drugs or electroconvulsive therapy (ECT). However, the incidence of further attacks and of more indefinite depressive invalidism has proved to be higher than that found in a long-term follow-up of elderly depressives without cerebral pathology[30] whose long-term prognosis is not very favorable either: A recent sample[34] was carefully followed over 3 years following discharge and received further treatment (social support, psychologic support, drug therapy or ECT) as necessary. In spite of this, only 26.1 percent of patients had made lasting recoveries, and a further 37 percent suffered further attacks; some depressive invalidism with or without further attacks occurred in 25 percent, and 11.9 percent remained clinically depressed throughout the follow-up period. However, critical evaluations of the long-term outcome of depressive illnesses of younger patients[23,30] have shown that this tends to be far less favorable than textbooks continue to suggest. At all ages, and whether or not cerebral failure is present, the treatment of affective symptoms may be effective only for a limited time, and most patients will require repeated or continuous psychiatric attention.

DEPRESSIONS WITH DOUBTFUL CEREBRAL FAILURE

There remains a group of elderly depressives with minimal neurologic defects and with some difficulties in memory and orientation of doubtful significance, in whose case the careful clinician may wonder whether the affective disturbance might not be a "reaction" to early dementia. Thus, in a series of 100 patients,[30] 23 were originally diagnosed as depressed in relation to one type of cerebral pathology or another. In four of these patients, follow-up over 8 years or to death demonstrated that no such pathology had in fact been present. One third of the remaining 81 patients had exhibited more isolated neurologic abnormalities such as tremors, rigidities, weaknesses, or reflex inequalities, but over 8 years these did not forecast beyond chance expectation the future development of cerebral deterioration or an unfavorable course of the affective illness. Similarly, doubtful intellectual impairment was recorded on clinical grounds in 41 of 100 patients, but in contrast to unequivocable impairment, this did not significantly influence long-term outcome. Since then, the same observation has been made by other workers[1] in the case of community subjects with mild functional psychiatric conditions. The lack of clinical significance of isolated neurologic findings in old people was fully documented some 40 years ago by Critchley, and his views have also been confirmed recently.[35] Doubtful electroencephalographic findings are equally of little value in giving an early warning of incipient cerebral pathologic events.[26]

The suggestion arises that in these cases of depression with doubtful early cerebral failure psychologic tests might be employed to decide the issue. The reader may, in fact, have begun to wonder why so far no mention has been made of ''tests of deterioration.'' The reason for this omission arises from the high level of agreement that has usually been found between the results of tests carried out by psychologists and the kind of thorough clinical assessment outlined in this communication. This agreement makes testing by a psychologist as a routine investigation quite unnecessary in clinically clear-cut cases. Where, on the other hand, the clinical assessment suggests doubtful cognitive impairment, psychologic testing usually produces equally doubtful results. Only occasionally is the psychologist able to allay the clinician's doubts by obtaining test results that definitely exclude cerebral failure. In any case, many of these emotionally disturbed, bewildered, retarded, or agitated patients prove to be ''untestable.''

It has been known for many years that some depressives, who later make good recoveries, may, at the height of their illnesses, exhibit a degree of intellectual impairment that suggests the onset of senile or arteriosclerotic dementia. It used to be thought that the depressive illness had mobilized a dementing process, which, on recovery from the depression, came to a halt or at any rate once again became imperceptibly slow. As we saw earlier, long-term follow-up studies have shown conclusively that this suggestion is fortunately no longer tenable. In fact, Madden and co-workers[24] discovered temporary intellectual impairment to be without prognostic significance in some 10 percent of 300 functional psychiatric patients over the age or 45, and they were probably the first among several later writers on the same subject to use the term ''depressive pseudodementia.''[31] As has been pointed out previously,[11] this transient cognitive impairment of depressed elderly patients cannot be simply put down to lack of cooperation, toxic factors, or ''inaccessibility.'' Moreover, some 16 percent of depressives over 60 were able to score normally on a number of clinical and psychologic tests, but failed specifically on a procedure that required them to learn the meaning of words previously unknown to them. Assessed on this Synonym Learning Test[21] in isolation of all other findings, they would have been misclassified as suffering from diffuse brain damage. In fact, their response to treatment did not differ from that of other patients.[32] These patients also did badly on some memory questionnaires, thus raising the clinician's suspicions of cerebral deterioration. They tended to have verbal I.Q.s below 95, and to be more often delusionally depressed than subjects performing normally.[21] Other learning and psychomotor speed tests[21] have shown similar transient declines in levels of performance, with improvement going beyond the effects of practice following remission of the depressive state. Kendrick[20] has recently demonstrated a method by which the test battery that has come to be known by his name may be used in retrospect to differentiate patients who had exhibited the phenomenon of depressive pseudodementia.

Earlier, it was stressed that depression should be treated vigorously even in the presence of unequivocally demonstrated cerebral deterioration. The presence of doubtful or even of pseudo-dementia should not deter the psychiatrist from employing active therapy. Contradicting some impressionistic views, the careful use of electroconvulsive therapies is not followed by lasting impairment of memory functioning,[22] and in many ways may be preferable to long courses of tricyclic or other antidepressant drugs.

SOME THEORETICAL ISSUES

It has been shown in the preceding sections that the difficulties of differentiating between the depressions and the dementias of late life should not be exaggerated. True, it may not be possible to distinguish an affective psychosis of sudden and acute onset from acute cerebral failure related to toxic–metabolic disorders developing suddenly and overwhelmingly, except after a period of observation, unless reliable independent observers are available and can give a clear history of the development of the illness. Much more frequently, however, depression or cerebral failure develops gradually, and, provided careful clinical assessment is carried out, there are only occasional difficulties in distinguishing these two conditions. In a small number of cases, both an affective disorder and cerebral disease may be present. Only in a few patients may genuine diagnostic doubts be raised by objectively demonstrated cognitive impairment. These doubts may continue to be entertained and may only be resolved by the course of the patient's current illness, his later progress, or the results of psychologic retesting in relation to a subsequent breakdown. Diagnostic doubts should not prevent energetic attempts at removing affective symptoms and distress, and the point cannot be made too strongly that depressive pseudodementia should no longer be regarded of immediate practical or remote prognostic significance.

However, in this final section it will be shown that with depressive pseudodementia as a starting base some important theoretical issues can be tackled. The first of these may be put as the following question: Why do depressions become more frequent and more severe in later life, and why do they tend to recur more frequently?

This problem would most logically be studied by comparing young and old depressives during their first attack and by following their progress over a number of years. However, organizing such a prospective study (the collecting of consecutive samples of patients alone) would take much time, and workers have taken a shortcut by investigating elderly depressives whose first attacks had occurred at different ages. First of all, there is general agreement[4,14,17,30,37,44] that elderly depressives whose first attacks had occurred before the age of 40–50 had a significantly greater incidence of affective family histories than patients with first depressions occurring at a later age. At the same time, the mean age of relatives of early-onset probands at the time of their first illnesses was only insignificantly lower than that of the affected relatives of late-onset depressives,[4] who therefore are unlikely to constitute a genetically differentiated subgroup (other than in terms of diminished loading with hereditary factors). Late-onset depressives also tended to have been physically more robust during adult life,[31] while early-onset depressives had been more often handicapped throughout adult life or earlier by neurotic and adjustment problems.[4] Previous claims[25] alleging specific personality defects of so-called involutional depressives have not been confirmed by more recent work.[4]

Constitutional predisposition to affective disorders would thus appear to be much weaker in late-onset depressive patients, and in keeping with the many kinds of emotional trauma to which the elderly are singularly exposed, it might be thought that in them external etiologic factors were more important. To put it simply and in accordance with common sense, elderly persons may be especially prone to depressions because they experience so much that is depressing. This assumption has, however, received only partial support. True, in from 60 to 80 percent of elderly depressives[4,34] the illness had been preceded by recent bereavement, sudden and unaccustomed physical illness, loss of home, retirement, the moving away of children, and so forth. However, such precipitating events tended to be found as frequently in early-onset depressives as in those who had experienced depressive illnesses solely in late life. There were only a few exceptions. Death of spouse was only insignificantly more often implicated in late-onset depressives, although it tended to occur earlier during the period of mourning than was the case in early-onset depressives.[4] Physical illness is also a more frequently ascertained etiologic factor in late-onset depressives, but only in male patients to a statistically significant degree.[38] Thus it appears that neither specific constitutional predisposition nor a greater importance of psychic trauma can satisfactorily explain the increased propensity of aging persons for affective illnesses, and incidentally toward suicide, suicidal attempts, and mild depressive swings. One is, therefore, impelled toward considering the role of the aging process itself.

Research that begun with the observation of pseudodementia in depressives over the age of 60 has, in fact, started to yield some support for the suggestion that age changes affecting the brain may facilitate the occurrence of depression. Before summarizing some results of these investigations, it is necessary to take a brief look at work on brain function in affective disorders.

Several strands are distinguishable in a development during which the affective psychoses, in spite of their official classification as functional disorders, have become increasingly linked with abnormalities of cerebral functioning. At the synaptic level, abnormalities have been demonstrated in catecholamine concentration, in the level of enzymes destroying them, and in mineral metabolism (especially potassium–sodium distribution). Contributions in this area and in the psychopharmacology of depression are well known but too numerous to refer to here. All the substances concerned have been shown to influence the excitability of nervous tissues. Interestingly, clinicians have for a long time suspected that some of the behavioral changes (especially slowing) in severe depressions were due to a lowering of cerebral activity and that some processes leading to "inhibition" were at work. Their mechanisms have been speculated on along both Pavlovian[7] and psychodynamic lines.[8,12] Experimental work on "arousal" (a problematic concept describing level of cerebral functioning) has been carried out by Shagass and his group,[41] as well as more recently by other workers,[28] by means of sleep- and sedation-threshold estimations. Thresholds (measured as milligrams of sodium amytal per kilogram of body weight to achieve "sedation" or "sleep") have been found to be lowered (that is, sensitivity to intravenous sodium amytal increased) in psychotic depressives and to a greater extent in dementing patients.[2,41] Thresholds tended to increase (that is, barbiturate sensitivity tended to decrease) in depressives after remission.[28,42] The interpretation is that in dementia permanently, and in depression reversibly, some aspect of brain function is altered so that less intravenous barbiturate is required to produce a given level of impaired awareness. Turning from physiologic to psychologic measures of cerebral function, we noted of course the phenomenon of pseudodementia in elderly depressives, but the occurrence of transient cognitive impairment in younger depressives has been more sparsely documented.[6,10]

Current investigations are aimed at (1) confirming a reduction in the level of cerebral functioning in elderly demented and depressive subjects, (2) at testing the role of an age factor, and (3) at unraveling some of the mechanisms at work. The general working hypothesis employed during these studies is presented in Table 6-3. In the center of the table are the two parameters used for the measurement of cerebral impairment, one psychologic and the other neurophysiologic. They comprised various tests of intelligence, learning, and psychomotor speed on the one hand, and estimations of sedation and sleep thresholds on the other (the methods employed have all been fully described elsewhere[3]). As indicated in Table 6-3, impairment of brain function is held to be produced differently in progressive cerebral disease and in depression. The sequence of events occurring in dementing patients would appear to be known in general outline; the mechanisms producing measurable impairment of cerebral functioning in depressives are still open to conjecture. For the purposes of this working hypothesis, it has been postulated that depression is always preceded by an affective state within the realm of normal experience, for which the term "emotional turmoil" has been used. As we saw, depressive illnesses are preceded by emotionally distressing events in the vast majority of patients, and there is good reason to believe that in the remainder covert emotional factors

Table 6-3
Suggested Sequence of Events in Elderly Dements and Depressives

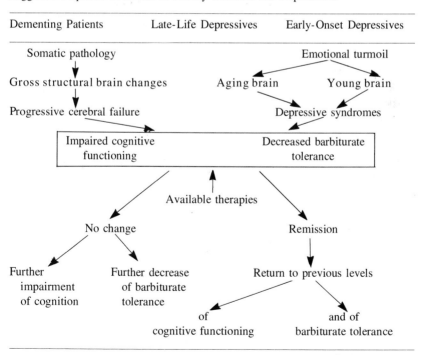

have been at work in a precipitating fashion.[34] There is some experimental evidence for the existence of a physiologic correlate to this postulated state of emotional turmoil,[9] which will be discussed later, but for the mechanisms by which it is translated into the clinical state of depression there is as yet only speculation.[7,8,12] What seems certain is that only persons with the relevant inherited or acquired predisposition will in fact develop a depressive illness,[34] but only one of many etiologic factors, the absence or presence of age changes in the brain, has been included in Table 6-3. The lower portion of Table 6-3 presents subsequent changes: Progressive cerebral failure will take its course until such a time as effective therapies are available, and cognitive functions will continue to decrease, as will tolerance of barbiturates. In contrast, depression should recover or improve. At the same time, any cerebral impairment should disappear, as shown by improved performance of psychologic tests and increased barbiturate tolerance. The working hypothesis depicted in Table 6-3 allows a number of predictions to be made. These, and the statistically significant results obtained on testing them, will be briefly summarized.

1. In the case of patients suffering from one of the dementing illnesses of old age, mean scores on psychologic tests and mean barbiturate threshold values were expected to be below those obtained in remitted elderly depressives. This was confirmed.[11]
2. In dementing patients, test scores and threshold values should decline further with the passage of time. On account of the experimental situation, patients were reassessed after only 6 weeks. A significant decline was therefore not observed, but neither was an increase.[11]
3. In depressives responding to treatment, improvements of psychologic scores and increases of sleep- and sedation-threshold values were predicted. Changes in the predicted direction, which were thought to reflect improvement of cerebral functioning, did in fact occur.[3] Moreover, the gains made correlated positively and beyond chance expectation with independent ratings of clinical change. As might have been expected, brain function had been lowered initially to a greater extent and rose more steeply after treatment in patients who had been graded as more severely ill, and as exhibiting symptoms and characteristics of psychotic rather than of neurotic depressions.[3]

By and large, changes in psychologic scores in comparison with those of physiologic measures correlated to a smaller although still significant extent with type of depression and outcome.[3] It may be added here that workers during a more recent investigation[5] using different psychologic measures found similar increases over 3 months in a group of older functional psychiatric patients, while during the same period the scores of dementing patients failed to register any significant changes. So far, then, findings have been in keeping with the working hypothesis, and in addition it has been demonstrated that the clinically observable phenomenon of depressive pseudodementia merely presents the proverbial tip of an iceberg, in that many more elderly depressives suffer measurable reductions of cerebral functions at a subclinical level.

We will now turn to the main argument, which runs as follows: Age changes in the brain, falling short of clinically identifiable pathologic processes, are responsible for the greater frequency and recurrency rate of depression in late life, and more particularly they are an important etiologic factor in subjects who (unlike early-onset depressives) have shown little predisposition to depressive illnesses earlier in life. It is suggested that, in many aging persons levels of cerebral functioning are reduced, and that this may under the impact of emotional turmoil facilitate further reductions to levels associated with clinical depression. This hypothesis would clearly fail if the last prediction arising from our working hypothesis turned out to be false.

4. Patients with late onset of their first depressive illnesses should after remission of their current illness yield lower psychologic test scores and lower barbiturate threshold values when compared with patients whose illnesses had started earlier in life. (Obviously, patients could not be assessed before they had become depressed, and the assumption was made that the values obtained after successful treatment closely approximated those theoretically obtainable before the illness; certainly the type of treatment employed, drugs or ECT, did not influence the posttreatment values.) This prediction was not negated: The higher the patient's age at the time of his first attack, the lower were his sleep and sedation thresholds after remission of the current illness.[3] For technical reasons arising from the distribution in this sample of verbal intelligence scores (which understandably correlated with learning and psychomotor speed scores), the prediction that age at first attack would also correlate negatively with posttreatment psychologic scores could not be tested. However, the suggestion that age changes in the brain may present an additional and important etiologic factor leading to an increased frequency and severity of depressive illnesses in the middle-aged and the elderly has found some support. Further confirmation of the etiologic role of aging has recently come from a different quarter: an age-wise increase of monoamine oxidase in the body has been reported.[36]

From these observations, a few speculations seem permissible. First, the findings of the investigations reported here seemed at first to contradict those of an earlier group of workers.[9] They had reported not increased, but decreased, sensitivity to barbiturates during depression, and increases in the course of remission. Their estimations of barbiturate sensitivity were carried out by electroencephalographic means, while large doses of pentothal (thiopental) were rapidly injected to produce deep anesthesia preliminary to the application of ECT. It was suggested that in depression subcortical arousal mechanisms were "set" at a higher level, and that for this reason greater amounts of barbiturates were required to suppress the outflow to the cortex and to evoke the electroencephalographic phenomenon of suppression burst patterns, which indicted that a certain stage of deep anesthesia had been reached. The role of emotional turmoil and anxiety in the genesis of depression, a theory that has been postulated by some writers, is thus seen to have a possible observable physiologic backing. By contrast, in our investigations[3,11] only "sedation" and light sleep were induced. The end points were determined by responses to auditory stimuli. Combining these two reciprocal sets of observations is in keeping with the suggestion that in depression there is heightened subcortical arousal (? reticular system) coupled with diminished (? inhibited) activity at higher levels of the CNS. Clinically, it is well recognized that in most patients anxiety and agitation (that is, heightened arousal) tend to be present to varying degrees simultaneously with depression and retardation. Moreover, anxiety symptoms not infrequently precede the phenomena of depression. We shall see presently that the reciprocal observations that have just been discussed fit in with a two-arousal hypothesis of cerebral functioning.

A further discrepancy arose from the fact that psychologic test scores changed in the predicted direction during remission of depressions to a smaller (albeit still significant) extent than did physiologic measures.[3] Also, in contrast to what was found in the case of patients with evidence for pathologic brain changes, in depressives psychologic and physiologic measures failed to correlate with one another.[3,11] Not perhaps surprisingly, the suggestion arose that the psychologic defects observed during a depressive illness were in many ways different from those occurring in structurally produced cerebral failure. So, the investigation was extended by the inclusion of further psychologic measures and additional dementing patients, and it was again confirmed that the depressives had some degree of learning defect. However, it was found that this was less severe and affected fewer of the tests than in demented patients. Also, the types of errors made by depressives differed from those exhibited by dementing subjects.[45]

Furthermore, attempts have been made to explain the discrepancy between changes in psychologic and in physiologic functions. The fact that these failed to occur in unison in the case of depressives (that is, failed to correlate with one another)[3] indicated that they were not related to an identical common mechanism, for example, to "arousal." Doubts about arousal being a unitary concept had been expressed earlier,[11] and it has been suggested[20] that our findings might fit in with a two-arousal hypothesis of cerebral function[40] based on the results of animal experiments. These were thought to yield evidence for the existence of an arousal system A probably related to the reticular activating system, which maintains arousal of the organism and provides organization for responses. A second arousal system B was related to the limbic system, and was thought to provide control of responses through incentive-related stimuli. These two mechanisms were found to be reciprocal, in that they inhibited one another and provided a regulating system. The special role of the limbic system (thought as mediating arousal B) for learning has been accepted for some time, but the additional suggestion was made that the way in which responses were laid down as memories was facilitated by the suppression of system A (reticular) by system B (limbic).

As a framework for further research, the following hypothesis, which is in keeping with the findings summarized in this chapter, may then explain the mechanisms operating in dementia and in depression, respectively: (1) Widespread cerebral damage affects both arousal systems as well as cortical functions, and this results in global mental impairment including that of memory. (2) In depression, there occurs greatly increased arousal A (reticular) and a reciprocal decrease of arousal B (limbic) resulting in far fewer and less severe changes in mental functions, especially those concerning learning ability and possibly psychomotor speed.

Finally, it is of interest to note the way in which ideas about depressive states in old age have changed in the course of the last 25 years. Initially, depression arising during the last period of life was generally regarded as an early phase of senile mental decay, although the occurrence of senile depressions with a good prognosis was also recognized (evidence summarized elsewhere[30]). Next it was shown that elderly depressives did not in fact develop senile, atherosclerotic, or other pathologic brain changes any more frequently than old persons did generally, and the increasing frequency and severity of depressions in late life were thought to be related to social and psychogenic factors that became increasingly stressful as people grew older. Now we are once again considering the role of impaired cerebral functioning in facilitating depression in late life, but the emphasis has shifted from definite brain pathology to brain aging.

ACKNOWLEDGMENT

My thanks are due to Dr. W. A. Lishman for his helpful criticisms of the final draft of this chapter.

REFERENCES

1. Bergman K, Kay DWK, Foster EM, McKechnie AA, Roth M: A follow-up study of randomly selected community residents to assess the effects of chronic brain syndrome and cerebrovascular disease. Excerpta Medica International Congress Series No. 274. Psychiatry (Part 2). Proceedings of the Fifth World

Congress of Psychiatry, Mexico, D.F., Nov. 25–Dec. 4, 1971, Excerpta Medica, Amsterdam

2. Caird WK, Laverty SG, Inglis J: Sedation and sleep thresholds in elderly patients with memory disorder. Gerontol Clin (Basel) 5:55–62, 1963

3. Cawley RH, Whitehead A, Post F: Barbiturate tolerance and psychological functioning in elderly depressed patients. Psychol Med 3:39–52, 1973

4. Chesser ES: A study of some aetiological factors in the affective disorders of old age: Unpublished dissertation. London, Institute of Psychiatry, 1965

5. Copeland JRM: U.K.–U.S. Diagnostic Project. Personal communication, 1972

6. Cronholm BC, Ottoson J-O: Memory function in endogenous depressives before and after E.C.T. Arch Gen Psychiatry 5:193–199, 1961

7. Davis DR: The psychological mechanisms of depression, in Davies EB (ed): Depression. Cambridge Univ Pr, 1964

8. Engel GL: Anxiety and depression withdrawal: The primary effects of unpleasure. Int J Psychoanal 18:84–97, 1962

9. Fenton GW, Hill D, Scotton L: An EEG measure of the effect of mood change on the thiopentone tolerance of depressed patients. Br J Psychiatry 114:1141–1147, 1968

10. Friedman AS: Minimal effects of severe depression on cognitive functioning. J Abnorm Soc Psychol 69:237–43, 1964

11. Hemsi LK, Whitehead A, Post F: Cognitive functioning and cerebral arousal in elderly depressives and dements. J Psychosom Res 12:145–156, 1968

12. Hill D: Depression, disease, reaction, or posture? Am J Psychiatry 125:445–457, 1968

13. Hodkinson BM: Mental impairment in the elderly. J R Coll Physicians Lond 7:305–317, 1973

14. Hopkinson FJ: A genetic study of affective illness in patients over 50. Br J Psychiatry 110:244–254, 1964

15. Isaacs B, Akhtar AJ: The set test: A rapid test of mental function in old people. Age and Aging 1:222–226, 1972

16. Karp HE: Dementia in systemic diseases. Postgrad Med 50:202–208, 1971

17. Kay DWK: Observations on the natural history and genetics of old age psychoses: A Stockholm material 1931–1937. Proc R Soc Med 52:791–794, 1959

18. Kay DWK: Outcome and cause of death in mental disorders of old age: A long-term follow-up of functional and organic psychoses. Acta Psychiatr Scand 38:249–276, 1962

19. Kay DWK, Roth M, Hopkins B: Affective disorders in the senium: (1) Their association with organic cerebral degeneration. J Ment Sci 101:302–318, 1955

20. Kendrick DC: The Kendrick battery of tests: Theoretical assumptions and clinical uses. Br J Soc Clin Psychol 11:373–386, 1972

21. Kendrick DC, Parboosingh RC, Post F: A synonym learning test for use with elderly psychiatric subjects: A validation study. Br J Soc Clin Psychol 4:63–71, 1965

22. Kendrick DC, Post F: Differences in cognitive states between healthy, psychiatrically ill, and diffusely brain-damaged elderly subjects. Br J Psychiatry 113:75–81, 1967

23. Lauter H: Phasenueberdauernder Persoenlichkeitswandel und persistierende Symptome bei der endogenen Depression, in Hippius H, Selbach H (eds): Das Depressive Syndrom. Muenchen, Urban & Schwarzenberg, 1969

24. Madden JJ, Luban JA, Kaplan LA, Manfredi HM: Non-dementing psychoses in older persons. JAMA 150:1567–72, 1952

25. Malamud W, Sands SL, Malamud I: The involutional psychoses. Psychosom Med 3:410–424, 1941

26. Pampiglione G, Post F: The value of electroencephalographic examination in psychiatric disorders of old age. Geriatrics 13:725–732, 1958

27. Pearce J, Miller E: Clinical Aspects of Dementia. London, Baillière & Tindall, 1973

28. Perris C, Brattemo CE: The sedation threshold as a method of evaluating antidepressive treatments—a preliminary report. Acta Psychiatr Scand Suppl 169:111–119, 1963

29. Post F: The outcome of mental breakdown in old age. Br Med J 1:436–448, 1951

30. Post F: The Significance of Affective Symptoms in Old Age. Maudsley Monographs 10. London, Oxford University Press, 1962

31. Post F: The Clinical Psychiatry of Late Life. Oxford, Pergamon Press, 1965

32. Post F: Somatic and psychic factors in the treatment of elderly psychiatric patients. J Psychosom Res 10:13–19, 1966

33. Post F: The factors of aging in affective illness, in Coppen A, Walk H (eds): Recent Developments in Affective Disorders. Br J Psychiatry Special Publication No. 2, 1968

34. Post F: The management and nature of depressive illnesses in late life: A follow-through study. Br J Psychiatry 121:393–404, 1972

35. Prakash C, Stern G: Neurological signs in the elderly. Age and aging 2:24–27, 1973

36. Robinson DS, Davis JM, Nies A, Ravaris CL, Sylwester D: Relation of sex and aging to monoamine oxidase activity of human brain, plasma and platelets. Arch Gen Psychiatry 24:536–9, 1971

37. Roth M: The natural history of mental disorders in old age. J Ment Sci 101:281–301, 1955

38. Roth M, Kay DWK: Affective disorders arising in the senium: II. Physical disability as an aetiological factor. J Ment Sci 102: 141, 1956

39. Roth M, Morrissey JD: Problems in the diagnosis and classification of mental disorders in old age. J Ment Sci 98:66–80, 1952

40. Routtenberg A: The two-arousal hypothesis: Reticular function and limbic system. Psychol Res 75:51–80, 1968

41. Shagass C, Jones AL: A neurophysiological test for psychiatric diagnosis: Results in 750 patients. Psychiatry 114: 1002–1010, 1958

42. Shagass C, Mihalik J, Jones AL: Clincial psychiatric studies using the sedation threshold. J Psychosom Res 2:45–55, 1957

43. Shapiro MB, Post F, Loefving B, Inglis J: "Memory function" in psychiatric patients over sixty, some methodological and diagnostic implications. J Ment Sci 102:233–246, 1956

44. Stenstedt A: Involutional Melancholia. Acta Psychiatr Neurol Suppl 127, 1959

45.   Whitehead A: Verbal learning and memory in elderly depressives. Br J
      Psychiatry 123:203–208, 1973

Commentary

Obviously, dementia and depression are important disorders that between them, produce a sizable portion of all mental disability. This is particularly true in later life, at which time the disorders have a number of similarities; differentiation may be quite difficult but is of obvious importance. While there are cases of depression in physically healthy elderly people in which the diagnosis of dementia has been incorrectly made (see Chapter 1), Felix Post has pointed out that the presence of relatively mild brain changes may well predispose to a depressive state in the elderly. It is imperative that depression and dementia, even when coexisting, be properly diagnosed, since both conditions are amenable to treatment, although the therapies are very different.

The following chapter will present clinical findings helpful in the diagnosis of both organic and psychogenic mental disorders, findings that are noted in the patient's verbal output. While emphasis in the following presentation has been toward the problems faced by the psychiatrist, the need for meaningful evaluation of verbal expression is just as great for neurologists and neurosurgeons. In fact, pertinent language evaluation must be considered part of every mental status evaluation.

D. Frank Benson, M.D.

7
Disorders of Verbal Expression

Psychiatry is unique among the medical specialties in that the psychiatrist depends a great deal on the verbal accounts of patients for diagnosis and, to a considerable extent, for treatment. History-taking, based on verbal accounts, is also important in the other medical specialties, but physical examination and laboratory studies are far more significant. The psychiatrist often bases his entire opinion on material the patient has presented verbally, demanding that he possess considerable sophistication in evaluating verbal output. Many psychiatrists do possess exceptional skills in this area finely attuned to interpreting the emotional and rational content of verbal expression. On the other hand, very few have experience in the recognition of speech or language disorders, which influence verbal output. The present paper will outline a number of disturbances of verbal expression that are likely to be seen in psychiatric practice.

Three categories of verbal output disorders will be discussed, first by definition and then by example. There are no hard and fast rules that define these varieties, but common sense and observation demonstrate that distinctions do exist. The definitions, then, are more practical and experiential than scientific. We will speak of three major disturbances of expressive output: speech disorders, language disorders, and thought disorders. This breakdown suggests that three separate psychophysiologic entities exist: speech, language, and thinking and, to a reasonable extent, this is true. It has long been accepted

This project was aided in part by Grant NB 209 from the National Institute of Neurological Disease and Stroke to Boston University School of Medicine.

that speech and thought are distinct entities.[17] Differentiation of language and thought is not so easily accepted but has been thoroughly discussed in the past (see especially Vigotsky[25] and Critchley).[8] The difference between speech and language is similarly obscure, and yet most authorities also regard this separation as real.

Speech disorders can be characterized as disturbances in verbal output produced by abnormal function of the efferent (outflow) pathways, the neuromuscular components necessary to produce verbal output. The patient with a speech disorder knows exactly what he wants to say, but mechanical disturbances interfere with output. A speech disorder, then, can be defined as a distortion of an otherwise adequate verbal output caused by neuromuscular disturbance involving the speech mechanisms. Writing may or may not be involved simultaneously.

In contrast to the rather simple definition of a speech disorder, the definition of a language disorder is much less exact. Clinically, language disorders may be characterized as abnormalities of verbal output in which the patient has difficulty manipulating the semantic and syntactic structures necessary to express his ideas. This breakdown in the ability to use symbolic and grammatical structures to express ideas may be considered a definition of language disorder.

The third category, thought disorder, is the most difficult to define. Clinically, thought disorder is said to be present when the mechanisms for both speech and language are intact but the ideas expressed in the verbal output are abnormal. Thought disorders, thus, represent abnormalities of ideation reflected in the verbal output.

Patients often have abnormalities in several of the above categories simultaneously and determining where the disorder fits may be difficult. Nonetheless, most abnormalities of verbal expression can be recognized and classed appropriately and this information often leads to appropriate treatment.

Although abnormalities of verbal expression also occur in childhood, the following discussion will be limited to disturbances of verbal output that are seen in adults. While much of what will be described in the following sections concerning adults can also be seen in children, disturbances of verbal expression in childhood are further complicated by the stage of development of speech, language, and thought at which the abnormality occurs plus variation based on congenital or developmental abnormality. Disturbances of verbal expression in childhood are even more complicated than those of adults.

SPEECH DISORDERS

A large number of fairly well-known diagnostic entities can be classed as speech disorders. Some are of known organic etiology; others appear to be manifestations of purely psychogenic dysfunction; and some can be called psychosomatic disorders. In the latter, the importance of the organic or the functional components is not clear and both components appear significant.

Stuttering can be considered the classic example of a speech disorder. Stuttering is a hesitation or interruption of speech, characterized by an uncontrollable tendency to repeat the initial syllable of a spoken word. The repetition may be once, twice, or more times, occasionally achieving a machine-gun-like quality. The patient's flow of speech stops while he attempts to produce one syllable. Occasionally, the attempt fails, and the stutterer must look for another word to express his idea. Stuttering is more common in males, is most common in the early years, particularly adolescence, and is aggravated by emotional stress and fatigue. The etiology of stuttering remains unknown despite innumerable attempts to build and test theories or models. Basically, three separate theories of etiology predominate; one suggesting severe emotional conflict (neurotic), a second postulating an underlying constitutional abnormality (organic), and the third implicating severe environmental pressures (developmental). There is no solid proof that excludes any of these theories. Many contemporary speech therapists consider that parental stress is a frequent cause, and treatment for stuttering often features family therapy. While this approach and other psychologically oriented therapies have not been universally successful, many stutterers do improve, suggesting that psychotherapeutic efforts can help.[1]

Cluttering is a comparatively rare speech disorder that can produce considerable disability. In this disorder, the patient speaks with such excessive rapidity that comprehension is difficult. The incomprehensibility is increased by a tendency to omit syllables from words and to run words together. Thus, a sentence such as "Yesterday we all ate lunch together at the Mayflower Hotel" might be given as "Yesirwe late lunchtherathe may flotel" and be totally impossible to understand. If the listener merely said "What?" the rapid fire presentation would be repeated, but if slowness was strictly demanded each syllable of the sentence could be presented properly. Treatment is by rigid exercises in slow, carefully produced speech, the elocution lessons of an earlier day. The etiology of cluttering is completely unknown; no organic lesion has been discovered and the significance of psychogenic factors in producing or maintaining the state is equally uncertain. Psychotherapy has not been notably successful but remains one of the accepted adjuncts to speech therapy.[1]

Stuttering, or a clinically similar disorder, can result from brain disease in an adult who has never previously stuttered. The mechanism underlying acquired stuttering is unknown but a partial shift of language dominance from left to right hemisphere is suspected. Most cases of acquired stuttering occur in individuals who have suffered damage to both hemispheres. Some patients with language disorder based on brain damage (aphasia, see later) speak in a rapid, mumbling manner somewhat similar to cluttering, but both the stuttering and the pseudocluttering produced by brain damage appear to be disorders of speech, not of language.

Palilalia is a rare speech disturbance in which there is an involuntary repetition of a word or phrase. Unlike stuttering, which usually involves the initial syllable, palilalia affects the final word or phrase. In true palilalia, the repetitions are multiple, accelerating in speed of output but decreasing in volume. The repetitions may be interrupted with an effort, by curses or other expletives, but more often simply die away. Traditionally, the basal ganglia pathology of encephalitis lethargia has been said to be the underlying cause of palilalia.[5] However, recent experience on our service with three patients with palilalic speech output suggests a broader view. One patient had a hereditary extrapyramidal disorder with choreiform movements and demonstrable calcification in the basal ganglia; the second was a left-handed individual who recovered from a severe right hemispheric infarction with speech output featuring both palilalia and agrammatism; while the third was a young, disorganized schizophrenic. At present, palilalia remains a speech disorder of uncertain etiology, but the presence of extrapyramidal disturbance should be considered.

Mutism is a rather unusual condition that can be caused by a variety of disorders. Inasmuch as some of the causes are organic, while others are functional, and inasmuch as the cause often cannot be determined, mutism may pose a difficult problem for the psychiatrist. By definition, mutism is a lack of verbal expression and in its most absolute state there is no verbalization. Often, however, the condition is incomplete and the patient is capable of some verbal expression. This may be limited to unvoiced whispers, hoarse whispering, or slow, soft, poorly inflected speech production. In all of these forms of output, the syntactic and semantic features are intact. The disturbance involves speech, therefore, not language. While some mutes suffer thought disorders, others do not, and mutism, per se, cannot be considered a disturbance of thinking.

Surgical procedures involving the supplementary motor area of the dominant hemisphere[9,16] produce a speech disorder that, at its worst, is a total mutism. This disturbance is usually transient (several days), and during recovery the patient produces a soft, dysarthric but grammatically correct verbal output. One of the complications of bilateral thalamotomy for Parkinsonism has been a change in verbal output.[19] When most severe, there is total mutism, but more frequently it is characterized by slow, grammatically intact speech of a soft, frail quality. The speech disorder following thalamotomy may remain permanently or may undergo slow improvement.

A lack of verbal output is one of the characteristics of the condition known as akinetic mutism. These brain-injured patients rarely talk or move, but there is neither paralysis nor change in state of consciousness to explain this lack of movement and verbalization. In one variety of akinetic mutism, the patient appears alert and follows movement with his eyes but does not move or speak. This has been called *coma vigil*. In a second variety, somnolent akinetic mutism, the patient appears to be asleep but can be alerted; he then shows akinesia, mutism, and disordered ocular movements. Intermediate combinations are seen. Neuropathologic correlation demonstrates that coma vigil occurs with lesions involving the posterior inferior frontal cortex, the so-called septal area, while the somnolent variety follows lesions involving the upper mesencephalon.[22]

A rare variety of abnormal speech output, in which the only disturbance is an inability to articulate, has been called *aphemia*[2] (also called cortical anarthria, subcortical motor aphasia, pure word dumbness). In this disorder, associated with either an acute lesion in the posterior inferior frontal cortex (Broca's area) or the efferent pathways from this area, the patient is fully alert, understands language perfectly well, can communicate his thoughts and ideas fully in writing, but is unable to speak. In some cases, there is no paralysis or other significant neurologic abnormality associated with the aphemia. Diagnosis can be difficult.

As can be noted from the above description, organic mutism may be produced by pathology involving rather variable areas. To be specific, mutism may result from pathology in the upper mesencephalon, the thalamus, the inferior and medial temporal area, the supplementary motor cortex, and, finally, from the dominant hemisphere speech area itself.

Elective mutism is a rare occurrence. In this situation, the patient, usually an adolescent, is said to speak normally to his peers, to his siblings, or even his parents but refuses to speak to others such as his teacher, other relatives, physicians, etc. Early reports of this condition[20] emphasized the transient nature and the need to counsel the parents, teachers, and so forth in methods for bringing the patient out of the defensive shell. Later reports,[18] however, noted that following "recovery" the individual demonstrated a verbal abnormality that had probably existed prior to the onset of the mutism. Elective mutism thus appears to be an organic disorder with a functional overlay.

Mutism may occur in severe psychotic states, particularly the stupor states of catatonic schizophrenia and severe depression. Almost never will a severe stupor state with mutism occur in a patient who has not had previous evidence of psychosis. In the known schizophrenic or depressive patient who has not undergone adequate treatment, the onset of mutism may be considered a part of the psychotic disease. The possibility of an underlying organic cause of the mutism should, however, be kept in mind.

Finally, mutism (or aphonia) is often thought to occur as part of a neurotic disorder and has been called "hysterical" mutism. The term hysteria is poor, since it fails to characterize or elucidate the underlying problem. Mutism may occur as part of a conversion reaction or be a manifestation of a dissociative reaction. Thus, while mutism may be considered a simple psychic defense mechanism, it is supremely demanding and, if maintained, usually indicates serious underlying psychic turmoil. A diagnosis of "neurotic" mutism often indicates the presence of a "psychotic" or prepsychotic condition.

Actually, evaluation of the vocal cords is one of the most important investigations in neurotic mutism (or in any other variety of mutism). The single most common cause of inability to talk is the aphonia produced by primary laryngeal disease. Acute laryngitis, laryngeal edema, carcinomatous or other nodule of the vocal cords can all produce an inability to phonate and demand consideration in cases of mutism.

Disorders of speech are relatively easy to discover, but the etiology may run the entire gamut of organic and functional disorders. Careful and continuing attention to the cause of the speech disorder is necessary. Abnormality of speech production may represent a psychic defense mechanism, but it often does not, and the psychiatrist must be continually on the lookout for additional findings indicating organic disease.

LANGUAGE DISORDERS

Aphasia is usually defined as a language disorder, and, by a circular route, language disorder is best characterized by aphasia. One definition of aphasia is an acquired language disorder caused by brain damage. With only a few exceptions, the presence of language disorder (aphasia) indicates disease or destruction of some part of the cerebrum. More specifically, aphasia indicates damage to the left hemisphere in the vast majority of people. Usually the diagnosis of aphasia is obvious and differentiation from psychiatric disorder presents little problem. There are significant exceptions, however, and the clinician needs some guidelines for these cases. The two best guides already noted are: (1) the presence of organic brain disorder and (2) involvement of the left cerebral hemisphere. When these simple guides do not offer sufficient information more sophisticated diagnostic techniques become necessary.

Evaluation of language function is not easy but by checking the competency of a number of language functions, demonstration of an aphasic disorder is almost always possible. Testing techniques will be reviewed briefly here; for more detailed information the reader is referred to recent publications.[3,11] The first step in evaluation, the analysis of conversational or spontaneous speech, utilizes differentiation of *fluent* and *nonfluent speech*. Nonfluent conversational speech contains very few words, and these are pronounced poorly. Although there is obvious effort to produce words, the number of words per phrase is consistently small, most often just one word, and normal speech melody is lost. The linguistic content of nonfluent output features meaningful substantive words with a notable omission of relational or filler words, the so-called *telegraphic speech*. By contrast, fluent aphasic speech is characterized by many words produced without effort, good articulation, normal phrase length and normal speech melody but paraphasic substitutions, pauses for word-finding, and a shortage of substantive words. Nonfluent output is readily recognized as aphasic; on the other hand, fluent output may be difficult to recognize and can be mistaken for other disorders characterized by abnormal verbal expression.

Comprehension of spoken language is difficult to test but is often a key aspect. Evaluation of comprehension depends on establishment of a consistently accurate response system. Verbal commands can be used but apraxia frequently interferes with the response. Yes–no responses are comparatively simple, but some aphasics cannot respond accurately because of perseveration or apraxia. Asking the patient to point (to objects, body parts, and so forth) is another simple resonse that can be used. In most aphasics, comprehension can be tested accurately by the use of these tests. Evaluation of comprehension is of particular importance for the patient with fluent output as it offers a ready differentiation between aphasic and schizophrenic verbal expression (see later).

Repetition of spoken language is tested by asking the patient to repeat numbers, words, multisyllabic words, phrases, and/or sentences. The failure to repeat accurately up to sentence level usually indicates either a depressed attention span or some structural abnormality in the perisylvian region.

Word-finding is most readily tested by pointing to objects, parts of objects, body parts or colors and requesting that the patient give the name. This is an evaluation of the patient's ability to present the word, not to recognize the object; only presentation of the correct word following a visual, tactile, or auditory stimulus can be accepted (see later for discussion of significance of word-finding difficulty).

Reading is evaluated in two parts: reading aloud and reading for comprehension. Either function may be abnormal while the other is not. Reading is tested simply by requesting that the patient both read aloud and interpret words and sentences written by the examiner. It is good to use material that the patient has already successfully comprehended by auditory means, but, in some cases, written language is comprehended better than spoken language.

Writing is probably the most fragile of all language functions and almost every aphasic demonstrates some degree of agraphia.[7] The patient should be asked to write his own name (both illiterates and aphasics can often write their own names but nothing else), but for full evaluation dictated words and sentences and construction of a sentence describing the weather, his job, and so on should be requested.

Certain aspects of language abnormality are of particular importance in the differentiation of aphasia from psychogenic disorders. Probably the most common source of confusion is word-finding difficulty *(anomia)*. Even normal individuals show a considerable variation in the ability to use names based on educational level, cultural background, specific vocational or hobby interests, reading habits, and so forth. Word-finding disability occurs in a number of organic disorders that do not fulfill the definition of aphasia (for example, toxic or postconcussion states). Similarly, difficulty in word-finding occurs in anxiety states, severe depression, catatonia, and other psychiatric states. Nonetheless, some degree of word-finding difficulty is demonstrated in every case of aphasia and the presence of a naming problem (anomia) should remind the examiner of this possibility. The conversational speech of individuals with aphasic anomia has frequent *pauses* and/or *circumlocutions*. The pauses most often occur when a specific, substantive word is needed. Often an attempt is made to define the missing word with a descriptive phrase. The descriptive phrase, however, depends on another substantive word that is also unavailable. An attempt is made to define this word, and so on, until the response has circled to a point remote from the original topic. Superficially, this circumlocutory output may be confused with the *circumstantiality*. Similarly, the high frequency and specific location of the pauses in anomic aphasia are readily differentiated from the *thought-blocking* of schizophrenia. When differentiation is not obvious on these bases alone, the tests of naming ability noted earlier will identify the patient with anomic aphasia. On the other hand, a diagnosis of aphasia based on word-finding defect alone is treacherous; in general, if anomia is the only language disability demonstrated, one must look carefully for other indications of whether the case is organic or functional.

Abnormalities of grammatical structure occur in many cases of aphasia. The most striking of these is the condition called *aggrammatism* seen in nonfluent aphasia. In essence, agrammatism is characterized by the ommision of relational and filler words in spoken sentences. The resulting telegraphic output is unique and difficult to mimic.

Hysterical imitations of language disorder are rare and most often appear in someone who has had considerable exposure to aphasic speech. Such hysterical pseudoaphasias often feature a disturbance of grammar, but one that is quite different and easily differentiated from true agrammatism. Thus, a functional "aphasic" may say "Me no got any money," whereas the aphasic is more likely to say (with considerable effort) " . . . . money" while shaking his head negatively. The functional output resembles the dialect attributed to the American Indian in movie productions.

Two striking abnormalities of language production, *echolalia* and *perseveration*, occur in both aphasic and nonaphasic disorders. *Echolalia* may be described as a strong but not mandatory tendency to repeat what has just been said. The reiteration is not a passive echo, however; the aphasic patient usually repeats only a part of the statement, almost invariably makes appropriate pronoun changes (that is, "I" for "you"), echoes only the language directed to him, fills in open-ended sentences and, in general, demonstrates recognition of the rules of language.[24] Echolalia is a prominent feature of several varieties of aphasia (the transcortical aphasias) and is associated with excellent ability to repeat. Echolalia may occur in catatonic schizophrenia; the phenomenon is usually transient, being present on one examination but not on the next. Echolalia is also seen in states of clouded consciousness, in some individuals of low-grade mental capacity and is almost a characteristic feature of early childhood autism. A discrepancy between a low level of language comprehension and a relatively advanced state of the speech output characterizes each condition underlying echolalia except for schizophrenia, in which comprehension is comparatively normal. Determination of the cause of echolalia in any individual depends on the patient's history and the related clinical findings. Echolalia is a symptom, not a diagnosis.

Perseveration denotes a state characterized by repetitious use of a word, phrase, action or thought. Goldstein[10] attributed perseveration to fatigue of a damaged nervous system and considered it a primitive mechanism to avoid the catastrophic reaction. Perseveration is common in severely brain-damaged individuals, both aphasic and nonaphasic. It is also seen in the mentally defective and in schizophrenic breakdown. The presence of perseveration is not diagnostic and the clinician needs other findings to differentiate organic and nonorganic causes.

Abnormal language (aphasia) with a fluent output, particularly when accompanied by considerable paraphasic substitution, offers the greatest diagnostic problem. For instance, a patient may be seen who has no apparent neurologic disturbance such as payalysis, sensory loss, and so forth, who produces many words in grammatically acceptable combinations and with good speech melody but whose output is incomprehensible and who fails to react to the examiner's verbalizations. In this situation, a psychotic breakdown with abnormal thought content is often considered. The description, however, characterizes severe fluent aphasia, a state that is often misdiagnosed as an acute psychosis. Accurate differentiation is necessary if appropriate treatment is to be offered. Before discussing this differentiation, we should analyze the third type of abnormality of verbal expression, that caused by thought disorder.

THOUGHT DISORDERS

Of all the abnormalities of verbal expression, disordered thought is both the most difficult to define and the most difficult to outline. The boundaries separating language and thought are particularly indefinite. From the clinical standpoint, however, there are some differences that stand out as self-evident and many others that appear significant.

As a first step in demonstrating that disordered thought produces disordered verbal expression, it is best to exclude abnormalities of speech or language. Absence of these difficulties, however, does not prove that abnormal verbal expression is based on disordered thinking. Positive diagnostic criteria are needed and, unfortunately, such criteria are only crudely available.

One step is to interpret the content of the patient's verbal expression. In doing this, the psychiatrist must remember to base his interpretation on the organizational qualities of the thought processes as well as the social or interpersonal factors influencing the content of verbal output. Defective ability to organize and process thoughts is manifested in disordered verbal output that becomes diagnostic. For further description of such defects, disease states with abnormal thinking will be described.

Dementia is a diagnostic category made up of many quite different entities that have a great variety of etiologies but that all feature an abnormality of thinking. Many abnormalities of higher function are present in dementia; such disorders as agnosia, apraxia, amnesia, personality change, and aphasia may be demonstrated, but the characteristic feature of dementia is deterioration in intellectual functioning. This deterioration is best demonstrated by special testing techniques (that is, proverb interpretation, calculations, determination of judgment) but is reflected in the patient's conversation and can often be suspected or even diagnosed by evaluation of the verbal output. In moderate-to-advanced cases of dementia, word-finding difficulty is usually present. Verbal output is empty and generalizations are frequent (words like "thing," "it," "they," instead of proper names). Attempts to describe a word that cannot be recalled diverts attention from the original thought to the definition. A rambling, circumlocutory output is produced that, while possessing many words and partial ideas, shows emptiness and lack of cohesiveness. This word-finding disability is similar to that seen in aphasia, but other aphasic abnormalities such as paraphasia, repetition defect, and so forth mentioned earlier are not seen.

The tendency of the demented individual to ramble is enhanced by memory disturbance. The patient is unable to retain the original line of thought through distractions, even his own distractions and changes from topic to topic. Often, while attempting to formulate an answer, the patient will forget the question or topic of discussion. Long pauses are frequent, usually awaiting further stimulation from the examiner.

Analysis of the verbal output of a demented individual shows inability to utilize abstractions. Language comprehension is performed only at the concrete level (for example, a bed is for sleeping but not for flowers); metaphor disappears from the verbal output except for overlearned cliches and even these may be used improperly. Proverb interpretation or other formal testing techniques may be necessary to document the loss of abstracting ability, but frequently the verbal output demonstrates this aspect by the concrete use of words. In fact, when the verbal expression is appropriately analyzed, the presence of dementia is usually obvious. Most of the verbal difficulties are based on abnormal thinking, and dementia can be considered a prime example of thought disorder.

In a quite different manner, *depression* can be considered a thought disorder characterized by abnormality of verbal expression. As already noted, in severe depressive states the patient may be mute or nearly so; it is far more common, however, for the depressed patient to have normal speech and essentially normal language production. The depressed patient is usually soft-spoken and limited in verbal output but characteristically shows a tendency for morbid, sad, deprecatory, and self-incriminating statements. Actual counts of words used by depressed patients demonstrates a sharp increase in morbid terminology when compared with normal output. Similarly, tests of memory function demonstrate that depressed patients are better at remembering material of a negative quality whereas normals are much better at remembering material of a happy nature.[12] Intelligence and memory, insofar as they can be tested, are unimpaired in depressive states. Thus, the verbal output accurately reflects the negative, gloomy quality of the thought processes.

In a similar manner, *mania* is well characterized by the abnormality of verbal expression. While mania does produce physical evidence such as restlessness and irritability, the most characteristic feature is the rapidity of the stream of thought, the pathognomonic "flight of ideas." Verbal output is incessant, apparently under the control of casual associations, similar sounds, puns, and so forth. At times, the output breaks into scattered sequences that reflect the extreme distractibility of the severely manic patient. In this situation attention is fleeting, the patient rarely finishing any task or thought before attention becomes focused elsewhere. Just as in cases of depression, intelligence and memory remain intact.

Schizophrenia is a disease state characterized by an abnormality of thinking that is primarily mirrored in the verbal output. Of the six primary psychologic abnormalities characterizing schizophrenia[14] five are totally or partially expressed verbally. Analysis of the verbal expression in schizophrenia reveals many diagnostic features that vary with the stage of deteriorating or improving symptomatology. Chapman,[6] in a retrospective study of acute schizophrenic breakdown, demonstrated a series of steps, most of which involved language disability. First, the patients noted intermittent episodes of word-finding difficulty. Increases in duration and frequency of this problem created difficulty in both the expression and reception of language. Next, the patients told of increasing difficulty in screening out unwanted words, eventually failing, so that improper words were expressed. Continuous monitoring of the verbal output was necessary, and as communication difficulties increased, it became easier to avoid speaking and to withdraw from social contact. In the most severe stages, Chapman's patients told of greatly decreased verbal output, involuntary echoing of what was heard and blocking during attempts to speak. While all of the above are disturbances of verbal output, they do not represent abnormalities of either speech or language. It is exceptional for a schizophrenic patient to have a breakdown of language (see below). Analysis of the verbal output of most schizophrenic patients demonstrates intact speech, intact language, a sizeable vocabulary, and correct use of grammatical and syntactical constraints. It is the bizarre content of schizophrenic output, not the abnormality of language production, that characterizes "schizophrenic language."

Many contemporary psychiatrists postulate a disturbance of attention as the basic psychopathologic abnormality in schizophrenia. Schilder[21] described the thought disorder of schizophrenia as an inability to maintain the determinative idea because of an inability to focus attention on it. Self-distraction is a commonly noted feature in schizophrenia. The verbal output often appears to be directed by alliterations, by analogies, by clang associations, by associations with events in the immediate environment, by symbolic meanings, or by the condensation of several contradictory ideas. In addition, the schizophrenic appears to be restricted to use of the concrete or high-frequency meaning of a given word, an inability to use abstract terminology.[13] On the surface, at least, this is similar to the difficulties with abstraction noted in cases of dementia.

While disturbed attention may be the basic disorder in schizophrenia, this cannot be described as a diminution of attention. In fact, a heightened sense of awareness, a degree of hyperalertness, is more characteristic of the acute schizophrenic and, again, is reflected by disorganization of verbal output. The patient appears to be overwhelmed by a flood of details and cannot completely express his thoughts because of distraction. In this manner, the acute schizophrenic appears similar to the manic patient.

The schizophrenic patient is often aware of his own problems with thinking and expression of his thoughts, and complaints about them offer some of the more pathognomonic signs of schizophrenia. Thus, thought withdrawal, thought insertion, thought broadcasting or extreme pressure of thoughts are often described during an acute psychotic breakdown. In fact, descriptions of thought disorders make up most of the first-rank symptoms of Schneider,[15] one of the more reliable guides to the diagnosis of schizophrenia.

Yet another clinical feature of schizophrenia that may be reflected in the verbal output is the hallucination. Schizophrenic hallucinations occur in the fully alert state and auditory hallucinations are far more common than visual. While nonverbal stimuli such as whistling, neologistic or nonsense expressions, and so forth may be noted, hallucinations consisting of voices talking to the patient, arguing with him, or attempting to direct his behavior are very common. Almost invariably, the schizophrenic patient is certain that these perceptions are real and in most instances is willing, even eager, to discuss the hallucinatory experience with the examiner. Hallucinations occur in many mental disorders and cannot be considered diagnostic of schizophrenia. However, when auditory hallucinations are present in a patient suffering some of the verbal difficulties noted above, a diagnosis of schizophrenia is reasonable.

Several other suggestive features are available by analyzing the content of schizophrenic verbalizations. During an acute break, the output is strongly related to the present and the immediate past; with improvement discussion of the future and the more remote past is again possible.[23] Similarly, with improvement the disorganization of thought processing diminishes and this improvement can be monitored by analysis of verbal output. The stages outlined by Chapman are reversed but remnants of the severe breakdown may remain well into the recovered stage.

Finally, some note should be made of the severe breakdown of verbal output, the so-called "schizophrenic word salad,"[4] which can mimic aphasia. Word salad is an outpouring of real words, phonemic substitutions, verbal substitutions and neologisms that combine to make an unintelligible output. This disorder was usually reported only in chronic schizophrenics who had been isolated on a back ward for a long period. At the present time, the condition is rarely reported, possibly a reflection of improved care for the chronic psychotic patient. The few patients referred to the author because of "word salad" have all eventually been demonstrated to have a true aphasia. In these cases, the "word salad" proved to be a fluent–paraphasic language disturbance and a specific brain lesion could be identified. This misdiagnosis is reasonable, since patients with severe posterior superior temporal lobe damage have an inability to understand spoken language and have a rapid output contaminated with many paraphasias. Several differentiating points are available. If the jargon output occurs in an adult patient of previously good mental health, the disturbance is almost undoubtedly aphasic and not schizophrenic. Even in the individual with known schizophrenia, the sudden development of an excessive, unintelligible verbal output would favor a diagnosis of aphasia. Only in the chronic schizophrenic with a long history of isolation should word salad be considered primarily, and even then, the possibility of aphasia deserves consideration. A short test of language comprehension will usually make the diagnosis clear. Fluent, paraphasic aphasia is almost invariably associated with defects in language comprehension and repetition. In contrast, even severely deteriorated schizophrenics usually show some appreciation of language, either by echoing, by incorporating the examiner's words in his own output, or by carrying out verbal commands. Thus, whenever word salad is

being considered, the possibility of an aphasia must be given careful consideration.

SUMMARY

This presentation has divided the abnormalities of verbal expression into
three categories: speech, language, and thought. While this division is not
novel and has been discussed many times on philosophic and psychologic
bases, the present paper is limited to clinical examples of classic disease types
that illustrate the separation of the three categories. For every practicing
physician, but particularly for the psychiatrist, an ability to recognize and
differentiate abnormalities of verbal expression is of obvious importance, and a
number of practical guides have been presented for this purpose.

REFERENCES

1   Ainsworth S: Methods for integrating theories of stuttering, in Travis LE (ed):
    Handbook of Speech Pathology and Audiology. New York, Appleton-
    Century-Crofts, 1971
2. Bastian HC: On different kinds of aphasia. Br Med J 2:931–936, 985–990, 1887
3. Benson DF, Geschwind N: Aphasia and related cortical disturbances, in Baker
    AB, Baker LH (eds): Clinical Neurology. New York, Harper & Row, 1971
4. Bleuler E: Dementia Praecox. New York, Internat Univ Pr, 1950
5. Brain R: Speech Disorders—Aphasia, Apraxia and Agnosia. London, Butter-
    worths, 1961
6. Chapman J: The early symptoms of schizophrenia. Br J Psychiatry 112:225–251,
    1966
7. Chedru F, Geschwind N: Disorders of higher cortical functions in acute confu-
    sional states. Cortex 8. 395–411, 1972
8. Critchley M: Aphasiology. London, Edward Arnold Ltd, 1970
9. Foerster O: Motorische felder und bahnen, in Bumke O, Foerster, O (eds):
    Handbuch der Neurologie. Berlin, Springer, 1936
10. Goldstein K: Language and Language Disturbances. New York, Grune &
    Stratton, 1948
11. Goodglass H, Kaplan E: The Assessment of Aphasia and Related Disorders.
    Philadelphia, Lea & Febiger, 1972
12. Lishman A: Selective factors in memory. Part 2: Affective disorders. Psychol
    Med 2:248–253, 1972
13. Maher B: The language of schizophrenia: A review and interpretation. Br J
    Psychiatry 120:3–17, 1972
14. Mayer-Gross W, Slater E, Roth M: Clinical Psychiatry (ed 3). London,
    Baillière, Tindall and Cassell, 1969

15. Mellor CS: First rank symptoms of schizophrenia. Br J Psychiatry 117:15–23, 1970
16. Penfield W, Roberts L: Speech and Brain-Mechanisms. Princeton, NJ, Princeton Univ Pr, 1959
17. Pick A: Aphasia. Springfield, Ill, Thomas, 1973
18. Reed GF: Elective mutism in children: A re-appraisal. J Child Psychol Psychiat 4:99–107, 1963
19. Riklan M, Levita E, Zimmerman J, Cooper IS: Thalamic correlates of language and speech. J Neurol Sci 8:307, 1969
20. Salfield DJ: Observations on elective mutism in children. J Ment Sci 96:1024–1032, 1950
21. Schilder P: On the development of thoughts. Z gesamte Neurol Psychiatry 59:250–268, 1920
22. Segarra JM: Cerebral vascular disease and behavior. Arch Neurol 22:408–418, 1970
23. Silverman G: Redundancy, repetition and pausing in schizophrenic speech. Br J Psychiatry 122:407–413, 1973
24. Stengel E: A clinical and psychological study of echo reactions. J Ment Sci 93:598–612, 1947
25. Vygotsky LS: Thought and Language. Cambridge, M.I.T. Pr, 1962

Commentary

Several points raised by this article should be noted. The most obvious one concerns the ability to use verbal expression as a diagnostic tool. It is probably true that the great diagnostic skill demonstrated by some of the "old-timers" was based on an almost instinctive ability to extract diagnostic clues from the verbalizations of their patients. Appropriate investigations should allow at least some of these diagnostic clues to be distilled and made available for all clinicians. While this article offers only a foundation for this kind of clinical research, it does direct our attention to a worthwhile but currently overlooked area.

A second and far different point suggested by this article concerns the differentiation of speech, language, and thought. For the philosophic theorist these three functions fuse into one another, and their differentiation has been considered difficult if not almost impossible. On the other hand, it is clear that, from the clinical and pathologic viewpoints, disturbances of these functions are readily differentiated and experience tells us that functional differentiation based on clinical and pathologic differences is real. Further study of the differential factors that can be gleaned from the verbal output of various pathologic states will certainly allow a better understanding of these three functions.

The next three chapters will investigate symptomatology related to specific parts of the central nervous system. In the development of the human brain, no portion has grown so rapidly as the prefrontal lobes. The vast increase in the size of the forebrain as compared to other areas has lead to considerable speculation, and a vast literature concerning the importance of the prefrontal lobes in the human existence. At various times, all of the ''higher'' and more strictly human behavioral functions have been attributed to the frontal lobe. Similarly, the frontal lobes have been implicated in many disorders of intellect and behavior. To say the least, much of the literature concerning frontal lobe functions is contradictory, confusing, and, in many instances, has been proved wrong. That the prefrontal lobes do have important functions cannot be denied, and there is at least some agreement as to what these functions are. In the next chapter, Drs. Hecaen and Albert review a major portion of this literature.

Henry Hecaen, M.D. and Martin L. Albert, M.D.

8
Disorders of Mental Functioning Related to Frontal Lobe Pathology

The "riddle" and the "problem" of the frontal lobes and the "unity and diversity" of frontal lobe functions have been the motivating forces behind scientists' attempts for nearly a century to try to unravel the "hidden secrets" of the relationship between the frontal lobes and human intellectual functioning. Before 1900, prior to the development of systematic analyses of frontal lobe functions, individual cases of striking behavioral alterations associated with frontal lobe pathology were reported. Often cited is the case of Velpeau and Delpech, reported by Lhermitte,[23] in which a 66-year-old man was admitted to Charity Hospital in Paris for treatment of a minor urinary tract disorder. The surgeons were astonished at his abnormal behavior: He was constantly expressing strange ideas and would make inappropriate remarks and jokes. Later, bilateral frontal lobe tumors were discovered at autopsy.*

Since the turn of the century, systematic analyses of behavioral alterations in humans with frontal lobe pathology due to trauma, tumors, infections (especially syphilitic), vascular accidents, and surgical interventions (lobec-

This investigation was supported by a grant from the Grant Foundation (Professor Hecaen).

*Another celebrated case is the one of Phineas P. Gage, "the American crowbar case," whose detailed history was quoted in 1878 by Ferrier. This young man had his prefrontal region completely pierced by an iron bar and lived for 12 years following the trauma. The change in his personality was considerable; his doctor summarized his posttraumatic state as follows: "A child in his intellectual capacity and manifestations; he has the animal passions of a strong man . . . ."

tomies, lobotomies, topectomies) have allowed the development of a semiology of frontal lobe syndromes.

A new period of experimental research on the frontal lobes was signaled by publications in the mid-1930s concerning the functions of the frontal association areas in nonhuman primates.[18,19] Studies of large numbers of brain-damaged subjects following the second world war permitted more detailed neuropsychologic analyses.

This chapter will deal primarily with humans. We will discuss clinical features of frontal lobe syndromes, data from neuropathologic material, pertinent neuropsychologic studies, and, finally, theories proposed to explain the phenomena observed in humans following frontal lobe damage. It should be noted that when we refer to "frontal lobes," we are speaking of the massive portion of the frontal lobes anterior to and exclusive of the precentral (Rolandic) gyrus.

CLINICAL "FRONTAL LOBE" SYNDROMES

This section describes some personal experience and provides a synthesis of clinical reviews.[1,4,9] Despite the specificity of known cortico–cortical connections involving different portions of the frontal lobes,[33] the nature of clinical material has been such as to prevent the development of a clinico-–anatomic specificity. We believe that it is premature to attempt to correlate specific behavioral deficits in humans with specific regions within the frontal lobes. On the other hand, it is possible to categorize or group the behavioral defects, correlating them with frontal lobe damage, without further specifying which area of the frontal lobe has been damaged. Lesions of the frontal lobes may be associated with personality disorders, alterations in motor activity, disorders of cognitive function, and paroxysmal disorders.

Personality Disorders

Frequently, one sees an apparent heightening of affective tone, with euphoria and lack of concern for the present or the future. This behavioral change does not necessarily reflect a true alteration of mood, however. Such patients, in the midst of apparent euphoria, will state that they are not at all happy. A puerile or silly attitude may be maintained, often with an inappropriate use of pretentious language. Erotic behavior, sexual exhibitionism, or lewd remarks are not rare. Euphoric excitation may take on an atypical hypomanic aspect, "moria": the patient, overexcited, manifesting erotic behavior, bothers the examiner with inappropriate jokes and caustic or facetious remarks (Witzelsucht).

The diverse aspects of excitation and euphoria are rarely permanent. In general, they appear episodically, superimposed on an underlying background of abulia and apathy. The euphoric periods may alternate with periods of apparent depression. True depression, however, is rarely seen; rather, a picture of asthenia and akinesia imitates a true depression. A disorder of activity, rather than of affectivity, is the hallmark.

Outbursts of irritability are common. These may be the first behavioral change noted; often these outbursts reach such a degree of violence that they force a family to institutionalize the patient.

Alterations of Motor Activity

Lack of initiative or spontaneity is a characteristic feature of frontal lobe pathology. These are linked to a general diminution of motor activity. The patient no longer voluntarily carries out the necessary daily activities of life, such as getting out of bed in the morning, washing or dressing himself, feeding himself, or even urinating or defecating in the toilet. These latter activities may be carried out at any time or place, without regard for the social consequences. The actual ability to carry out the various activities of daily living is not impaired—the patient is neither paralyzed, apraxic, nor confused. When he is vigorously urged to do something, he can do it. What is impaired is the ability to initiate spontaneously a desired or an automatic motor task.

It is this rupture between the patient and the external world, this diminution of activity in manipulating real objects, this reduction of interpersonal exchange that appear to be a loss of interest on the part of the patient. Whether there is a true loss of interest or an apparent loss of interest due to an impairment of spontaneous initiation of activity, the effect on the examiner remains the same.

Disorders of Cognitive Function

Loss of the "esthetic" sense or loss of "abstracting" ability are considered to be early signs of frontal lobe dysfunction. Underlying these cognitive defects, one finds disorders of attention and memory. From the first examination of the patient, the disorder of attention is noticeable; it is necessary to repeat questions and orders several times to obtain a response.

The disorder of memory may be of two types. One type is primarily a disorder of recent memory, similar to that seen in the Korsakoff syndrome, in which remote events may be better preserved and recalled than recent events. The other type of memory defect is more a forgetfulness than a true memory disorder. In this situation, the patient "forgets to remember" certain information that he has preserved in his memory. This defect seems to be one of lack of initiative to recall elements that have not truly been forgotten. In many ways, this defect is similar to the lack of spontaneity or initiative seen in the motor system. If these patients are given enough time, or if they are urged with sufficient vigor, they will recall items and events of which they had previously denied knowledge.

Paroxysmal Disorders

Paroxysmal disturbances of mental functioning are rare. Occasionally, one sees abrupt and transitory periods of disorientation. Rarely, brief episodes of visual or olfactory hallucinations have occurred following frontal lobe damage. This may be related to lesions of the olfactory or optic nerves. Patients have infrequently complained of periods during which they were only able to think about, and seemed to be forced to think only about, a single idea, thought, or topic. These paroxysmal disturbances may represent epileptic equivalents or auras.

NEUROPATHOLOGIC STUDIES

Tumors

The history of systematic studies of clinico–anatomical correlations of behavioral disorders with frontal lobe tumors has shown a clear trend. The earliest reports[3,34,38] were efforts to describe general psychiatric syndromes associated with cerebral tumors. Symptoms and signs included torpor, irritability, and depression. No attempt was made to define specific "frontal lobe" behavior. It was noted, however, that "general mental symptoms" did seem to occur earlier in the course of the illness if the tumor were frontal.

Subsequent research tended to isolate specific behavioral abnormalities, such as memory disturbance, euphoria, loss of initiative, and so forth and relate these behavioral abnormalities to frontal lobe change rather than to general cerebral dysfunction.[10,22] Finally, attempts were made to localize within the frontal lobes the various clinical abnormalities found.[8,26,31]

A summary of the various studies relating frontal lobe tumors to behavioral abnormalities would include the following. Disorders of mental functioning occur in 60–90 percent of cases in which cerebral tumors involve the frontal lobes. It is not yet possible to correlate specific behavioral syndromes with tumoral invasion of specific regions of the frontal lobes. The general defects of behavior following frontal lobe damage by tumors may include any combination of signs or symptoms described above in the clinical sections.

However, the rate of growth of the tumor does have an effect on symptomatology. Slowly growing frontal tumors are characterized primarily by apathy, akinesia, and loss of spontaneity or initiative. Personality changes may be quite marked. Rapidly growing frontal tumors are more often associated with torpor or with confusional states.

Trauma

In his famous textbook of "brain pathology," Kleist[21] describes alterations of mental functioning following frontal lobe trauma. He includes, in particular, psychomotor disturbances: loss of initiative, lack of "motor spontaneity," depression, and mutism. Goldstein[13,14] cites defects of attention and memory, affective indifference, and akinesia. Jarvie[20] considers the chief feature of frontal lobe trauma to be a disinhibition that permanently alters the patient's personality in such a way as to reduce his control of socially acceptable behavior.

To the above we would add the not infrequently observed syndrome of akinetic mutism that appears following bilateral frontal lobe trauma. In this syndrome, also referred to as coma vigil, the patient is able to move but does not; he is able to speak but does not. He lies in bed, mute and immobile, with eyes open and with wandering eye movements. For brief periods, the eyes may fix on a moving object and follow it. Rare spontaneous or responsive movements may be made; rare sounds and single words may be heard. We have observed remarkable recoveries, especially in younger patients, following several years in this state.

Neurosurgical Intervention

FRONTAL LOBECTOMIES

Ordinarily, one expects valuable clinico–anatomical information from lobectomies. In the case of the frontal lobes, however, the information has been contradictory. Several authors report no deficit whatsoever, following unilateral frontal lobectomy; others note "inability to concentrate," "impairment of synthetic or organizational ability," and "loss of initiative."[1] Rylander,[36] in a good review of the topic including 32 of his own cases, concluded that frontal lobectomies are associated with behavioral modifications in almost every case: reduction of affective response inhibition, tendency to euphoria, emotional instability, impairment of attention, and reduction of initiative. In a follow-up study,[37] he indicated that disorders of mental functioning are clearly more marked following frontal lobectomy than following ablation of any other lobe.

FRONTAL LOBOTOMIES

From the moment of their introduction by Moniz and Lima in 1935, frontal lobotomies for the treatment of mental illness created a storm: first a storm of enthusiasm, then a storm of rejection in which the procedure nearly became taboo, and now in recent months, especially in the United States, a new storm of controversy has arisen over the political, medical, and social implications of psychosurgery. From a strict neuropsychologic point of view, little useful scientific information relating frontal lobe lesions to human behavior can be gleaned, chiefly because of the preexisting mental disorders in patients undergoing frontal lobotomies.

Depending on the precise region of the brain attacked (orbital or orbito –frontal regions, cingulum, and so forth), one could nevertheless expect to see certain behavioral characteristics of the lobotomized patient: loss of initiative, apathy, some euphoric tendencies, simplification of social interactions, loss of concern for the future.[11,15,27,30]

Proposed Mechanisms Underlying the Functional Deficits (Based on Anatomo-Clinical Correlations)

Many authors have used anatomo–clinical correlations as a basis for theories of frontal lobe function. Vincent[41] and Hebb[17] believed that a "disorganization" created by the presence of the frontal lobe lesion was responsible for the mental abnormalities. Total removal of the lesion, by unilateral or bilateral frontal lobectomy, would return the patient to normal.

Most authors, however, felt that the presence of a lesion or ablation of a frontal lobe produced the same effect. Brickner[5] believed that the basic disorder in the frontal lobe syndrome was a deficit in the highest levels of associative processing, a reduction in the capacity for synthesis, upon which all other abnormalities depended.

Kurt Goldstein[13,14] thought that the fundamental disorder underlying the features of the frontal lobe syndromes was an inability to grasp the entirety of a complex situation or to differentiate one complex situation from another. This apparent identity of differing complex situations produced indifference and a pathologic alteration of emotional reactions. For Goldstein, the observed disorders of motor activity and social conduct resulted from a response by the patient to fragments of a situation and not to the whole. The inability to comprehend the whole situation caused a failure to recognize the key features of that situation: an impairment in the capacity to extract the essential figures from a background. The end result was a regression from the abstract attitude toward the concrete.

Other authors wrote about disorders of vigilance[16] or of inhibition.[2]

Angelergues et al.[1] warned against the imposition of a priori theoretical conceptions, preferring to refine the clinical descriptions, thus providing a solid clinical base for detailed neuropsychologic analyses.

NEUROPSYCHOLOGIC STUDIES

Functional Deficits Following Frontal Lobe Lesions in Animals

It is not our intention to review here the vast literature in experimental neuropsychology concerning the frontal lobes. A summary of this material reveals the following main functional deficits: deficient delayed response, impaired delayed alternation in space, perseveration, distractibility and hyperactivity, deficits of sensory–motor integration. Undoubtedly, some or all of these abnormalities underlie the behavioral alterations found in humans with frontal lobe pathology.

Given our current level of knowledge, it is not unreasonable to add certain anatomical information obtained from animal studies.[24,32] There appears to be a direct behavioral association with the frontal–limbic–hypothalamic–midbrain axis. This behavioral–anatomical axis is comprised of two parallel circuits of activity. One of these circuits involves connections of medial frontal regions to cingulate gyrus to hippocampus to fornix to mammilary bodies to anterior thalamus and back to frontal lobes. The other circuit involves connections of orbito–frontal regions to medial temporal areas to amygdala to dorsomedial thalamus and back to frontal lobes. Both of these parallel circuits have centrifugal connections to the hypothalamus and midbrain. Each of these circuits communicates with the other by way of septal, preoptic, lateral hypothalamic, and midbrain connections. The medial frontal–hippocampal circuit and the orbital–frontal–amygdalar circuit have sufficiently distinctive pathways to allow for the carrying out of different behavioral activities. To attempt the correlation of these data with data from human studies, however, is still premature.

Functional Deficits Following Frontal Lobe Lesions in Man

Basing their work on the techniques and results of experimental (animal) neuropsychology, researchers have attempted to find the fundamental neuropsychologic defects underlying the behavioral alterations in humans with frontal lobe pathology. Results have been contradictory and difficult to interpret. Thus, Ghent, Mishkin, and Teuber[12] could not find a deficit in delayed reaction among subjects with frontal lobe trauma. Chorover and Cole[6] did demonstrate disturbed performance in humans on a test of delayed alternation; however the deficits were present with any cerebral lesion and not specifically frontal.

On the Wisconsin Card Sorting Test, on which the subject must repeatedly change his principal line of reasoning in order to solve a problem, the performance of 25 subjects with frontal lobe resections, right or left, was significantly inferior to that of control subjects. The frontal deficit was manifested by an inability of the subject to overcome a previously established response pattern. A tendency to perseveration, previously demonstrated in ''frontal'' animals, was thus shown to be present in humans with frontal lobe lesions.[28]

Milner subjected large numbers of subjects with cerebral ablations for epileptogenic cortical scars to a series of verbal and nonverbal tests.[29] She indicates that subjects with frontal lobe lesions have difficulty distinguishing the degree of recency of an item among a series of presented items. Prisko (cited by Milner[29]) had previously shown that frontal lobectomy impaired the subject's ability to perform on a delayed paired-comparison task. In this task, the subject must suppress the memory of earlier trials and compare the present stimulus only with the one that immediately preceded it. Prisko's data suggested that frontal lesions prevent the subject from keeping the different trials apart. On verbal and nonverbal recency tasks Milner and Corsi[29] established that frontal lobectomy produces a disturbance in the temporal ordering of events, but that the impaired performance, verbal or nonverbal, is different according to the side of the lesion. Lesions of the left frontal lobe produced a deficit on the verbal tests; lesions of the right frontal lobe, a deficit on the nonverbal tasks.

Milner had previously demonstrated other hemispheric asymmetries following frontal lobe lesions: left frontal lobe lesions were associated with deficits on a verbal fluency task, while right frontal lesions were associated with deficits on a maze-learning task. In regard to verbal fluency tests, Ramier and Hecaen[35] have found deficits following either right or left frontal lobe lesions; however, the deficits were much more marked when the lesion was on the left. Milner tentatively concluded that a common defect underlies the various functional abnormalities observed: impairment of the ability to suppress the interference effect of a previous action on a current task.

Proposed Mechanisms Underlying the Functional Deficits Based on Neuropsychologic Studies

Among the many valuable theoretical contributions to our understanding of frontal lobe functions in man, those of Teuber and of Luria stand out and will be cited here.

For Teuber, the frontal lobe contributes to the control of behavior by originating anticipatory discharges (corollary discharges) that attain sensory structures, preparing them for the motor activity that is about to occur. Because of the reception of these corollary discharge signals, the sensory systems can compare the expected results of the action with the intention of the subject. This theory would account for observed functional deficits in frontal lobe animals; the absence of comparable deficits in man would be explained by his capacity for verbal mediation as an additional regulator of motor activity. In man, the frontal lobe deficits would be manifested not only as problems of control of reflexive movement or posture but also as deficits in the regulation of their voluntary control. By such a hypothesis the grasping or groping reflexes seen after frontal lesions could be explained.

Teuber based his theoretical analyses on a series of studies carried out by his group on subjects with war-missile-induced cerebral lesions. In these studies, there were 90 subjects with frontal lesions, 142 subjects with other cerebral lesions, and 118 normal controls. The subjects with frontal lobe lesions were specifically impaired on four perceptual–motor tasks involving posture and movement. These tasks were a visual–spatial task requiring appreciation of verticality; a study of reversible figures, the double Necker cube; a test of visual searching; and a test of personal body orientation in space.[39]

The interpretation proposed by Luria as an explanation of frontal lobe dysfunction is somewhat similar to that of Teuber.[25] For Luria, frontal lobe lesions provoke a disturbance in the programing of one's diverse activities; there is impairment in the final intended action because of a lack of information provided during the elaboration of the action. Thus, the frontal lobes regulate the "active state" of the organism, control the essential elements of the subjects' intentions, program complex forms of activity, and constantly monitor all aspects of activity. The regulatory function of the frontal lobes is effected by a constant comparison between the effect of an action and its program of origin: if there is a correspondence, the action is completed; if there is no correspondence, the action continues until the desired effect and the necessary correspondence are obtained. This mechanism is based on a system of "feedback afferents." Consequently, frontal lobe signs do not represent a disorder of sensation or perception, of language, or of primary motor or reflex activity. Rather, they represent disorders of regulation of activity and correction of errors.

Disorders of regulation of activity are manifested clinically by apathy and akinesia. In milder cases, instead of responding correctly to the command, the subject cannot maintain his attention and the desired program of action is replaced by a stereotyped motor response. The physiologic basis for these observations can be demonstrated by a study of the autonomic components of the orienting reaction. In the case of a lesion other than frontal, these autonomic responses evaluated by plethysmography and electrodermal reaction, may be disturbed, but any verbal command gives the stimulus a new signal value and brings about a reappearance of the orienting reaction. On the other hand, in the case of a frontal lesion, the autonomic components of the orienting reaction are suppressed or diffused, and verbal instructions do not bring about their reappearance. In similar fashion in frontal lobe patients, electroencephalographic expectation waves (contingent negative variations) do not appear following verbal instruction.

Additional clinical manifestations of the loss of frontal lobe regulatory control are the phenomena of motor impersistence and perseveration. For example, it may be difficult for a patient to repeatedly open and close his eyes or to open and close his fist; on the other hand, once started, it may be difficult for the patient to stop these activities. Luria concludes that these phenomena are indications that the subject has "ceased to be controlled by the prescribed program and has passed under the influence of nonpertinent factors." It becomes impossible for the patient to create a complex and selective system of connections to control the active movement. The necessary program is replaced by inert stereotypes.

With a series of ingenious motor tests of increasing motor responses to a conditioned signal, conditioned choice reaction, reactions in conflict, complexity (simple and successive actions in direct or alternating series), Luria has been able to demonstrate the impairment of regulation of voluntary acts that are no longer subject to verbally formulated programs.

Certain aspects of perceptual and intellectual activity may also be impaired following frontal lobe lesions. If a visual or tactile perceptual task is relatively simple, it may be carried out accurately. However, if the perception requires a preliminary analysis during which the subject must make a correct choice among several reasonable possibilities, the disorder becomes manifest. Such is also the case for disorders of arithmetic, other tasks of problem-solving and other intellectual activities.

As for memory disorders, these are demonstrated most clearly when two memory tasks are given one after another in a short period of time. The items and associations from one task interfere with those of the other. For Luria, the frontal lobe memory disorders are related, at least in severe cases, to defects of attention, temporal–spatial disorientation, and confabulation.

Problems are posed by the clinical material Luria used for his studies, and for these reasons a certain prudence is warranted before accepting his hypotheses. Most of his observations are based on cases with massive frontal tumors that quite possibly extend beyond the limits of the frontal lobes both in depth and on the cortical surface. Several of his patients must have had increased intracranial pressure, confounding the clinical and experimental picture. In addition, many of the experimental results put forth by Luria to support his arguments are of a purely qualitative nature. No comparative studies with normal controls or with brain-damaged subjects with nonfrontal lesions are presented. Denny-Brown, in a review of Luria's work, was struck by the significant role played by perseveration in the impaired performance of Luria's patients. The perseveration was of a sufficient severity to have accounted for many of the reported behavioral abnormalities. Yet, perseveration cannot be considered an abnormality limited exclusively to frontal lobe lesions. It remains to be proved that posterior cerebral (nonfrontal) lesions produce a perseveration that affects different behavioral functions than that produced by frontal lesions.

These criticisms in no way reduce the intrinsic value of the interpretive analyses or examining techniques presented by Luria. Rather they are intended to stimulate an experimental evaluation of his theories. In order to confirm a general hypothesis of frontal lobe function it will be necessary to apply systematically a standardized battery of tests to large numbers of subjects with relatively limited and well-localized cerebral lesions in various locations.

REFERENCES

1. Angelergues R, Hécaen H, Ajuriaguerra J: Les troubles mentaux au cours des tumeurs du lobe frontal. Ann Med Psychol 113:577–642, 1956
2. Arnot R: A theory of frontal lobe function. Arch Neurol Psychiatry 67:487–495, 1952
3. Baruk H: Les troubles mentaux dans les tumeurs cérébrales. Paris, Doin, 1926
4. Benson DF, Geschwind N: Psychiatric aspects of neurologic disease, in Reiser, M. (ed) American Handbook of Psychiatry. New York, Basic Books, 1975
5. Brickner R: An interpretation of frontal lobe function based upon the study of a case of partial bilateral frontal lobectomy. Res Publ Assoc Res Nerv Ment Dis 13:259–351, 1934
6. Chorover S, Cole M: Delayed alternation performance in patients with cerebral lesions. Neuropsychologia 4:1–7, 1966
7. Cohen L: Perception of reversible figures by normal and brain-injured subjects. Arch Neurol Psychiatry 81:765–775, 1959
8. Cushing H, Eisenhardt L: Meningiomas. Springfield, Ill., Thomas, 1938
9. Denny-Brown D: The frontal lobes and their function, in Modern Trends in Neurology. London, Butterworths, 1951
10. Frazier C: Tumor involving the frontal lobe alone. Arch Neurol Psychiatry 35:525–571, 1936
11. Fulton J: Frontal Lobotomy and Affective Behavior. New York, Norton, 1951
12. Ghent L, Mishkin M, Teuber HL: Short-term memory after frontal lobe injury in man. J Comp Physiol Psychol 55:705–709, 1962
13. Goldstein K: The mental changes due to frontal lobe damage. J. Psychol Neurol Psychol 17:27–56, 1936

14. Goldstein K: The mental changes due to frontal lobe damage. J. Psychol
     17:187–208, 1944
15. Greenblatt M: Studies in Lobotomy. New York, Grune & Stratton, 1950
16. Halstead W: Brain and Intelligence. Chicago, University of Chicago Press, 1947
17. Hebb D: Man's frontal lobes: A critical review. Arch Neurol Psychiatry
     54:10–24, 1945
18. Jacobsen CF: Studies of cerebral functions in primates. Comparative Psychol
     Psychiatry 33:558–559, 1935
19. Jacobsen CF: Studies of cerebral functions in primates. Comparative Psychol
     Monographs 13:1–68, 1936
20. Jarvie H: Frontal lobe disinhibition. J Neurol Neurosurg Psych 17:14–32, 1954
21. Kleist K: Gehirnpathologie. Leipzig, Barth, 1934
22. Kolodny A: Symptomatology of tumors of the frontal lobe. Arch Neurol
     Psychiatr 21:1107–1127, 1929
23. Lhermitte J: Le lobe frontal. Encephale 24:87–118, 1929
24. Livingston K: The frontal lobes revisited; the case for a second look. Arch Neurol
     20:90–95, 1969
25. Luria A: Higher cortical functions in man. New York, Basic Books, 1966
26. Messimy R: Faits expérimentaux et cliniques concernant les fonctions des lobes
     préfrontaux, Ann Méd 49:69–85, 1948
27. Meyer A, Beck E: Prefrontal leucotomy and related operations: Anatomical
     aspects of success or failure. Springfield, Ill., Thomas, 1954
28. Milner B, Teuber HL: Alteration of perception and memory in man, in Weis-
     krantz L (ed): Analysis of Behavioral Change. New York, Harper & Row, 1968
29. Milner B: Interhemispheric differences and psychological processes. Br Med
     Bull 27:272–277, 1971
30. Moniz E: Prefrontal leucotomy in the treatment of mental disorders. Am J
     Psychiatry 93:1379–1385, 1937
31. Morsier G, Rey A: Le syndrome psychologique dans les tumeurs des lobes
     frontaux. Monatsschrift für Neurologie und Psychiatrie 110:293–308, 1945
32. Nauta W: Neural associations of the amygdaloid complex in the monkey. Brain
     85:505–520, 1962
33. Nauta W: The problem of the frontal lobe: A reinterpretation. J Psychiatr Res
     8:167–187, 1971
34. Pfeifer B: Les troubles psychiques dans les tumeurs cérébrales. Arch Psychol
     47:558–591, 1910
35. Ramier A, Hécaen H: Role respectif des attaintes frontales et de la lateralisa-
     tion lesionalle dans les déficits de la "fluence verbale." Rev Neurol 123:17–22,
     1970
36. Rylander G: Personality changes after operations on the frontal lobes. Acta
     Psychiat et Neurol. London, Oxford Univ Press, 1939, Suppl 20
37. Rylander G: Mental Changes after Excision of Cerebral Tissue. Copenhagen,
     Einar Munsgaar, 1943
38. Schuster W: Psychische Störungen bei Hirntumoren. Stuttgart, Enke, 1902
39. Semmes J, Weinstein S, Ghent L, Teuber HL: Correlates of impaired orientation
     in personal and extrapersonal space. Brain 86:747–772, 1963

40.   Teuber HL, Mishkin M: Judgment of visual and postural vertical after brain injury. J Psychol 38:161–175

41.   Vincent C: Diagnostic des tumeurs comprimant le lobe frontal. Rev Neurol 1:801–884, 1928

Commentary

It is obvious from the previous presentation that the frontal lobes subserve many separate functions and that many different approaches to the study of frontal lobe function can be fruitful. This multiplicity of activities obviously adds to confusion concerning symptomatology secondary to frontal lobe disorder. A notable example of such confusion concerns the "frontal lobe personality." Organic personality alterations are of particular concern for the psychiatrist for several reasons: (1) organic personality changes are frequently misdiagnosed as depressive, hypomanic, or psychopathic states; (2) the effects of psychosurgical lesions are best understood by the study of the effects of frontal and temporal lobe pathology on personality; (3) animal studies have been of limited value in the study of organic personality disorders so the physician's knowledge in this field must come from the study of his own patients.

In the following chapter, the "frontal lobe personality" is discussed together with and in contrast to the "epileptic personality" that appears to be associated with irritative lesions of the temporal lobe. More of the rationale for the latter association and a more global picture of the range of personality and behavioral changes with temporal lobe epilepsy is given in Chapter 10. It would appear that almost all significant organic personality disorders occur with disease in either the frontal or temporal lobe.

Dietrich Blumer, M.D., and
D. Frank Benson, M.D.

9
Personality Changes With Frontal and Temporal Lobe Lesions

It is well recognized that disorders affecting the brain can produce changes in personality. The specific alterations in personality brought about by brain disease depend on a number of factors. In widespread disease (dementia or delirium), impairment of intellect and memory or florid psychosis are the foremost characteristics. Depressive, manic, paranoid, or catatonic states may occur in previously well-adjusted individuals; lability of emotional expression may be seen; altered states of awareness are common in acute toxic states; loss of social inhibition is a frequent occurrence in both acute and chronic disturbances. An ancient dictum states that the personality traits seen in organic brain disease are exaggerations of preexisting traits. In some instances this is true. Thus, in senility a previously reserved and parsimonious individual may become miserly and paranoid with the diseased personality representing a caricature of his prior traits. The opposite may also occur, however. With brain disease, a quiet, cautious individual may become garrulous, grandiose, and free-spending, an apparent reversal of previous personal habits. Many variations exist between these two extremes, and for clinical purposes it is widely recognized that it is a *change* in the personality, not the specific personality traits produced, that suggests organic brain disease.

Two types of localized brain disorders, however, produce characteristic personality changes. Lesions affecting the frontal and temporal areas tend to leave intellectual functions intact while causing prominent alterations in personality. It is important to note that the localization is not the only important factor; frontal personality disorders result from destructive lesions, whereas temporal personality changes are the product of irritative (epileptic) disorders. The personality alterations noted with these special conditions of etiology and focus will be the topic of this presentation.

THE "FRONTAL LOBE PERSONALITY"

Damage to the premotor frontal lobes does not produce clear-cut neurologic changes, but such patients do suffer "psychologic" changes. Frontal disease can often be suspected by the characteristic alterations of personality and behavior; recognition of such changes should avert one of the more serious errors of diagnosis made by psychiatrists. The earliest symptom of frontal lobe tumor is usually an alteration in behavior that is often considered to be of psychogenic origin. Obviously, it is important to make an early diagnosis of operable brain tumor; even demonstration that a tumor is inoperable provides little consolation to the psychiatrist who has mistakenly provided psychotherapy for many months.

Over the years, a fair understanding of the characteristic mental changes associated with lesions of the frontal lobes has been developed by neurologists and neurosurgeons. Much knowledge has stemmed from study of war-injured military personnel from the two world wars. In addition, the experiences gained during the era of psychosurgery stimulated considerable interest in the mental changes related to frontal lobe disease. It is surprising, therefore, to note how little of this accumulated information can be found in current psychiatric curriculum, textbooks, or literature. A brief review of this background will help establish the characteristics of the frontal lobe personality.

Background

An early report documenting a change in personality following frontal lobe injury dates back to 1835.[22] A 16-year-old adolescent of morose, shut-in character and limited intellect shot himself in the lower midforehead. He suffered extensive damage to the mesial–orbital parts of his frontal lobes and lost his sight entirely. Not only was he unconcerned over his blindness but assumed a gay, vivacious, and jocular disposition.

Several decades later, the case of Phineas Gage[12] aroused great interest. He survived, without gross neurologic disability, an explosion that blasted a pointed iron bar (3 ft, 7 in. long, 1 1/4 in. at its widest point) through his head. After the injury, however, he was "no longer Gage." Although untrained in school, he had possessed a well-balanced mind, was "very energetic and persistent in executing all his plans of operation." His posttraumatic personality is described as follows:

The equilibrium or balance, so to speak, between his intellectual faculties and animal propensities seems to have been destroyed. He is fitful, irreverant, indulging at times in the grossest profanity, manifesting but little deference for his fellows, impatient of restraint or advice when it conflicts with his desires, at times pertinaciously obstinate, yet capricious and vacillating, devising many plans of operation, which are no sooner arranged than they are abandoned in turn for others appearing more feasible. A child in his intellectual capacity and manifestations, he has the animal passions of a strong man. . . .

The injury affected the left frontal lobe from the mesial–orbital part upward to the convexity between the midline and the precentral cortical area.

The first correlation of personality changes with frontal lobe lesions documented by postmortem examination[29] occurred in a furrier who fell 100 ft from a window, suffering a compound fracture of the frontal bones and severely injuring the right frontal lobe. He was never unconscious, and was confused only briefly. Previously good-natured, sociable, and gay, he became cantankerous, nasty, and threatening. Eventually, he resumed his trade and, although slower, he was still a capable worker. During the entire posttraumatic period, his intellect appeared intact. Autopsy, 1 year later, showed a deep scarring of the orbital part of both frontal lobes, more extensive on the right.

Among the many excellent psychiatric studies of brain lesions[4,8,14,16,19,23] Kleist's efforts to relate localized brain lesions to behavior and personality changes are noteworthy.[17] He confirmed Welt's thesis of the significance of lesions to the orbital brain, and related changes toward immoral, unfaithful, deceitful, thievish, and defiant behavior to orbital lesions. Kleist also noted puerile and facetious behavior in patients with orbital lesions. Euphoria was observed as a frequent early mental change in patients with frontal–orbital injuries; the euphoria was usually transient and at times changed to a dysphoric mood. Kleist presumed that the unity of personality and man's self-determination were related to the orbital brain and its connections. In contrast, lesions of the upper portions of the frontal lobes (convexity), were associated with lack of psychic and motor initiative. Lack of thought formation (impoverished and stereotyped modes of thinking) characterized these patients.

The term "moria" was employed by Jastrowitz[16] for the childish, cheerful excitement of patients with frontal lobe lesions, and Oppenheim[23] referred to a similar attitude as "Witzelsucht" (facetiousness). Urinary and rectal incontinence have been reported with marked regularity. Holmes[14] referred to three general types of changes associated with frontal lobe injury: (1) apathy and indifference; (2) depression, intellectual enfeeblement, automaticity, and incontinence; and (3) restlessness, exuberance, euphoria, irritability, childishness, facetiousness, and marked egoism.

Brickner[3] discussed the functions of the frontal lobes of one patient who had undergone amputation of the larger part of both frontal lobes. Almost the entire spectrum of "frontal lobe changes" was present.

Goldstein[8] described differences in the everyday behavior of frontal lobe patients: "Their faces are usually rigid, they lack expressive movements, they are slow and dull. In contrast to this usual behavior, they may suddenly react in an abnormal way and become abnormally excited." Goldstein felt that their mental condition could be understood as an impairment of the "abstract attitude."

The Russian psychologist Luria has studied frontal lobe disorders of both war-injured and neurosurgical patients.[20] The characteristics of frontal lobe disorder, Luria emphasizes, are disturbances of attention and concentration plus an inability to perform complex actions in sequence. The former produces the well-recognized apathy, while the latter causes an immediacy (concreteness) in both expression and action.

Another source of material highlighting the effect of frontal lobe injury on personality comes from the reports of frontal psychosurgical procedures. In one early lobotomy series,[9] patients treated for chronic pain became uninhibited, euphoric, and tended to be restless and purposeless. A second group showed slowing of thinking and acting, dullness, lack of emotional expression and display, plus a striking reduction in interest and drive. Admixture of the two occurred. Inappropriate or misplaced emotional reaction characterized all patients after lobotomy. In a review of the effects of "total bilateral frontal lobotomy," Greenblatt and Solomon,[10] listed four major results: decreased drive, decreased self-concern, depression of outwardly directed behavior and social sense, and shallower affective life. Modern psychosurgical procedures are less extensive and personality alterations are infrequent, but when they do occur they tend to confirm Kleist's thesis. Following tractotomy of the posterior orbital pathways bilaterally, Ström–Olsen and Carlisle[27] reported personality alterations in 2 percent in the form of irritability, aggressiveness, outspokeness, and spitefulness. On the other hand, bilateral cingulotomy appears to produce personality traits of relative apathy and unconcern. It would appear that the final result of a psychosurgical procedure that disconnects frontal centers depends on the premorbid personality traits and the extent and location of the surgery performed.

Illustrative Cases

CASE 1

A 45-year-old female physician felt markedly listless. Several years earlier, at a time of stress in her family life, she had required psychotherapy, and her current difficulty was initially considered a recurrent depressive reaction. When out-patient psychotherapy was unsuccessful, she was admitted to a psychiatric hospital. Three months later, the need for a pulmonary check-up prompted transfer to a general hospital where, somewhat fortuitously, a brain scan was ordered leading to the diagnosis of a large brain tumor. Her husband had noted an increasing listlessness about 1 year earlier when she had started to take refresher courses. She would often sleep in classes, would frequently stay in bed until noon, and generally experienced difficulty in getting going. She became slow in answering questions. About 6 months prior to hospitalization she became incontinent of urine and displayed a remarkable lack of concern. Her psychiatrist overlooked the fact that she never complained of depressed feelings, almost never cried, and lacked the morbid thoughts customary in the depressed. Her appetite had remained good, sleep was actually excessive, and she had stopped having dreams. She had remained affectionate toward her husband and was sexually responsive. She became extremely apathetic, never spoke on her own, was slow in response, and gave only brief answers when queried. She described her state of mind as a lack of enthusiasm and energy for almost anything. Electroencephalogram, brain scan, and preoperative ventriculography indicated a vascular tumor involving the anterior portion of the corpus callosum. The meningioma that was removed at right frontal lobectomy weighed almost 125 g.

CASE 2

A 54-year-old male had been very successful, amassing a considerable fortune. Almost 4 years before he received proper medical attention, personality changes in the form of irritable and aggressive behavior began. He became careless concerning money, even with his income tax. His business associates and his wife abandoned him, and his enterprises began to fail catastrophically. Regardless, he remained totally unconcerned and apparently happy. He lost his entire fortune—business, farm, horses and all—and was finally arrested for passing a forged check. He appeared confused to the judge and was sent to a state hospital instead of to prison. After 3 months of hospitalization, a diagnosis of an organic condition was made when it became apparent that he could not remember. He was transferred to a general hospital where bilateral papilledema, symmetrically hyperactive deep tendon reflexes, and intermittent incontinence of bowel and bladder were noted. Brain scan revealed a large, midline frontal mass, which appeared to be arising from the floor of the frontal fossa, and arteriography showed marked posterior displacement of both anterior cerebral arteries. Upon craniotomy, a large bilateral olfactory groove meningioma was removed.

CASE 3

A 32-year-old white male was admitted for behavioral evaluation. History revealed that he had sustained a gunshot wound in Vietnam 5 years previously. A high-velocity missile had entered the left temple and emerged through the right orbit. Infection necessitated surgical removal of most of the orbital surface of the right frontal lobe. On recovery, he was neither paralyzed nor aphasic but suffered a remarkable change in personality.

Prior to injury he had been quiet, intelligent, proper, and compulsive. He was a West Point graduate and spent the ensuing years as a military officer attaining the rank of captain. Both as a cadet and later as an officer, he was known to be quiet, strict, and rigid. He was considered a good commander, trusted by his men, but never shared comaraderie with his troops or with his peers.

Subsequent to injury, he was outspoken, facetious, brash, and disrespectful. There was no evidence of self-pity, although he frequently made rather morbid jokes about his condition (for example, "dummy's head"). On admission to the hospital, he had just failed at an extremely simple job.

He was not aphasic but misused words in a manner that suggested inability to maintain specific meanings. For instance, when asked whether the injury had affected his thinking his response was, "Yeah—it's affected the way I think—it's affected my senses—the only things I can taste are sugar and salt—I can't detect a pungent odor—ha ha—to tell you the truth it's a blessing this way." When the examiner persisted, "How had it affected the way you think?" his response was "Yes—I'm not as spry on my feet as I was before." He was never incontinent, but did show a messiness in attire. His remarks to the nurses and other female personnel were open and frank but were never blatantly sexual. His premorbid IQ was reported at about 130. Present examination showed a full-scale IQ of 113.

CASE 4

At the age of 46, a successful salesman sustained a compound depressed fracture of the left frontal bone in a traffic accident. Treatment included debridement and amputation of the left frontal pole. Recovery was slow, and 9 months after the injury he was referred for long-term custodial management. By this time, he had recovered motor function with only a minimal limp and slight hyperreflexia on the right side, had normal sensation, no evidence of aphasia, and normal memory and cognitive ability (IQ 118). Nonetheless, he remained under hospital care because of marked changes in personal habits.

Prior to the accident, the patient had been garrulous, enjoyed people, had many friends and talked freely. He was active in community affairs, including Little League, church activities, men's clubs, and so forth. It was stated by one acquaintance that the patient had a true charisma, "whenever he entered a room there was a change in the atmosphere, everything became more animated, happy and friendly."

Following the head injury, he was quiet and remote. He would speak when spoken to and made sensible replies but would then lapse into silence. He made no friends on the ward, spent most of his time sitting alone smoking. He was frequently incontinent of urine, occasionally of stool. He remained unconcerned about either and was frequently found soaking wet, calmly sitting and smoking. If asked, he would matter-of-factly state that he had not been able to get to the bathroom in time but that this didn't bother him. Because of objectionable eating habits he always ate alone on the ward. His sleep pattern was reversed; he stayed up much of the night and slept during the day. He did not resent being awakened or questioned. He could discuss many subjects intelligently, but was never known to initiate either a conversation or a request. He could give detailed accounts of his life prior to the accident, of the hospitals he had been in, the doctors and treatment he had had but there was an unreality to his conversation. When asked, he would deny illness, state emphatically that he could return to work at any time, and that the only reason he was not working was that he was being held in the hospital by the doctors. At no time did he request a discharge or weekend pass. He was totally unconcerned about his wife and children. Formerly a warm and loving father, he did not seem to care about his family. Eventually, the family ceased visiting because of his indifference and unconcern.

These four patients with bilateral frontal lesions presented two strikingly different types of personality alterations. The hyperactive, irritable and insouciant attitude of Cases 2 and 3 contrasts with the listless indifference and slowness of the other two. The pathology involved the orbital lobes in the euphoric cases, and the frontal lobe convexity in the apathetic patients.

Discussion of the "Frontal Lobe Personality"

PSYCHOPATHOLOGY

The two types of personality changes occurring after frontal lobe lesions may be described as: (1) toward apathy and indifference ("pseudodepressed") and (2) toward puerility and euphoria ("pseudopsychopathic"). Admixtures of the two are more common than the pure types.

Patients who suffer the "pseudodepressed" type of frontal lobe personality alteration appear to have lost all initiative. They respond in an automaton-like fashion, but the responses are usually proper and intelligent. In fact, in testing situations where the initiative is provided by the examiner, these individuals characteristically produce normal test scores, even though they are unable to function independently in daily life. In the same manner, one patient of ours was able to perform sexual intercourse as long as his wife told him, step by step, what he had to do. Slowness, indifference, and apathy are the personality traits that overshadow the near-normal intellect; they characterize the personality alterations produced by prefrontal convexity lesions, the condition we term "pseudodepressed."

A similar, if not identical, clinical picture is seen in some subcortical disorders. Bilateral caudate nucleus atrophy (as seen in Huntington's chorea), bilateral thalamic destruction (surgical treatment of Parkinsonism) or atrophy (Steele–Richardson syndrome) can all produce a slowing of speech, thought, and movement that profoundly alters the personality. This has been termed "subcortical dementia"[1,21] but would appear to be closely related to the characteristic personality alterations of prefrontal convexity pathology. There is a close anatomical relationship between these subcortical centers and the prefrontal convexity, and, in fact, separation of these connections in the early massive prefrontal lobotomies produced the "vegetative states" that were reported. The "pseudodepressed" personality thus appears to result from destructive pathology affecting the prefrontal convexity, certain subcortical centers (particularly the basal ganglia and thalamus) and their connections.

The "pseudopsychopathic" type of frontal lobe personality is best characterized by the lack of adult tact and restraints. Such patients may be coarse, irritable, facetious, hyperkinetic or promiscuous; they often lack social graces and may, on impulse, commit anti-social acts. Paranoid or grandiose thinking may be present. While they may flare with anger, they do not bear a grudge. Outwardly at least, their behavior resembles that of the sociopathic personality. The history of personality change occurring with organic brain disease and the presence of related symptoms, particularly incontinence, however, suggests that the disorder is "pseudopsychopathic". As noted in the review of the literature and from our own cases, the "pseudopsychopathic" personality traits apparently follow injury to the orbital frontal lobe or pathways traversing this region.

DIFFERENTIAL DIAGNOSIS

The apathy of a patient with a frontal lobe lesion may be mistaken for the psychomotor retardation of the depressed. But the ideation of a frontal lobe patient with apathy is that of empty indifference, while the depressed patient reveals a morbid preoccupation with worrisome thoughts. Apathy also results from lesions of other parts of the brain (thalamic, hypothalamic, and other subcortical regions). Brain-stem lesions, such as those of encephalitis lethargica, may be responsible for hyperactive and antisocial types of behavior as well as for akinetic behavior.

The "pseudopsychopathic" type may resemble, superficially, a manic or hypomanic patient. The affect is shallower in the organic case, but one may have to consider the course of the illness, the premorbid personality and the presence or absence of previous episodes. Differentiation from an antisocial character disorder will be less of a problem. Antisocial acts that are in marked contrast to the previous behavior demand careful scrutiny for organic etiology.

Incontinence occurs frequently with frontal lobe lesions, while seizures are less common. Both incontinence and seizures are strong indicators of an organic lesion.

ETIOLOGY

A fairly strong argument can be made in relating the "pseudodepressed" type to lesions of the convexity of the frontal lobes and the "pseudopsychopathic" type to lesions of the orbital surface. The common admixture of the two personality types would be related to the relative rarity of pure lesions of the convexity or of the orbital surface, respectively. Bilateral pathology is probably necessary to produce the personality changes.

A great variety of lesions, including those of psychosurgery, may produce the frontal lobe type of personality alteration. Postraumatic frontal lobe personality changes are often transient but may be permanent. In the case of tumors, the frontal lobe syndrome is supplanted in time by signs of more diffuse brain disease, in particular with increased intracranial pressure. In the past, general paresis was a frequent cause of the frontal-lobe-type personality; both Huntington's chorea and multiple sclerosis can also produce this type of mental change.

TREATMENT

There may be a treatment for the underlying disease but there is no specific therapy for the frontal lobe personality. For patients with the "pseudodepressed" type of change, however, early and steady rehabilitation efforts are important. These patients should not be allowed to sit around; they should be activated by occupational therapy and similar approaches as soon as possible. Patients with the "pseudopsychopathic" alteration tend to be very difficult for their family members who may need support and counseling.

THE "EPILEPTIC PERSONALITY"

For over a century, physicians have listed personality traits that they considered characteristic of the epileptic. The epileptic personality has become a controversial subject; opinions have varied, shifting with the expertise of the reporting clinician and by the variety of epilepsy studied. Most significantly, however, there have been dramatic changes in the descriptions of the "epileptic personality" that reflect changes in the opinions of both physicians and the public concerning epilepsy. Thus, early descriptions of the epileptic personality featured the presence of evil spirits, devils, and so forth. Later, other characteristics included slow-wittedness, apathy, and incompetence, and probably reflected the inadequacy of the early treatment regimes. Next came an era when most grand-mal epileptics could be well controlled and could lead normal lives. The mention of "epileptic personality" became an anathema, a symbol of society's prejudice against epileptics. Nonetheless, descriptions of "epileptic personality" persisted but now related the abnormal behavioral traits to psychomotor epilepsy. Recently, this description has been modified to emphasize the impulsivness, aggressiveness, and violence that some investigators suggest characterize temporal lobe seizure patients.

In the present section, we will review some of this background, present illustrative cases and attempt to delineate personality changes that are unique to epileptics, specifically those with temporal lobe seizure foci.

Background

In Europe, psychiatrists have traditionally studied epilepsy in their efforts to arrive at precise descriptions and classifications of mental illness. Discussion has never centered around the concept of the "epileptic personality" but has concerned broader mental manifestations occurring in the course of epilepsy. Samt,[24] Kraepelin,[18] Gruhle,[11] and Schorsch[25] present the views on epilepsy of German psychiatrists over the past 90 years. They describe and discuss typical symptoms including the personality aberrations of the disease. By contrast, Freud[5] and Szondi[28] attempt to elucidate the dynamic interaction of typical mental changes—to understand the epileptic.

Samt, a psychiatrist at the Charité Hospital in Berlin deserves mention for his early descriptions of "forms of epileptic insanity." Under this title, he published two papers in 1875 and 1876 describing the habitual peculiarities in the character of epileptics as follows:

I have seen such religious martyr-faces, epileptics who speak "frankly and freely from the bottom of my heart"; who beat their chests: "As true as I live, from my heart I speak for emperor and king, dear God is with me"; epileptics who act like the most pious sufferers, who kneel down and swear as to their angel-like innocence: "Yes, I am sometimes a bit mean, but I don't attack, I want a pistol to my head if I do, but I love to live"; who if they are in the wrong, want to be "crucified and condemned"; epileptics who see "dear Jesus" in dreams and recognize a message from "God the father" in a drawing on the wall, and who steal, strike and curse in a most vulgar manner—enough, those poor epileptics, such as one might meet in every institution, who have a prayer book in their pocket, dear God on their tongue, but an excess of viciousness in their whole body.

The last sentence in this paragraph is frequently cited in German psychiatric textbooks. While most authors assert that the picture fits only a few cases, Samt's drastic description of the two-faced epileptic has exerted a fascination for almost 100 years.

Kraepelin[18] emphasized that the intellectual processes of epileptics combined slowness, circumstantiality, and persistence. Religious ideas are cultivated. In advanced cases, memory suffers and thinking becomes impoverished. Kraepelin comments: "The most drastic changes brought about by epilepsy are in the emotional sector, even in cases where no impairment of the intellect can be recognized. Almost always an intensification of angry irritability occurs . . ." Epileptics like to work; they may be slow but are often pedantically precise. They frequently show an awkward helpfulness.

About 30 years later, Gruhle[11] described certain personality traits of the epileptic: "He is enormously circumstantial, it takes him a long time to get to the point, he uses expletives as well as an excessive number of polite expressions, fills in with quotations, and tries to insure himself in advance against any possible misunderstanding."

More recently, Schorsch[25] presented a comprehensive summary of the modern knowledge of epilepsy including the "epileptic personality changes."

He noted that the formal course of mental processes is changed by the illness "toward slowness, adhesiveness, perseveration," toward the well-known viscosity: "The patients lose their versatility, become awkward, circumstantial, pedantic. The difficulty in working through impressions and a delayed ability to react may well be of significance for the tendency toward penting up of affects and resentment." Yet most patients are basically good-natured, childlike-dependent, and conscientious in their work. Emotional lability, with sudden surprising changes of attitude, is frequently noted. "Such contradictory behavior is due to the illness and therefore cannot be assessed in the same way as the insincerity, hypocrisy, and bigotry of healthy persons."

Freud[5] in his paper "Dostoevsky and Patricide" (1928) renders a coherent picture of the contradictory personality of the famous epileptic: the threat of repetitive, uncontrollable acts of murderous or near-murderous violence; the guilt and the need for atonement; seeking forgiveness and help from God; the attempt to adhere to a strict moral code; proving onself as the "mildest, kindliest, most helpful person possible." Although Freud doubted that Dostoevsky could be thought of as a true moralist, he did not refer to him as a hypocrite. A hypocrite is a person who merely plays the role of a moral and pious person; Dostoevsky's religiosity and moral strivings appear to be of a genuine nature.

Szondi[28] agreed with Freud about the psychodynamic factors in epilepsy, but he considered the "epileptic reaction" to be a genuine phenomenon that cannot be explained in terms of the sexual, sadomasochistic drives. He sees the "epileptic reaction" as a pathologic variant of a general biologic mechanism, whose goal is to rescue the individual from a dangerous situation by the paroxysm of a sudden, surprising action. In this mechanism, by necessity, there is a close correlation of psychic–emotional and physical–motor factors. The dynamic factor in this mechanism has the quality of a drive. Three phases can be differentiated in the drive process: "First, the energies of the crude affects are pent up; rage or hate, anger or vengeance, envy or jealousy are incited. . . . Then follows the explosive discharge in some form of fit. . . . Finally the phase during which the person tries to make-up, the hyperethical, often hyperreligious phase." As an example of this process the author cites the case of an 18-year-old epileptic, who, prior to an attack, would throw lighted matches in his mother's face or would throw her clothing in a stove; after the seizure, he would be exceedingly obedient, helped his mother wherever he could and overwhelmed her with signs of his affection. In the phase of explosive discharge, the pent-up energy is either turned actively outward or passively inward, against the self: A real or suspected enemy is attacked, or the person is "seized by an attack." Either way it is not merely anger, but anger at its pathological extreme: the murderous intent.

After discussing the views of various authors Szondi remarks: "It is astonishing to note how often the gluey-viscous affectivity was considered the core of the mental make-up of epileptics, and to which degree so many authors stayed stuck themselves to this syndrome of adhesiveness, and with how many Greek words the same phenomenon was labeled.''

More recently, Geschwind[7] has detailed the personality traits that tend to follow the onset of illness in temporal lobe epilepsy. He characterized the overall picture as that of a profound deepening of the patients' emotional responses. All events are serious to these patients; there are no trivial occurrences. They may become excessively concerned with moral issues and involve themselves with the rights and wrongs of rather trivial affairs; excessive religiosity may be a striking feature of the temporal lobe epileptic. A surprising number among them begin to write extensively. Paranoid ideation may be present. Interictal aggressiveness is a common feature but is relatively well tolerated by many of the families, probably because of the marked emotional warmth customarily displayed by these same patients toward the family members. Both the exaggerated aggressiveness and the unusual emotional warmth are seen as contrasting aspects of the deepened emotional responses. Changes in sexual behavior are a striking feature in many cases.

Illustrative Cases

CASE 5

A 53-year-old white male had suffered from psychomotor and generalized seizures since age 13. The EEGs demonstrated two separate right temporal spike foci. A right temporal lobectomy at age 40 was followed by decreased frequency of psychomotor seizures and disappearance of grand-mal attacks.

Following graduation from high school he worked steadily, but despite superior intelligence he never sought advancement. The seizures were chiefly nocturnal and remained a well-guarded secret. In 20 years' work as a stock clerk in the same company no one knew about his epilepsy.

At age 30, he married for companionship after showing little interest in dating. The couple had intercourse only a few times during the first eight years of the marriage and never after.

Prior to the operation he had been irritable and moody, often for days. His wife threatened to leave him and he made two suicidal attempts. He then chose to undergo surgery for his epilepsy. Despite the incomplete control of the seizures, the moodiness gradually subsided and he became easier to get along with. He assumed an exuberant, enthusiastic attitude and participated regularly in a number of community and church activities. He became eager to help others and volunteered for many causes. However, there were occasional periods of anxiety, depression, and hypochondriacal concern. He remained without friends, not because of his seizures, which were nocturnal and unknown, but because he seemed so different to others and knew himself to be different.

He was examined regularly after the operation. He never betrayed anger and always presented himself in a most compliant manner. He eagerly volunteered for any new test or study and kept his physician informed by regularly forwarding a log of daily events, which included his dreams. He was both verbose and meticulous in his statements. For example, when asked what he would do if he saw a fire in a theatre, or if he found a stamped envelope in the street, he gave traditional answers but made sure that all possibilities were covered; for instance, he considered whether or not the stamp was cancelled and whether the fire was large or small, had just begun, or had been going for some time. Characteristic of his communications is the following squirrel story, an excerpt of one of his regular reports.

When we moved from an upstairs apartment to a first floor one (Dec. 1, 19--), the squirrels I feed night and morning followed right with us. The squirrels are very tame and cute. They would feed out of my wife's and my hands. While I watch the door for a man to pick her up for work while she got ready I would prop the screen door open about 4 inches and feed them from inside by opening the inside door about an inch. They would come through the screen door opening and feed as I gave them food through the crack in the inside door. They would sit on the door sill and eat it (most of the time). It was winter and this way I could feed them while inside. When I went walking I would prop the screen door open and place some food in a dish on the door sill and they would feed from that. One day I did not put the dish there, they had enough, and went walking. When I came back the screen door had not gone completely shut and they had chewed about one third of the door away. I repaired this with water putty and painted it. Then to teach them to stay away from I rubbed some Red Pepper on the repair with my finger. As I watched the next day one of them must have got into it. He just stood on the porch. You could see he was in awful pain, he quivered, cried and dripped from the mouth. It was awful to witness but they have not bothered the door since. The next day (June 5) I took a dish of peanuts out on the porch to feed them. They all acted normal until I saw one coming from the side to get in the dish. He upset it and I went to brush him away with my hand. As I did he gave me a good bite on the outside of the right hand at the little finger. I washed it good with soap and water and put on some Merthiolate. I have been taught to watch the animal. If it has Rabies it will die in 10 to 14 days giving time to start the Pasteur treatment. Also the further from the head the bite is the longer it takes. Rabies is a virus of the nerves following the nerves from the bite to the head where it is fatal.

Our squirrels are fed clean food and water. They do not get into any dead or rotten food. They all are as healthy as can be. Have a pretty coat and the cutest habits you would want to see. The litter they had this spring were the most domesticated I have ever seen. *Wouldn't you fight anything you knew treated you like he was with red pepper?* Squirrels are like other forms of life. One alone you can train and it will respond without any trouble. But when another one or two show on the scene they are always fighting each other and chasing each other from the source of food. Also one always wants to be a bully. You should hear them growl and chase each other away when more than one tries to feed from the same dish.

I was a little alarmed about the bite because we have some neighbors who are scared of any animal at all. All they can say is "you know they can give you Rabies." Knowing circumstances I managed to conquer my nerves for a month and the squirrel was here and healthy as ever. After 2 weeks I felt safe, free and my nerves were quiet again. . . . . . .
August 12 a squirrel came to the door. I thought it was a meek one. I held a piece of

Graham Cracker toward it. It looked at me and went for my hand as if to take the cracker. It ignored the cracker and bit my finger instead. This time it was the little finger of the left hand. Within 10 seconds the bottom of my stomach hurt, I got a headache and the base of my throat started to hurt and feel tight. As I write this it is bringing back memories and I can feel it again.

I stood it as long as I possibly could. The worry was making a wreck of me. Then I went to Dr. R. August 17. He is treating me as you did. Reassuring me it was my nerves. Proving my thoughts and worries wrong and in my own thoughts. He told me to increase my Valium to half a tablet at 8:00 a.m. and half at 4:00 p.m. He also told me something I had read and forget. The state is considered Rabies free. There has not been a case I think he said in 5 or 7 years. This program of having dogs injected to prevent Rabies is purely political to make money and keep a record of dogs for licensing. Now I remember reading that in the paper when they started the program a few years ago.

Also do not feed the squirrels by hand. Toss the food to them or put it on a plate for them. They are wild animals and while no Rabies has been reported for a long time they can chew you up bad then infection maybe. He also reminded me that Bats are the ones that are full of Rabies. This I knew from childhood. Now I feed the squirrels in a dish on the porch. *No more by hand*. I slowly got ahold of myself again.

All details are meticulously recorded. The depth of feeling for what went on between the patient and the squirrels is remarkable, and at least remotely reminiscent of *Crime and Punishment*.

CASE 6

A 43-year-old successful businessman of superior intelligence had run away from a home void of affection in his early teens and made his career without further schooling. He had become a sponsor of the fine arts and was recognized for his cultivated taste. His home life was less happy. He had remained loyally attached to a spouse who was little able to show affection, and the marital relationship was stormy. A closed head injury suffered in a car accident at age 20 was followed by seizures and personality changes that played a significant role in the vicissitudes of his interpersonal relationships.

Shortly after the head injury, he was noted to react with excessive anger to minor provocations. A few years later he first suffered generalized seizures. Excessive irritability would be present for hours or days preceding the grand-mal attacks. At such times of heightened irritability, he reacted in a paranoid manner and fought with friends or strangers "over nothing." Anxiety or feelings of unusual strength and inspiration would frequently precede an attack. The EEGs occasionally showed temporal lobe abnormalities but more often were within normal limits.

After the head injury, he developed a peculiar difficulty in communication. He had always been talkative but very much to the point; he became verbose and bogged down with irrelevant details. His conversation was so detailed that he was in danger of losing the train of thought and became concerned about the competence of his memory. He would elaborate unnecessarily on secondary (and tertiary) facts before coming forth with the primary fact. For instance, he would dwell at some length on "Friday noon" before coming to the point of a particular doctor's appointment (on Friday noon). While he was aware of this tendency he was unable to maintain a fluent and relevant speech. Only at times when angry or speaking of a matter close to his heart could he proceed properly from point to point.

His wife confirmed that he talked too much with exaggerated emphasis on details—literally spending hours on little things and repeating himself over and over again. This tendency even more than his irritability contributed to a near breakdown of their communication. The wife noted that his inability to "let something go" would worsen during the heightened tension of the prodromal phase of a seizure.

He would get depressed to the point of neglecting his work during a period of marital separation. It should be noted that he owned deep and very special religious feelings. He confessed to a deep awe of some force larger than himself and in the course of his conversation impressed friends by his mysticism.

Discussion of the "Epileptic Personality"

PSYCHOPATHOLOGY

A complex syndrom of personality and behavior changes follows (or rarely, precedes) the onset of temporal lobe seizures, or of generalized seizures with presumed involvement of the temporal lobes. While sexual arousal and response tend to be reduced, there is often a profound deepening of emotional responses.[7] This deepening includes penting up and episodic discharge of anger and rage on the one hand, and intensification of ethical–religious feelings on the other. The need to be goodnatured, helpful, and God-fearing is much more prominent than the highly publicized violence-proneness.

The deepening of emotional responses affects much of the patient's psychic life. The so-called epileptic "viscosity" may be viewed as a result of the intensified ethical sense: there are no trifles; the right or wrong of every item needs to be considered along with all ramifications; no issue can be easily dropped; these patients become long-winded in speech and often feel the need to put down their thoughts in lengthy writings; they tend to be remarkably without humor, in general, and without appreciation of sexual humor in particular.[6]

To others, these individuals are patently different. They also feel different and tend to withdraw from ordinary social intercourse. While they are good-natured and cooperative when they feel appreciated, they are often difficult to bear for those about them daily. Angry outbursts can be triggered by issues that others consider irrelevant but to the patient are important considerations of right or wrong.

Paranoid attitudes are not infrequent and the schizophrenia-like psychoses of temporal lobe epileptics are well known.[13,26] Other patients are prone to depression; manic mood swings or chronic hypomanic states may occur. Anxiety, hypochondriacal, and hysterical reactions are not uncommon in temporal lobe epileptics. As a point of fact, this very vulnerability of epileptics to most of the well-known, functional mental changes has blinded observers to the presence of the personality and behavioral changes that are unique to epileptics. It may be helpful to refer to the former traits as secondary symptoms and to the latter as primary symptom of mental disorder in epilepsy.

DIFFERENTIAL DIAGNOSIS

Patients with the personality and behavior changes described above may suffer from temporal lobe seizures that have not been recognized. The diagnosis of temporal lobe seizures usually can be made clinically, based on the documentation of the characteristic brief repetitive events. These vary considerably between patients but usually remain stereotyped for a given patient. Seizures are characteristically followed by a postictal confusional–amnestic phase.[2,15] Cases of temporal lobe epilepsy with persistently negative EEG findings do exist but are rare. Multiple EEGs with recording during sleep and with special leads may have to be obtained to demonstrate the abnormality. Generalized seizures are frequent in temporal lobe epileptics, and their presence may make the diagnosis of epilepsy obvious.

The presence of the "epileptic personality" has been described in patients with epileptogenic foci in the temporal lobes who have no overt seizures. The significance of EEG changes alone in patients with explosive personality disorders or with global hyposexuality is not established. Much additional evidence will be necessary before a temporal lobe EEG focus without overt seizures can be related to the personality aberrations of temporal lobe epilepsy.

Hysterical seizures are frequent among epileptics, and the recognition of hysteria does not exclude the diagnosis of epilepsy. The schizophrenia-like psychoses that tend to occur in some patients after years of temporal lobe epilepsy are characterized by comparative intactness of affect, ability to relate to others and by lack of schizophrenic deterioration. Otherwise, any of the symptoms of schizophrenia may be present.

While unique personality and behavioral changes have been described above, only exceptionally will the entire spectrum of characteristic primary mental changes be present in one individual patient. A combination of several of these traits, however, is common. The addition of secondary behavioral symptomatology may make diagnosis very difficult.

ETIOLOGY

Temporal lobe seizures can result from tumors, scars of brain trauma or birth injury, sclerosis of Ammon's horn (presently attributed to prolonged infantile seizures), infections or vascular lesions. Personality changes are exceptional in the early stages of temporal lobe epilepsy but are common in chronic cases. Some patients with generalized seizures may develop the traits of the epileptic personality earlier or later, probably depending on the primary or secondary involvement of the temporal lobe structures.

TREATMENT

Of primary importance is the treatment of the epilepsy. Temporal lobe epilepsy does not respond very well to anticonvulsant drugs, but if control of seizures can be achieved, there may be a concomitant recovery from the global hyposexuality and from the heightened irritability. Dilantin, phenobarbital, Mysoline, and Tegretol are the anticonvulsant drugs of choice for temporal lobe epilepsy.

Some patients, on the other hand, become more disturbed when the seizures are suppressed. They may become irritable, paranoid, depressed, and may even become psychotic. It is sometimes necessary to lower the anticonvulsant level and allow occasional seizures to improve the mental well-being of the patient.

Unilateral anterior temporal lobectomy, performed in patients with primarily unilateral epileptogenic foci who have not responded to medication, may have a beneficial effect on some of the behavioral changes. If the seizures are abolished, the sexuality and episodic aggressivity tend to become normalized. The so-called "vicosity," however, appears irreversible. Various secondary symptoms of mental disorder in temporal lobe epilepsy may abate following successful surgery, but paranoid and schizophrenia-like changes tend to persist.

Psychotropic drugs may be tried in epilepsy but, in general, are of limited effectiveness. The phenothiazines, however, are not contraindicated and may be helpful in paranoid, agitated, and schizophrenia-like states.

Psychotherapy is of limited value and usually must be of the supportive type. The viscous type of verbal expression often represents a significant obstacle for psychotherapy. The patients tend to respond much better to a kind and understanding approach than to strict limit setting. Family members may need much support and help in understanding the patient.

CONCLUSION

Severe and unique personality changes can be described in certain patients with frontal lobe lesions on the one hand and some patients with epilepsy on the other. The terms "frontal lobe personality" and "epileptic personality" should only be used with implicit reservations. A frontal lobe lesion probably needs to be bilateral before it results in a personality change; lesions to the frontal convexity produce a different personality change from lesions to the orbital area; and certain subcortical lesions may lead to similar personality changes. The "epileptic personality," far from being characteristic for most epileptics, appears to be associated with chronic involvement of temporal-limbic structures. A more precise etiology of the described organic personality changes will have to be established by careful neuropsychiatric studies. The contrast between the two organic personality types is very striking. The frontal lesions are destructive in type and lead to immediate personality changes, while the temporal–limbic lesions are of an irritative–epileptogenic type and result only in gradually developing personality changes with peculiar psychodynamics of their own. The relative simplicity of the "frontal lobe personality" contrasts with the wealth of primary and secondary mental changes that may be associated with the "epileptic personality."

REFERENCES

1. Albert ML, Feldman RG, Willis AL: The sub-cortical dementia of progressive supranuclear palsy. J. Neurol Neurosurg Psychiat 37:121–130, 1974
2. Blumer, D: Neuropsychiatric aspects of psychomotor and other forms of epilepsy, in Livingston S: Comprehensive Management of Epilepsy in Infancy, Childhood and Adolescence. Springfield, Ill, Thomas, 1971
3. Brickner RM: The Intellectual Functions of the Frontal Lobes. New York, Macmillan, 1936
4. Faust C: Die Psychischen Störungen nach Hirntraumen, in Gruhle HW, Jung R, Mayer-Gross W, Müller M (Eds): Psychiatrie der Gegenwart vol 2. Berlin-Göttingen-Heidelberg, Springer, 1960
5. Freud S: Gesammelte Werke, vol 14. London, Imago, 1948
6. Ferguson SM, Schwartz ML, Rayport M: Perception of humor in patients with temporal lobe epilepsy—a cartoon test as an indicator of neuropsychologic deficit. Arch Gen Psychiatry 21:363, 1969
7. Geschwind N: The clinical setting of aggression in temporal lobe epilepsy. In Fields WS, Sweet WH (eds): The Neurobiology of Violence. St. Louis, Warren H. Green, 1975
8. Goldstein K: Aftereffects of Brain Injuries in War. New York, Grune & Stratton, 1948
9. Greenblatt M, Arnot R, Solomon H: Studies in Lobotomy. New York, Grune & Stratton, 1950
10. Greenblatt M, Solomon HC: Studies of lobotomy, in The Brain and Human Behavior, Proc. Assoc. Res. Nerv. Ment. Dis., 36, New York, Hafner, 1966
11. Gruhle HW: Epileptische Reaktionen und epileptische Krankheiten. Handbuch der Geisteskrankheiten, Bumke O. (Ed.) vol 8, Berlin, Springer, 1930, pp 669–728
12. Harlow JM: Recovery from the passage of an iron bar through the head. Publications Mass Med Soc 2:329–346, 1868
13. Hill D: The schizophrenia-like psychoses of epilepsy. Proc. R Soc 55:315–316 (Discussion) 1962
14. Holmes G: Mental symptoms associated with cerebral tumours. Proc R S Med 24, 1931

15   Janz D: Die Epilepsien. Stuttgart, Thieme, 1969
16. Jastrowitz M: Beiträge zur Localisation im Grosshirn and über deren praktische Verwerthung. Dtsch Med Wochenschr 14:81, 1888
17. Kleist K: Gehirnpathologie. Leipzig, Barth, 1934
18. Kraepelin E: Psychiatrie, Leipzig, Barth, 1904
19. Kretschmer E: Die Orbitalhirn-und Zwischenhirnsyndrome nach Schädelbasisfrakturen. Allg Z Psychiat 124:358–360, 1949
20. Luria AR: Frontal lobe syndrome, in Vinken PJ, Bruun GW (eds): Handbook of Clinical Neurology, vol 2. Amsterdam, North-Holland, 1969
21. McHugh PR, Folstein MF: Subcortical dementia. Address to the American Academy of Neurology, Boston, April, 1973 (unpublished)
22. de Nobele E: Annales de medecine Belge. Fevr. 1835
23. Oppenheim H: Zur Pathologie der Grosshirngeschwülste. Arch Psychiat 21:560, 1889
24. Samt P: Epileptische Irreseinsformen, Archiv Psychiatrie 5, 1875 and idem 6, 1876
25. Schorsch G: Epilepsie: Klinik und Forschung, in Gruhle HW et al (eds): Psychiatrie der Gegenwart, vol 2. Berlin, Springer, 1960
26. Slater E, Beard AW: The schizophrenia-like psychoses of epilepsy. Br J Psych 109:95–150, 1963
27. Ström-Olsen R, Carlisle S: Bi-frontal stereotactic tractotomy: A follow-up study of its effects on 210 patients. Br J Psychiat 118:141–154, 1970
28. Szondi L: Schicksalsanalytische Therapie. Bern, Huber, 1963
29. Welt L: Ueber Charakterveränderungen des Menschen infolge von Läsionen des Stirnhirns. Dtsch Arch Klin Med 42, 1888

Commentary

The two types of personality changes noted following frontal lobe disorders correspond to separate localizations of pathology. This appears clear-cut in the examples, but it must be remembered that in most cases of frontal lobe disorder the pathology fails to respect anatomical boundaries and some admixture of symptoms is the rule. Division into pseudodepressed and pseudopsychopathic types, however, will aid the clinician in diagnosing and understanding frontal lobe personality problems. Some studies have suggested differences based on right or left hemisphere involvement, anterior or posterior involvement, medial or lateral involvement, and so on. Most of these studies are inconclusive at present, but, without question, we have evidence that demonstrates distinct personality abnormalities produced by organic disease and that these vary depending on location and type of pathology.

The next disorder to be discussed was at one time considered entirely a psychiatric problem. With the advent of specific medical treatment, however, the management of epilepsy has been taken over almost totally by the neurologists. While most neurologists and psychiatrists are satisfied with this division of labor, the patient does not always receive the best care. A sizable number of patients with seizure disorders also have significant psychiatric problems. Sometimes the two problems can be separated, and the epileptic will need both a neurologist and a psychiatrist for optimum treatment. Frequently, however, the psychiatric and epileptic problems are inseparable. Whichever specialist handles such a patient must not only be aware of both problems but also be equipped to care for both. The management of epilepsy has improved greatly when compared to the past, but many epileptics still suffer considerable disability that could be corrected by a combined therapy.

Dietrich Blumer, M. D.

10
Temporal Lobe Epilepsy and Its Psychiatric Significance

More than most other disorders, epilepsy requires both a neurologic and a psychiatric approach. Epileptics make up a substantial portion (from 3 to 10 percent) of the total number of mental hospital admissions.[58] In what must be considered a conservative estimate, one sixth to one quarter of the outpatients with epilepsy suffer from conspicuous psychiatric disorders; and about 10 percent have been admitted at some time to mental hospitals.[50,51] Neurologists, by nature of their interest and training, tend to pay little attention to the psychologic symptoms in epileptics. Psychiatrists, on the other hand, tend to overlook the epileptic nature of certain mental changes, or—once the diagnosis is known—often shun epileptics as cases from an alien field.

During the earlier decades of this century, much was written about the psychiatric aspects of epilepsy. With the advent of the EEG, more effective anticonvulsant therapy, and advanced physiologic and biochemical knowledge of seizures, epileptology has become established as a neurologic science. When it was determined that a majority of epileptics could lead useful lives free of seizures and mental disorder, the smaller but substantial number of epileptics with various emotional troubles was soon overlooked, or their difficulties were attributed to society's ostracism, to ''brain damage,'' to excessive doses of anticonvulsants, to the effects of institutionalization, or to the nonspecific psychologic effects of any chronic illness. Their existence at times almost seemed an embarrassment to many who fought against the public's prejudice toward epileptics. Paradoxically, a brilliant progress in medicine had led to a significant gap in health care.

171

This gap is particularly apparent in the United States where the battle against the view of epilepsy as a form of insanity has been waged most successfully. The notion that certain personality or behavioral traits may be characteristic of epileptics has been discarded, and there has been only sporadic interest in epilepsy on the part of psychiatrists. Epileptics with mental disturbance (often with poorly controlled seizures) find it most difficult to lead a normal life and need special attention, but, in fact, they are a neglected lot.

INCIDENCE OF PSYCHIATRIC COMPLICATIONS IN THE EPILEPSIES

Among the various epilepsies, psychomotor or temporal lobe epilepsy —the form of focal epilepsy involving the limbic system—has been singled out as being associated with the interictal mental changes that formerly were felt to be characteristic of epileptics in general. Early reports by Gibbs[21] noted the high incidence of psychiatric disorders among psychomotor epileptics (40%–50%) when compared to other epileptics (less than 10%); the disorders, however, were said to be variable and nonspecific. Gastaut and co-workers documented the presence of rather specific behavioral changes in temporal lobe epilepsy.[14–16] In clinical practice, neurologists tend to note a higher frequency of behavioral abnormalities in patients with temporal lobe seizures than in patients with other types of epilepsy of equal severity.[54]

Several often-quoted investigations, on the other hand, have cast doubt on the unique association between mental disorders and temporal lobe epilepsy. The report of Guerrant et al.[24] is based on a cross-sectional psychiatric and psychologic assessment of psychomotor and grand-mal epileptics and a control group with chronic medical illnesses; while laden with statistics, it gives scant consideration to qualitative differences between the groups.*

Similarly, Stevens[62] virtually ignored qualitative differences; she simply compared the incidence of psychiatric hospitalization in a series of 100

---

*Each of the three groups had roughly a 90 percent incidence of "functional emotional disorder warranting diagnosis," and the specific hypothesis of the study, that emotional disturbances were more common in psychomotor epileptics than in persons with other chronic illnesses, was "not confirmed." However, the psychomotor group showed a greater proportion of psychotic subjects than the other two groups and a very high incidence of "impotence and frigidity" (17 of 31 cases versus 8 of 24 in the grand-mal group and 9 of 26 in the medical illness group). Statistically significant differences between the combined epileptic group and the medical illness group concerned the former's maladaptation in the areas of sex, in relationships with parents, siblings, and boss; these differences were viewed as the results of superstition, fear, and prejudice to which the epileptic is exposed.

epileptics.* With little basis in facts,[20] she denied that temporal lobe epilepsy specifically predisposed to psychosis *or* personality disorders.

Small and co-workers[59-61] failed to document a difference in emotional disturbances between psychomotor and non-psychomotor epileptics. They found a very high frequency of emotional disturbances in both temporal lobe and nonfocal epilepsy. In only 18% of the epileptic outpatients no outstanding psychopathology was found! Epileptics and matched nonepileptic psychiatric patients, however, were found to have "different kinds of mental disorders" (that is, a much higher incidence of chronic brain syndromes, mental deficiency and "undiagnosed psychiatric illnesses" in the former; more functional psychoses, psychoneurotic reactions, and alcoholism in the latter).

From the studies reviewed, one would have to conclude that most patients with epilepsy were prone to mental disturbances. Was the method of inquiry inadequate? In order to establish what relationship if any exists between psychopathology and various forms of epilepsy, careful multidisciplinary and longitudinal (historical) studies must be carried out. While some of the psychiatric changes in epilepsy are stable (for example, hyposexuality and "viscosity"), others are episodic (for example, mood changes and irritability). Repeat observations must be combined with careful data gathering from next of kin. A relationship of trust results in more valid information and facilitates exploration of intimate spheres, such as sexuality. The investigator must have a broad psychiatric experience plus a familiarity with behavior and personality changes characteristic of epileptics.

The failure of controlled investigations to document *any* specific psychiatric significance of temporal lobe epilepsy may be due not only to shortcomings in their method of psychiatric inquiry, but also to sample selection. Here the possibility of temporal lobe epileptic abnormalities in "generalized epilepsy" is of fundamental importance.

There is a fair agreement that focal epilepsies involving the neocortex ("Jacksonian" epilepsies) are rarely associated with significant mental changes. On the other hand, patients with generalized seizures and bilateral synchronous EEG discharges often show mental changes; in such cases, either a primary or a secondary involvement of the temporal lobes may be present ("secondary bilateral synchrony" or "secondary temporalization").

---

*Stevens reports a very high frequency of psychiatric hospitalizations in both psychomotor epileptics (17 of 54) and grand-mal epileptics (10 of 34); but only 1 of 12 patients with focal motor or sensory epilepsy had been briefly hospitalized. The author mentions in passing that an accurate history of onset of psychosis could be obtained in 18 patients: 10 of 13 temporal lobe epileptics decompensated during a relative remission from seizures that was often induced by drug therapy; by contrast, in four of the five grand-mal patients for whom a reliable history was obtained, the mental symptoms appeared during the postictal state or at a time of seizure exacerbation (see p. 191).

Niedermeyer[46] has clarified the definition of *common generalized epilepsy in its pure form** presenting with grand-mal, petit-mal, and rarely with myoclonic attacks *in the absence of brain damage*. The picture of common generalized epilepsy may be *imitated* not only by temporal lesions giving rise to secondary bilateral synchrony and generalized seizures, but also by frontal, hypothalamic, and mesencephalic lesions and by metabolic disturbances such as renal disease and hypoglycemic conditions. Common generalized epilepsy in its pure form is a basically benign condition, but if its course is complicated by additional temporal lobe abnormalities (secondary temporalization) then seizures tend to become uncontrollable, and personality and behavior changes characteristic of primary temporal lobe epilepsy may develop.†

Since temporal lobe seizures tend to be poorly controlled, while common generalized epilepsy in its pure form tends to be well controlled, any attempts to match temporal lobe epileptics to patients with generalized seizures of equal severity are likely to result in the control group containing many "impure" generalized epileptics with primary or secondary temporal lobe involvement and consequently a high incidence of mental disorders. This appears to be true of the "well-controlled" series reviewed above. Gastaut's psychiatric and psychologic studies of psychomotor epileptics,[14-16] while not well controlled, carefully excluded patients with any organic cerebral involvement and/or secondary generalization from the contrast group designated "generalized epileptics." He noted that important interictal behavior and personality changes were characteristic for the group of psychomotor epileptics with discharging lesions of the temporal–limbic system, and he noted that very opposite behavioral changes were characteristic for destructive lesions, i.e.: the classic temporal lobe ablation studies on animals (Klüver–Bucy syndrome).[3] Gastaut's findings are more convincing, since they can be reconciled with the psychopathology described as characteristic for epileptics by many psychiatrists (see Chapter 9). Indeed, a majority of institutionalized epileptics are patients with temporal lobe seizure disorders.[37,52,53]

The hypothesis that temporal lobe seizure disorders are essential for the

---

*Niedermeyer outlines the following criteria for this form of epilepsy: (1)strictly generalized or bilateral synchronous seizure discharges, predominantly consisting of 3 to 4/second spike-wave complexes and multiple spikes; (2) no significant admixture of focal EEG abnormalities; (3) absence of neurologic deficits and neuroradiologic abnormalities; (4) no evidence of focal or lateralized epileptic seizures; and (5) no evidence of previous brain damage.

†The high incidence of Ammon's horn sclerosis among intramural epileptics has been stressed since 1825[17]; it may be a primary etiologic lesion in epilepsy but also may represent a secondary lesion, resulting from grand-mal-induced hypoxic changes. Niedermeyer believes that electrophysiologic abnormalities within the limbic "low-threshold areas" of amygdala and hippocampus may represent a "pick-up" of abnormal activity from remote sources of seizure activity, and that it may be often not necessary to invoke a sequence of neuropathologic events in order to explain the development of secondary temporalization.[46]

gradual development of the psychopathology characteristic for epileptics remains plausible. It has to be recognized, however, that anterior temporal lobe foci of similar appearance may have somewhat variable effects on behavior and personality. Apart from considerations related to the individual premorbid personality, factors such as age of onset and duration of illness, sex and age of the patient, laterality of lesion, its precise location, the preferential spread of epileptic discharge, and other still unidentified variables may play a role. In addition, the modifying role of more or less extensive brain damage beyond the medial temporal structures needs to be considered.

Our knowledge of the psychopathology of temporal lobe epilepsy has been advanced by the study of patients who were investigated prior to temporal lobectomy and for several years thereafter by teams of investigators. Broader longitudinal neuropsychiatric studies with full awareness of the potential complexities are required. Epileptic populations need to be matched at the *onset* of their illness and each individual's course needs to be charted and compared. The disadvantage of reliance on second-hand information can be minimized by careful scrutiny of all sources available. In order to avoid the bias of selective samples, a controlled epidemiologic approach is required.

Various types of epilepsy may transform into temporal lobe epilepsy. Apart from the infantile epileptic encephalopathy (West syndrome) and the childhood epileptic encephalopathy (Lennox–Gastaut syndrome),[8,19,46] which both entail deterioration of intellect, temporal lobe epilepsy is the most malignant form of epilepsy because of its chronicity and high risk of mental changes. This chapter deals primarily with the neuropsychiatric problems of temporal lobe epilepsy and refers briefly to those in other forms of epilepsy.

THE PSYCHOLOGIC IMPACT OF SEIZURES

The psychologic effects of recurrent seizures on the patient vary greatly with the type of seizure, personality of the patient, and with the reaction of the environment. These effects are usually understandable in a given case, and little can be said of general significance. It is not suggested, however, that the psychologic effects of episodic sudden loss of control should be underestimated.

In spite of broadening public understanding, the tendency to conceal one's attacks from the eyes of others is almost instinctive and has changed little since the time of the Hippocratic writings. Indifference in this respect may be feigned, or in some cases may indicate presence of hysterical seizures.

Two of our adult patients with temporal lobe epilepsy made serious suicidal attempts at the time their previously minor seizures became a public embarrassment. Hyposexuality and estrangement from his wife was a contributing factor in one of the two patients.

We know of a patient who since onset of his epilepsy had refused to leave his house; this reaction is highly idiosyncratic, since his attacks consist of mild and totally unobtrusive twitching in one hand. More understandable is the fact that the peculiar nature of certain temporal lobe seizures may lead patients to conceal them for fear they would be judged insane (see Case 1).

With habitual seizures, on the other hand, secondary gain may become invested in the attacks. Hysterical seizures are common among chronic epileptics, and neglect to take the anticonvulsant medication may be based on similar motivation.

The overt seizures are the chief target of therapy in epilepsy. But, in certain patients who become very difficult when their attacks are fully controlled, a need for tension-releasing seizures is evident and freedom from seizures may have to be sacrificed in the overriding interest of emotional well-being. Patients who are candidates for surgical removal of an epileptogenic focus and patients whose seizures are questionable in nature may require a period of observation in a hospital while off all anticonvulsants. Thus, the fear of the seizure, on the part of the patient, family members and physicians, may have to be tempered by broader considerations.

TEMPORAL LOBE EPILEPSY, TEMPORAL LOBE SEIZURES, AND THEIR RECOGNITION

Temporal lobe epilepsy is the most common form of focal epilepsy. Its prevalence has been reported in from 20 to 30 percent of all epileptics, with a higher percentage among the older than the younger. It may begin at any age, but the onset peaks in the second decade of life and around puberty or menarche.[32]

Birth trauma is a cause of temporal lobe epilepsy but has at times found exaggerated emphasis; prolonged infantile convulsions must be considered an important etiologic factor. CNS infections may be of significance during childhood in particular. Head injuries assume an important etiologic role beginning with late childhood years. Tumors and vascular disorders can be cited as important causes of temporal lobe epilepsy, the latter almost exclusively in advanced age. While brain damage to the temporal area plays an obvious role, an organic causal factor often cannot be established. The importance of heredity for temporal lobe epilepsy has been well documented by a number of investigators. The incidence of epilepsy increases from 0.4 to 0.5 percent in the average population to 2.6 percent among relatives of temporal lobe epileptics, to 5.4 percent among relatives of patients with combined grand-mal and petit-mal epilepsy.[32] In particular, heredity may favor the development of temporal lobe epilepsy by predisposing to convulsions in infancy.

The proportion of individuals with pure temporal lobe seizures to those with combined generalized seizures has been reported as 36 to 64 percent; in about one third of the cases temporal lobe seizures begin only after generalized seizures have occurred.[32]

The smaller number of patients with pure temporal lobe seizures may represent a diagnostic problem. The subjective and objective manifestations of a temporal lobe seizure tend to be pathognomonic and must be carefully documented by interviewing the patient and observers, or sometimes by direct observations. More or less elaborate EEG studies will confirm the clinical diagnosis in most instances; however, there are exceptional cases with persistently negative EEGs, and rarely the EEG has remained unremarkable even at the time of a clinical seizure. The diagnosis may still be made even in this latter group, if the descriptions by patient and observer are sufficiently characteristic (see Case 2).

Temporal lobe attacks are produced in a few patients without warning. They may remain unaware of their seizures unless told by others, or they may recognize a characteristic aftermath such as confusion, or may simply be aware of a memory lapse. The subjective experience of the seizure is referred to as aura or warning, but actually represents the very beginning of the attack and may be termed as the ''primictal'' event. The objective, observable events of the temporal lobe seizure, as a rule, follow the subjective events and are not recalled by the patients.

Among the *subjective events*, peculiar epigastric sensations are the most common; they may be described as rising sensations, at times rising up to the head whereupon consciousness is lost. Peculiar sensations in the region of the heart or in the head are reported, but occasionally almost the entire body may be involved. Well known are olfactory or gustatory hallucinations, described by the patients as very specific yet undefinable sensations of odor or taste (''uncinate fits''). Auditory or visual illusions or hallucinations may occur, or dizziness is reported. Illusions of memory in the form of déjà-vu (familiarity of the unfamiliar) or jamais-vu (unfamiliarity of the familiar), memory flashbacks, decreasing awareness, or changes in self-awareness represent peculiar paroxysmal psychic experiences that led to the introduction of the term ''dreamy state'' (Jackson) for such temporal lobe attacks. Dreamy states are often accompanied by psychic changes such as uncanny fear, or even despair; pleasurable, elated, or orgasmic feelings are less common. ''Forced thoughts'' that are unmistakably the same with each attack may occur, yet they often cannot be spelled out. Very often these seizure events occur in combination with each other.

Among the *objective events*, the arrest of ongoing activity may be noticed first. Awareness of the environment becomes impaired, the eyes may be widened, and there is often an expressionless stare. Highly characteristic are ''oral automatisms'' in the form of lipsmacking, licking, chewing, swallowing, choking, or vomiting. Various muscles may stiffen (tongue bites result not rarely from temporal lobe seizures), grimacing may appear, or there may be a loss of tonic reflexes. Speech utterances, dysphasic speech or speech arrest may occur. Autonomic changes may take place: pupillary dilatation (or more rarely constriction), pallor (or flushing), perioral cyanosis, salivation, sweating, tachycardia, hypertension, gastrointestinal motility changes, incontinence of urine (and rarely of feces), changes of respiratory rate or even apnea. Supple turning of eyes, head, trunk, or the entire body may be observed. Stereotyped repetitive motions occur, such as scratching, rubbing, stamping, or kicking about. More complex stereotyped behavior may occur during the attack in an occasional patient—perhaps in reaction to an experience that is never recalled—but what are commonly referred to as "psychomotor automatisms" are the not-so-stereotyped and more prolonged events of the postictal phase.

The *postictal phase* may be almost imperceptible in some patients but is usually more prolonged than the ictal phase. The patient is initially confused and relates to the environment in a gradually more organized fashion. He may become able to carry on a simple conversation and to appear coherent in his actions yet will be unable to recall the events of this latter part of the postictal phase (see Case 3).

Table 10-1 lists the characteristics of the ictal and postictal phases in temporal lobe epilepsy, and proposed subdivisions of both phases.[5,25,32]

While some of the cited seizure events are by themselves almost pathognomonic, the wealth of temporal lobe seizure phenomena is enormous. Individual seizures tend to be highly complex, and it would be difficult to find even two patients with precisely the same type of seizure. The clinical diagnosis of temporal lobe epilepsy can usually be made by consideration of the following facts:

1. In every given patient, the sequence of seizure events tends to be stereotyped, although it may not always run its full course and more than one pattern may occur.
2. The compulsory sequence of seizure events lasts for seconds to perhaps 1½ minutes,[1] then usually is followed by a gradually clearing confusional-amnestic postictal phase of 2–10 minutes' duration.[32] Temporal lobe seizure status exists but is very rare.
3. As with head injuries, there is a shrinking retrograde amnesia and a more prolonged permanent postical amnesia[5] (see below).
4. A peculiar undefinable nature is common to many subjective seizure events, which, however, are recognized as very specific and distinctly the same at each recurrence.
5. The seizures tend to occur in combination with characteristic interictal personality and behavioral changes (see below).

Table 10-1
Symptomatology of Temporal Lobe Seizures

ICTAL PHENOMENA

Stereotyped sequence of events: expressionless stare, passive experience, not related to environment. Duration seconds to 1½ minutes.

Primictal events (aura): Recalled
  "Dreamy state"; Déjà-vu, jamais-vu, illusions, hallucinations, mood changes, fear
  "Oral-digestive type": Visceral sensations, olfactory-gustatory sensations
  "Adverse type": Dizziness, crescendo sensations, auditory or visual hallucinations

Ictal events: Not recalled
  "Oral-digestive type": Oral—alimentary and respiratory automatisms
  "Adverse type": Supple turning of eyes, head or trunk
  "Speech utterances": Euphasic or dysphasic

Other phenomena: Repetitive motions, autonomic changes, tonic-atonic alterations

POSTICTAL PHENOMENA

Increasingly more variable and more complex events: looking about, more active, more related to environment; usually not recalled. Duration 2–10 minutes (0–60 minutes).

Simple repetitive motions
Scenic behavior
Attempts at reorientation

The following cases illustrate diagnostic problems in temporal lobe epilepsy.

CASE 1

A 52-year-old widowed housekeeper had suffered from episodes of loss of awareness over the past year and had then experienced a single major seizure that led to her hospitalization.

The patient reported some stereotyped and peculiar experiences. For the past 5 months, about once a week, the following would happen: She would feel a "breeze," like someone was brushing past her, then a very pleasant, smooth, silky feeling would come over her, from the head down to the toes and then would leave her. She claimed she did not lose awareness, would look around to see who may have brushed past her, and enjoyed the sensation. "If this is bad nerves," she said, "then it is still good to have!"

A relative who had witnessed about half a dozen of her spells described them as follows: She would suddenly, perhaps with a lull in the conversation, make a couple of utterances ("ok...hm"), would have her hands folded and rub them. After about 30 seconds, she would gradually come out of it, answering slowly at first, but unaware that something was wrong with her. On one occasion, she found herself in a different part of the building she worked in, without knowing how she got there, yet she denied having suffered a lapse of memory.

It was only after good rapport was established that she admitted the following: For the past 15 years she had heard her own first name called in a calm, even voice (she couldn't tell if it was the voice of a man or a woman) as often as two to three times per week. If this happened during the day she would look around. At first she was frightened because nobody would be there. At times the calling of her own name would wake her out of sleep. She had never told anybody about this weird experience, for fear of being judged insane.

An EEG showed sharp activity in the left frontal, anterior temporal area and some contralateral slowing. She was started on anticonvulsants and the attacks ceased.

CASE 2

A 28-year-old engineer had suffered from minor seizures for several years. Repeat EEGs were negative and even during an attack no electrical abnormality was apparent.

He described an aura consisting of an indescribable smell, experienced as he would breathe in, but perhaps also coming from the mouth like a taste. He compared the sensation to that of someone who eats Oriental food for the first time and is unable to give his experience a name. More recently, the olfactory or gustatory sensation was less prominent and he would merely "sense" that he was going to have an attack, a sensation like drifting out of touch. He denied ever having lost awareness or being aware of a memory lapse. His wife reported the following stereotyped observable seizure events of which the patient himself was not aware: he would stare, sigh, the eyes would water slightly and he would swallow. If he talked, his speech would be slurred.

The wife reported that following the onset of the seizures he gradually became more impatient and, in the course of two angry outbursts, he had struck blows, once at the icebox and the other time at her. She still described him as a generally quiet and easygoing person. The patient himself was evasive when asked about increased irritability. He readily admitted a marked decrease of his sexual arousal over the past couple of years from daily to once every 2 or 3 weeks. He also stated he had become more "gabby." During the interview, he was slow, meticulous, and circumstantial in his speech.

The clinical findings were considered characteristic of temporal lobe epilepsy, both the attacks and the gradually developing behavioral and personality changes. The patient kept working, but the seizures increased in frequency to several per day, and all anticonvulsants including Tegretol proved totally ineffective. It was therefore decided (in spite of negative EEG, brain scan, and angiography) to investigate with depth electrodes and pneumoencephalography in the hope of demonstrating a surgically treatable lesion. He was found to suffer from a right temporal astrocytoma.

MEMORY DISORDERS IN TEMPORAL LOBE EPILEPSY

Transient Memory Disorders: The Problem of the Amnesias

The memory disorders associated with traumatic head injuries—or with other acute transient brain disease involving the temporal–limbic structures —have been well studied, and it is recognized that they follow a distinct pattern.[63,65,70] There is, of course, no memory for the period of unconsciousness caused by the cerebral insult; after consciousness is regained, a period of *anterograde (posttraumatic) amnesia* usually extends beyond the time when confusion has cleared and alert and rational intellect and behavior are reestablished; a period of *retrograde amnesia* gradually shrinks, but a portion (pertaining to the most recent events preceding the trauma) usually remains permanent, and is shorter than the posttraumatic amnesia; finally, as long as some damage persists, there may be a "partial posttraumatic amnesia," which more correctly is referred to as a posttraumatic *impairment of recent memory*. The organic amnesias are not sharply demarcated, and the marking of onset of retrograde anmesia as well as of termination of posttraumatic amnesia tends to be more or less arbitrary. By its general pattern, organic amnesia is easily distinguished from functional amnesia.

The memory disorders associated with ECT, or with spontaneous seizures, are comparable to those associated with trauma to the brain. In both, the damage to the temporal–limbic area is of paramount importance. A significant memory impairment is observed if the mesial temporal lobe structures are bilaterally involved.

As already stated, the recalled subjective experience of a temporal lobe seizure (aura, warning, or primictal event) is followed by observable events for which there is usually no recall *(ictal amnesia)*. In a few patients, the seizure is only experienced as a memory lapse, a forgetting of what was just talked about.

Most patients following a temporal lobe attack are unable to resume the thread of the preceding conversation and often express puzzlement over how they got to the place they find themselves in. This confusion tends to clear gradually, as the *retrograde amnesia* shrinks. An occasional patient may report a persistent gap in his memory pertaining to a period preceding the seizures, during which orderly activity took place. Such activity was indeed normal, and perhaps so routine in nature that there was "no interest" in registration of its memory, resulting in an inflated retrograde amnesia. This cannot be termed an automatism just because there is no memory for it.

Analogous to posttraumatic amnesia, *postictal amnesia* often extends beyond the period of confused behavior, and may cover a period of fairly organized and rational behavior. Again, use of the term automatism is best avoided, unless one would redefine automatism as an event for which there is no recall. The postictal phase, then, consists of a period of confusional automatism followed by a more orderly phase of "postictal pseudoautomatism," for which there is no recall. The postictal phase tends to be more prolonged with more severe seizures and is particularly prominent in patients with bitemporal foci.

CASE 3

A 26-year-old single male with bilateral temporal lobe seizure foci suffered a minor seizure while being seen by his physician. When his actions and speech became orderly, he was advised to increase his anticonvulsant medication and acknowledged the new instructions. The patient and his family then departed on a vacation at the seaside, where the patient, on two occasions, almost drowned when he suffered seizures while swimming. His mother, who had been present in the doctor's office, then questioned if he was taking the higher dose of medication. She was amazed to find that the patient had no recollection of the doctor's instructions. In the postictal phase, no registration had taken place.

Jackson[29] reported the self-description of Z., a physician who suffered from temporal lobe epilepsy from age 20 until his apparent suicide at age 43. From age 36 on, Z's dreamy state, consisting chiefly of a feeling of remembrance (déjà-vu), was followed at times by prolonged periods of "automatic behavior without consciousness." Z. describes how he experienced a minor seizure while one of his patients, brought in for pulmonary symptoms, undressed for a physical examination. "I remember taking out my stethoscope and turning away a little to avoid conversation. The next thing I recollect is that I was sitting at a writing table in the same room, speaking to another person, and as my consciousness became more complete, recollected my patient, but saw he was not in the room." Later he found the patient in bed and the diagnosis which he, the doctor had written ("pneumonia of the left base") was found to be correct on reexamination. This is the most famous documentation of well-organized "postictal pseudoautomatism."

Prolonged "fugue states" with orderly behavior and amnesia are almost invariably nonorganic in nature. But the epileptic origin of such a state cannot always be excluded. Gastaut[18] has documented temporal lobe seizure status electrographically (consecutive independent discharges separated by 5- to 10-minute intervals) in a female patient who was completely conscious, answering questions and performing complicated orders, yet who was found to be amnesic for all questions and orders. This same patient had experienced a "fugue" lasting 30 days without errors of conduct but with complete amnesia. No further details are reported in this case.

In hysterical amnesia, the forgotten events tend to be painful, producing shame, sorrow, despair, guilt, or panic; they are inaccessible to voluntary recall yet may influence the individual's conscious thoughts or behavior or may appear in dreams; attempts to remove the amnesia are resisted (with anxiety or mutism, by changing of topic or abrupt leaving).[44] There may be a "hypermnesia" for the beginning and for the endpoint of the amnestic period, like the hyperemic zone around an area of necrosis.

CASE 4

A 22-year-old single Catholic woman found herself pregnant, yet was adamant in her statement that she had not had any sexual intercourse since she broke off with her fiancé a couple of years previously. When informed about her pregnancy, she remembered that around the time when conception probably occurred she had attended a party and was unable to account for what had happened during a quarter hour interval when she retired to a room with a young man. A few months later she recalled now very distinctly how she left for the upstairs room with the young man when the 11 o'clock TV news began and how he began to tell her about his stay in California when they were alone; next, she recalled very distinctly again, that they returned to the downstairs area when the weather report was in progress. Even when it was obvious what must have happened during the period of amnesia, the young lady of high moral standards was unable to recall the critical event.

Apart from such instances of simple amnesia, the phenomena of alternating amnesia or multiple personalities have been described as types of more complex functional or hysterical amnesia. Two or more states of consciousness alternate with one another, during each of which there is no memory of events that occurred in the other or to the other identity. It is clear that in brain disease the sense of one's own identity is lost totally only with advanced states of dementia. Patients recuperating from seizures will often be temporarily disoriented about place; even more prominent will be their loss of orientation in time; they may be unable to identify persons they had just met, but they will not be confused about their own identity. Individuals who complain about a loss of awareness of their former identity will show no signs of organicity. In my experience, these are patients with conflicting asocial trends who, at a time of severe stress, assume a delusional role-playing, thus perhaps rescuing themselves from suicide.

Finally, an interesting clinical syndrome has been described by Fisher and Adams[13] as *transient global amnesia*. It consists of the abrupt onset of disorientation due principally to a loss of recent memory, with retention of a remarkable degree of alertness and responsiveness. An episode usually lasts for a few hours, full recovery takes place, and often there is no recurrence. It is observed in middle-aged or elderly individuals. This age preference, the presence of a shrinking retrograde amnesia, and persistent inability to recall the events of the episode (and presumably some of its aftermath) suggests that one has to deal with an organic amnesia. The etiology remains obscure, although both an unusual type of temporal lobe seizure and a transient ischemia of the hippocampal–fornical–hypothalamic system have been implicated. Such isolated episodes require careful differential diagnostic considerations of the characteristics of both the organic and the functional amnesias.

It should be noted that emotional factors may play a role in organic amnesias, accounting for excessive and atypical loss of memory.

Permanent Memory Disorders

Relatives of a temporal lobe epileptic may state that he has a poor memory but may in fact refer to memory deficits at the time of his seizures, or perhaps to a period of time when seizures occurred frequently with consequent memory impairment. The latter phenomenon may be duplicated by closely spaced ECT.

A truly chronic memory impairment is difficult to document in temporal lobe epileptics. Patients may complain of a poor memory yet may be able to carry on their daily activities without difficulties and, on psychologic testing, show no significant memory impairment. It is possible that chronic subclinical seizure activity in both temporal lobes may interfere with memorizing, and that more sophisticated testing of memory functions (for example, under various distracting conditions) may document mild deficits.

The presence of subtle laterality–specific memory impairments can be documented in temporal lobe epileptics with unilateral focus. A dominant temporal lobe epileptogenic focus is associated with a very mild impairment of verbal learning,[38,69] while a similar nondominant lesion results in a very mild deficit of memory for nonverbal-patterned stimuli (tunes, faces, nonsense drawings).[33,41] These deficits have been demonstrated when matched groups of left versus right temporal lobe patients were compared. They are enhanced following unilateral temporal lobectomy. Verbal learning tasks may differentiate not merely groups but individuals who underwent a left temporal lobectomy from individuals with right temporal lobectomy.[5] Tests sensitive to right temporal damage are less powerful, perhaps because of the fact that even with use of nonsensical figures a verbal coding of the pictures cannot be totally prevented.

Occasionally, a patient will show a severe global impairment of memorizing after unilateral temporal lobectomy. These are usually patients who had surgery on the dominant side. While it has been shown that contralateral temporal lobe damage has been present in these cases,[40] the possibility of a highly dominant role for memory of one temporal lobe in an exceptional case cannot be totally excluded. Preoperative intracarotid sodium amytal injection (anesthetizing one hemisphere and thus simulating the absence of the temporal lobe structures on one side) followed by testing for memory may alert the neurosurgeon to the possibility of global amnesia after unilateral temporal lobe resection.[39]

Some cases of bilateral ablation of mesial temporal structures, performed before its damaging effect on memory was established, have been extensively studied.[42] They show no impairment of attention and no loss of preoperatively acquired skills or of intelligence as measured by standard tests. They can recall events from the remote past, and immediate recall is excellent (as measured, for instance, by the digit span task), but as soon as their attention is diverted to a new topic they no longer remember what went on before. They show a continuous ''anterograde amnesia,'' together with some permanent retrograde amnesia for the period immediately preceding the bilateral temporal lobe procedure. However, the loss is not absolute; the acquisition of motor skills, for instance, is relatively unaffected.

The individual permanently deprived of mesial temporal structures appears to show a memory impairment analogous to that of the patient who just experienced a seizure affecting both temporal lobes.

BEHAVIOR, PERSONALITY AND PSYCHOSIS IN TEMPORAL LOBE EPILEPSY

Chapters 9 and 11 deal with the important behavioral and personality changes in temporal lobe epilepsy (except for the psychoses) and include illustrative cases. The present section will sketch the psychopathology of temporal lobe seizure activity. It is emphasized that an understanding of the previously discussed "neurologic" aspects of temporal lobe epilepsy is indispensable for a proper understanding of the "psychiatric" aspects.

Psychiatric changes rarely precede the onset of overt seizures. There is age specificity to the sequence of some events: In childhood temporal lobe epilepsy, episodic rages and hyperkinesis may occur concomitant with the first seizures; past the third or fourth decade of life, hyposexuality may develop early or may even precede the onset of clinical seizures. In general, the behavioral and personality changes become manifest about 2 years following onset of the epilepsy, but there may be a more prolonged latency period. Epileptic (schizophrenia-like) psychoses occur at various stages, but on the average follow the onset of seizures by more than a decade. While hyperkinesis is limited to prepubertal age, the "viscosity" develops only after puberty.[8] Episodic rages are of decreasing incidence with advancing age, while depressive mood changes become increasingly prominent.[56]

There is an intimate association between episodic memory disorders and the seizures. Among the behavioral changes in temporal lobe epilepsy, sexual arousal and response is most closely related to presence or absence of seizure activity, while the personality changes of viscosity and deepening of emotional response, once they are established, tend to be fixed and show little or no fluctuation with variation of seizure activity. Episodic irritable and violent behavior shows a somewhat complex relationship to seizures and seizure activity. Dysphoric episodes and the epileptic schizophrenia-like psychoses tend to occur with lessening of seizure activity and may clear when seizures reoccur.

The wealth of psychopathologic changes in temporal lobe epilepsy is indeed remarkable. Beyond those already referred to, one may observe practically any of the so-called functional psychiatric symptoms among temporal lobe epileptics. This has led some observers to question the very existence of a psychopathology typical for epileptics. It appears necessary to differentiate between *primary mental changes, which are either unique for epileptics or can be shown to be closely related to presence or absence of seizure activity,* and secondary mental changes that occur less regularly and may be viewed as evidence for a vulnerability of individuals with temporal lobe lesions to a broad range of mental changes.

Primary Mental Changes

SEXUAL CHANGES

The most consistent behavioral change following onset of temporal lobe seizures is a *global hyposexuality* affecting both libidinal and genital arousal. While this change occurs in a private sphere of life and has remained almost unnoticed, several recent investigations[4,26,49,66] have confirmed the original finding by Gastaut and Collomb.[15] Patients with onset of temporal lobe epilepsy prior to or at the time of sexual maturation develop the secondary sex characteristics and display no endocrine abnormality but experience little or no sexual arousal and response. They do not complain and often remain single. With later onset of temporal lobe epilepsy, the subsequent loss of sexual arousal may prompt complaints, but the condition is identical to the (primary) global hyposexuality of early-onset temporal lobe epilepsy and should not be termed impotence. Male and female patients are equally affected.

The close relationship between sexual arousal and medial temporal seizure activity is well documented by the *normalization of sexual arousal and response* observed if the seizure discharges are abolished by either anticonvulsant medication[49] or surgical intervention.[4] Some patients who previously had been markedly hyposexual became hypersexual after surgery with onset in the second postoperative month and hyposexual again upon recurrence of the seizures.[7]

In the confusional–amnestic postictal period, temporal lobe epileptics may undress themselves, and on occasion such patients have been charged with exhibitionism.[28] More specifically, some temporal lobe epileptics consistently experience *sexual arousal in the postictal period,*[7] at a time when seizure discharges have cleared. Such arousal rarely occurs during the confusional-amnestic phase, but if so it may lead to inappropriate action; more often it takes place minutes later and is clearly remembered by the patient. Postictal sexual arousal is probably not rare, but is usually not reported.

Chronic temporal lobe seizure activity tends to inhibit sexual arousal. Nonetheless, there is clear evidence of a sexual–excitatory effect of temporal lobe seizure discharges. A few patients experience a sexual climax combined with other temporal lobe seizure events, as their customary seizure pattern.[2]

Such *sexual seizures* occur in both sexes and, as is typical for ictal events, they run their stereotyped course without regard for the environment. However, they are often triggered by sexually arousing stimuli. Similarly, the experience of sexual climax may lead, in an occasional patient who is free from spontaneous attacks, to a spreading seizure discharge with clinical (partial or generalized) seizure.[27]

Deviant sexual behavior has been noted in some temporal lobe epileptics.[6] A causal relationship is indicated, if the paraphilia occurs: (1) in association with hyposexuality (as transvestism, fetishism, homosexuality) and clears as the seizures are abolished; (2) in the course of and limited to the postoperative hypersexuality (as homosexual behavior); and (3) if the necessary trigger of a sexual seizure acquires the quality of a fetish.[43]

The *treatment* of the sexual changes is strictly directed toward control of the seizure activity. Anticonvulsants have been unjustly blamed for the sexual insufficiency of epileptics; to the contrary, the drugs may have an ''aphrodisiac effect'' if they eliminate the seizure activity. Hypersexuality following surgery for epilepsy may require hospitalization, treatment with antiandrogens[9] in the male and with tranquilizers or discontinuation of anticonvulsants in the female.

IMPULSIVE-IRRITABLE BEHAVIOR: THE PROBLEM OF VIOLENCE

Impulsive–irritable behavior in the form of outbursts of angry, verbally, or even physically abusive behavior develops gradually in many temporal lobe epileptics. While the excessive angry arousal of temporal lobe epileptics has been noted frequently, its relationship to seizure activity is not as close as that of the (usually diminished) sexual arousal. A seizure problem is often suspected when there is excessive violence, but it is a quite specific type of violent behavior—rather distinct from ''criminal violence'' and cold-blooded aggressiveness—that can be observed in temporal lobe epileptics.[3,47] The outbursts of violence tend to be limited to periods of increased penting up of anger, hatred and envy, lasting hours or days. They are not totally unprovoked, and can usually be avoided by a considerate, patient, and gentle approach. Unfortunately, this kind of approach is difficult to maintain, and irritability is the main reason for psychiatric hospitalization of the (nonretarded) epileptic.[37,52] Serious injury is uncommon during these outbursts; the patients are almost invariably remorseful for their behavior and the episodes of irritability usually alternate with more prolonged periods of very good-natured behavior. The families are hesitant about institutionalization and may tolerate the difficult behavior for a long time. A suspicious and almost paranoid attitude toward certain people may be revealed but is not predominant.

The outbursts of violence occur on provocation, are directed toward the environment, lack stereotypy, are not associated with seizure phenomena, and are recalled (although amnesia may be alleged): thus they lack all the criteria of a temporal lobe seizure. While these outbursts have a paroxysmal quality and are often referred to as ''a fit,'' they are not known to occur as ictal events. The common episodic impulsive–irritable behavior is a *phenomenon of the interictal phase* and, in certain patients, may be *accentuated in the preictal phase,* as a prodrome to an attack.

Postictal rage behavior, on the other hand, is not common.[34] An occasional patient may react aggressively during the confusional–amnestic postictal phase, and on rare occasions this may reach forensic significance. Amnesia is not feigned and such a patient may be judged insane at the time.

Treatment: The initial therapeutic effort is directed at the control of the seizure activity which, if achieved, may also improve the interictal impulsive-irritable behavior. The control of the overt seizures by means of medication, however, frequently leads to a worsening of the behavior disorder in epilepsy, and to prolonged periods of heightened irritability. This is well known in children but also occurs in adults. It may be necessary to lower the dose of anticonvulsants and to sacrifice seizure freedom to improve behavior. Such a procedure must be carefully explained to the patient and those about him. A need for occasional seizures in the interest of emotional well-being is apparent in patients who display a protracted prodromal phase marked by increasing angry explosiveness terminated by seizure. Major seizures tend to have a more beneficial effect on behavior than minor seizures, as can be observed with ECT. Successful anterior temporal lobectomy (for intractable, chiefly unilateral seizure disorders) may sometimes improve this behavior dramatically and immediately following surgery; more often there will only be a gradual and moderate improvement of the heightened irritability following surgery.[31,55,67]

Prior to the lowering of the anticonvulsant medication, a trial with tranquilizing drugs may be undertaken. Phenothiazines are not contraindicated for epileptics and may be helpful in some violence-prone cases. Tegretol is an interesting anticonvulsant drug, effective in temporal lobe epilepsy and perhaps with a beneficial psychotropic effect.

As a patient begins to recover from a seizure, he should not be restrained; if restraint is necessary it must be gentle. During the postictal confusional state patients may react with violence. Patients who become dangerously aggressive without any provocation in the postictal phase are rare; hospitalization may be necessary in such cases.

GOOD-NATUREDNESS AND RELIGIOSITY

Sole emphasis on the angry–explosive nature of temporal lobe epileptics does injustice to most of them. Many are surprisingly free from any irritability and remain good-hearted and helpful to others; many more show these positive traits predominantly, with only occasional moodiness and angry outbursts.

Predominance of irritable phases is the exception rather than the rule. Many temporal lobe epileptics differ from normals chiefly by the display of opposite extremes of "good and bad," or of a "Jekyll and Hyde personality."[10,32,64]

Temporal lobe epileptics tend to be not only hyperethical, but often hyperreligious. To them, their own ministers may lack deep religious conviction, and religious conversions are not rare among epileptics.[12]

Their mood may change dramatically, if their heightened sense of justice or religious conviction seems to be challenged. More common is a subtle alteration of moods unprovoked by external events. Just as a highly irritable phase may precede an overt seizure, the highly good-natured phase may follow the discharge.

CASE 5

A 40-year-old male had suffered from temporal lobe seizures since puberty. When he finally married, he showed no sexual interest, but became increasingly religious, and every few weeks he suffered periods of marked moodiness lasting several days. As gentle, friendly, and deferent as he usually was, he could be sarcastic, hostile, and arrogant during his bad days. The following incident led to his first psychiatric hospitalization: He had spent a weekend in the country in the company of his wife and stepson, listening all day to a radio station that continuously transmitted religious sermons. On the way home, he debated with his wife, arguing that she was not saved, while his soul was saved. When his stepson asked him how this was possible, he slapped both the youngster and his wife, shouting: "For a nickel, I will kill you both!" His angry outbursts, although limited to verbal threats and hostile glares, were always frightening, but within days he would revert, without explicit apologies, to his usual self.

No treatment efforts should be directed toward the extreme good-natured behavior, which is clearly preferable to the alternative. If temporal lobe patients are approached with patience and consideration, they will almost invariably respond with their good-natured self and will be very cooperative.

DEEPENING OF EMOTIONAL RESPONSE AND
VISCOSITY: "THE EPILEPTIC PERSONALITY"

The traits of the characteristic "epileptic personality" have been discussed in Chapter 9. The tendency to anger and rage (irritability) and to make up for it (good-naturedness) fluctuate somewhat with the seizure disorder but represent the basic ingredients of a remarkably fixed personality make-up in many epileptics with temporal lobe involvement. These basic traits account for a deepening of emotional response[20] with overemphasis on the qualities of good and evil, right and wrong. Nothing is trivial, every detail must be considered from all angles and weighed carefully. Humor is absent. All of this leads to a slow, pedantic, circumstantial, almost perseverative and verbose manner of speech. The petty details of daily life assume such importance that detailed written records full of trivialities may be kept. These writings also include less mundane topics (that is, religion), are overemphatic, circumstantial and verbose, constituting the characteristic hypergraphia of temporal lobe epilepsy.[68]

The formal aspects of this personality make-up have been variously referred to as the viscous, enechetic, glischroid, ictothymic (and so forth) personality type characteristic of epileptics and cannot be equated with "organicity" of unspecified etiology. This personality type is more or less pronounced in many temporal lobe epileptics of some severity and duration of disease. It is less well known that there may be a rather different type of personality change present in patients with generalized seizures without brain damage. Gastaut et al.[14] described them as quick, hyperactive, and emotionally labile; Janz[32] similarly outlined a rash, suggestible, excitable and emotionally labile personality type as characteristic of this group.

EPISODIC MOOD CHANGES AND EPILEPTIC (SCHIZOPHRENIA-LIKE) PSYCHOSES: THE PROBLEM OF ALTERNATING MENTAL CHANGES

The observation that epileptics, after years of seizure disorder, may develop chronic paranoid psychoses was made in the latter part of the 19th century by French and German psychiatrists.[11] More recently, Slater and co-workers[57] have shown that a schizophrenia-like psychosis may become manifest chiefly in temporal lobe epileptics whose seizure disorder has lasted, on the average, for over a decade. Any of the symptoms of schizophrenia may be present in such patients, with predominance of paranoid traits, at times with catatonic phenomena, and not rarely with religious delusions.[22] Yet they are able to maintain a good rapport and warmth of affect—they are schizophrenic without being "schizoid." Also, they do not tend to deteriorate as may be expected in long-standing schizophrenics, but they show more signs of an organic cerebral impairment, while the schizophrenia-like state may become less prominent. These states are generally considered as symptomatic schizophrenic psychoses in epilepsy and may be referred to simply as *epileptic psychoses*. They have received much interest recently but are much less common than any of the previously discussed mental changes in temporal lobe epilepsy.

Experienced observers have noted that the epileptic psychoses tend to occur in individuals who had developed epileptic personality and behavior changes. The psychotic patients continue to show traits such as irritability, hyposexuality, religiosity, circumstantiality, and pedantry.[32,58]

The epileptic psychoses, furthermore, cannot be considered in isolation from the *episodic mood changes* (epileptic dysphoric episodes) that are common in temporal lobe epileptics. The most prevalent mood change is the already noted episodic irritability. However, mood fluctuations of the depressed or, more rarely, of the elated type, or of a combined type, with sudden onset and lasting for hours or days, are also observed frequently. They are often marked by paranoid ideation. These mood changes may occur in the interictal period, often preictally, resolved by a seizure. They are characterized by a fairly sudden onset.

Glaus,[23] in 1931, reviewed over 6000 psychiatric cases for the combined occurrence of schizophrenia and epilepsy and drew the following conclusions: (1) true combinations of schizophrenia and epilepsy were rarer than expected; and (2) most frequently the schizophrenic picture developed with lessening or arrest of seizures—the two conditions tended to occur in alternation and, in particular, no worsening effect was noted of one on the other. Landolt[35] then documented by frequent serial EEG examinations that both the schizophrenia-like disorders and the episodic mood changes in epileptics tended to occur at a time of lessening or normalization of the electrographic seizure discharges. He referred to this phenomenon as *"forced normalization,"* occurring spontaneously or on suppression of seizure activity by anticonvulsants. He regarded this EEG normalization as an excessive reaction of the normal cerebral tissue to a circumscribed pathophysiologic cerebral condition at the expense of the mental condition, and therefore giving a forced impression. Before Landolt, Gibbs had reached the conclusion that "the epileptic and psychiatric components of psychomotor epilepsy are physiologically antithetic."[21]

The epileptic psychoses can be described as alternating psychoses—that is, alternating with epileptic abnormalities—and they often terminate with an overt seizure. They can be clearly differentiated from three other types of psychoses occurring in epilepsy:

1. *Postictal psychoses of generalized seizures:* Confusional or delirious states, lasting hours to a day or more, may follow generalized seizures and are marked by diffuse slow activity of the EEG.[35,36] If there has been a flurry of seizures, the psychosis may persist for many days up to a few weeks. There may be a lucid interval or a mildly obtunded state of one or two days' duration following the seizures and preceding the florid psychosis.[48]
2. *Petit-mal status:* Stuporous episodes lasting often for hours may be diagnosed by the characteristic spike and wave EEG pattern and have been called "spike–wave stupor."[45] The severity of the stupor may fluctuate.
3. *Toxic psychoses:* States associated with nonepileptic impairments, such as overdosage of anticonvulsant medication producing marked diffuse slowing of the EEG, and other reversible conditions of a dementialike nature, often of an obscure etiology.[35]

The older literature is rich in references to the postparoxysmal or post-epileptic mania or twilight states (postictal psychoses).* With effective anti-convulsant therapy, the postictal psychoses have become so much rarer, that even experienced neurologists hesitate to make this diagnosis, while psychiatrists tend to diagnose them as schizophrenia. The schizophrenia-like psychoses, on the other hand, have recently become a well-recognized if little understood entity. They do occur spontaneously, but more often manifest themselves when anticonvulsants are normalizing the seizure activity. Historically, the introduction of phenobarbital as an anticonvulsant was opposed by many clinicians well into the 1920s because it often produced marked mental changes.[35] While Glaus,[23] in 1931, reported the coincidence of schizophrenia and epilepsy in the same patient as rarer than expected, Slater et al.[57], in 1963, could state that the coincidence was much greater than expected. It is probable that the modern schizophrenia-like epileptic psychoses are largely iatrogenic in nature, caused by modern ability to control seizures.

Treatment: It is apparent that in temporal lobe epilepsy the seizures may represent a very minor problem compared to the mental disorder. Moreover, seizures may be needed to restore better mental health. Controlled seizures by ECT[58] may be preferable if a patient risks injury to himself by his spontaneous attacks. Otherwise, the most effective therapy consists of lowering the anticonvulsant level. Once an epileptic psychosis has lasted for some time, it may become irreversible; therefore, it may be preferable to stop anticonvulsants early in the course as the risk of harm by seizures may be the much lesser evil.[32] For episodic mood changes that become difficult, a simple lowering of anticonvulsants may suffice. The understanding and cooperation of the patient and family must be secured for such an unorthodox therapeutic approach.

Psychotropic medication may generally be given as needed without fear of its epileptogenic effects. The antagonism between seizure and psychosis appears reflected in the fact that anticonvulsants may cause psychosis in epileptics, while antipsychotic drugs (the phenothiazines in particular) may promote seizures.

CASE 6

A 40-year-old single male had suffered an hours-long convulsion at age 2½ when he had pneumonia and began to suffer from frequent minor seizures at age 11. They were initially labeled "dizzy spells," then were described as "funny attacks of lack of memory," or as brief "sensations of butterflies (or a funny feeling) in the stomach" followed by loss of consciousness of about 2 minutes' duration without falling. He also

---

*Jackson[30] listed the ways in which mental disorder is related to epilepsy as follows: "There is not only (1) the sudden and transient mental disorder after one or a few fits, but also (2) more lengthy infirmity after a rapid succession of numerous fits, and again (3) the persistent deterioration (imbecility), the results of fits repeated for months or years."

described attacks experienced as a feeling of anxiety with fluttering in his throat, or as a feeling as if he was in a very familiar place, without loss of consciousness. He often experienced a strong feeling of fear at the time of an attack. Attacks would occur up to four times daily, then none for a few days or a few weeks. From age 15 on, he suffered rare generalized convulsions. Some attacks were followed by loss of memory lasting 30–40 minutes.

He was described as easy-going and good-hearted and did well in school in spite of his attacks, completing four years of college. Subsequently, he began to suffer from frequent episodes marked by suspiciousness, paranoid feelings, and outbursts of anger. He worked as a clerk or an attendant in health clubs, and lost about a dozen jobs–sometimes because of his epilepsy, but more often because of his outbursts of temper. On several occasions, he became physically aggressive but then would be very good-natured again. From age 28 on, he was admitted to psychiatric hospitals on several occasions, for stays of a few weeks' duration. For instance, when walking through a park he felt some women were talking about him; he yelled at them, then went to his boss and behaved in an abusive, aggressive manner and had to be hospitalized. Later, he was more often depressed, and made some abortive suicidal attempts. At age 40, he slashed his throat seriously when he felt depressed and paranoid and had been unable to go to sleep for several days.

He kept very active in athletics. There had been only one girl he had cared for and whom he had dated for 6 years in his 20s, but never dated again. He lived with his mother. He had been very religious, but became disenchanted when a minister in whom he had great faith walked out on his congregation.

When it became apparent that his episodes of marked mental disturbance occurred at times of freedom from seizures, he was treated with fewer anticonvulsants and did much better. The addition of Mellaril helped him by regulating his sleep and by further decreasing his suspiciousness. He remained childlike, friendly, somewhat vague in his talk and outlook, at times sarcastic and contrary, easily discouraged, self-derogatory, and anxious.

The EEG showed bitemporal sharp wave activity. He had been variously diagnosed as "chronic brain syndrome associated with epilepsy and psychotic reaction" or "schizophrenia with recurrent decompensation" or "undiagnosed psychiatric disorder with recurrent episodes of decompensation manifested by acute anxiety, depression, and hostile behavior." More accurately, he suffered from epileptic dysphoric episodes with paranoid state so marked that the diagnosis of schizophrenia-like psychosis alternating with the epilepsy may be equally appropriate.

Secondary Mental Changes

Almost any of the well-known functional psychiatric symptoms may occur in temporal lobe epilepsy. Hysteria, depression, hypochondria, hypomania, paranoia and other symptoms should be listed as secondary mental changes, unless there is a marked episodicity with noticeable relationship to presence or absence of seizure activity. Phobic and obsessive–compulsive symptoms are rare.

Hypochondriacal complaints are probably related to the frequent depressive mood of temporal lobe epileptics. Hysterical seizures may occur in any form of epilepsy and can usually be differentiated from epileptic seizures—and almost invariably from temporal lobe seizures—by the experienced observer. In their presence, the existence of a true epileptic disorder is easily overlooked, and it has to be emphasized that a great majority of patients with hysterical seizures also suffer from true epileptic seizures.

CONCLUSION

In temporal lobe epilepsy, we can detect an impressive series of psychiatric correlates to seizure activity, its aftermath, its elimination, and its suppression. The picture presented has been based on personal clinical experience and references from the literature; an approach to therapy has been offered. Additional neuropsychiatric studies are needed to confirm, to differentiate further, or to correct the present conclusions.

Temporal lobe epileptics tend to be difficult patients for conventional psychotherapy once they develop a significant degree of deepening of emotional response or "viscosity." They are often inflexible and do not easily change their point of view. But usually they become cooperative and are most appreciative of a relationship of trust with a physician.

The general rule still applies for the psychiatrist: Treat a patient who has seizures as you would any other patient. Awareness is needed, however, of the specific considerations discussed in this chapter which may apply in a given patient.

REFERENCES

1. Ajmone-Marsan C, Ralston BR: The epileptic seizure. Its functional morphology and diagnostic significance. Springfield, Ill, Thomas, 1957
2. Bancaud J, Favel P, Bonis A, Bordas-Ferrer M, Miravet J, Talairach J: Manifestations sexuelles paroxystiques et épilepsie temporale. Rev Neurol 123:217–230, 1970
3. Blumer D: The temporal lobes and paroxysmal behavior disorders. Beiheft Schweizz Psychol Anwendungen (Szondiana VII) 51:273–285, 1967
4. Blumer D, Walker AE: Sexual behavior in temporal lobe epilepsy. Arch Neurol 16:37–43, 1967
5. Blumer D, Walker AE: Memory in temporal lobe epileptics, in Talland GA, Waugh, NC (eds): The Pathology of Memory. New York, Academic Press, 1969
6. Blumer D: Transsexualism, sexual dysfunction, and temporal lobe disorder, in

Green R, Money J (eds.): Transsexualism and Sexual Reassignment. Baltimore, Johns Hopkins Press, 1969

7. Blumer D: Hypersexual episodes in temporal lobe epilepsy. Am J Psychiatry 126:1099–1106, 1970

8. Blumer D: Neuropsychiatric aspects of psychomotor and other forms of epilepsy, in Livingston, S: Comprehensive Management of Epilepsy in Infancy, Childhood, and Adolesence. Springfield, Ill, Thomas, 1971

9. Blumer D, Migeon C: Hormone and hormonal agents in the treatment of aggression. J. Nervous Mental Dis, 160:127–137, 1935

10. Bräutigam W: Zur epileptischen Wesensänderung. Psyche 5:523–544, 1951

11. Buchholz A: Ueber die chronische Paranoia bei epileptischen Individuen. (Habilitationsschrift) Leipzig, Pries, 1895

12. Dewhurst K, Beard AW: Sudden religious conversions in temporal lobe epilepsy. Br J Psychiaty 117:497–507, 1970

13. Fisher CM, Adams RD: Transient global amnesia. Acta Neurol Scand 40 (Suppl 9):7–83, 1964

14. Gastaut H, Roger J, Lesèvre N: Différenciation psychologique des épileptiques en fonction des formes électrocliniques de leur maladie. Rev Psychol Appl 3:237–249, 1953

15. Gastaut H, Collomb H: Étude du comportement sexuel chez les épileptiques psychomoteurs. Ann Med Psychol (Paris) 112:657–696, 1954

16. Gastaut H, Morin G, Lesèvre N: Étude du comportement des épileptiques psychomoteurs dans l'intervalle de leurs crises; les troubles de l'activité globale et de la sociabilité. Ann Med Psychol (Paris) 113:1–27, 1955

17. Gastaut H: État actuel des connaissances sur l'anatomie pathologique des épilepsies. Acta Neurol Psychiat Belg 56:5–20, 1956

18. Gastaut H, Vigouroux M: Electro-clinical correlations in 500 cases of psychomotor seizures, in Baldwin M, Bailey P (eds): Temporal Lobe Epilepsy. Springfield, Ill, Thomas, 1958

19. Gastaut H, Roger J, Soulayrol R, Tassinari CA, Regis H, Dravet C: Childhood epileptic encephalopathy with diffuse slow spike-waves (otherwise known as "petit-mal variant") or Lennox syndrome. Epilepsia 7:139–179, 1966

20. Geschwind N: The clinical setting of aggression in temporal lobe epilepsy, in Fields WS, Sweet WH (eds): The Neurobiology of Violence. St. Louis, Warren H. Green, 1975.

21. Gibbs FA: Ictal and nonictal psychiatric disorders in temporal lobe epilepsy. J Nerv Ment Dis 113:522–528, 1951

22. Glaser GH: The problem of psychosis in psychomotor temporal lobe epileptics. Epilepsia 5:271–278, 1964

23. Glaus A: Ueber Kombinationen von Schizophrenie und Epilepsie. Z Gesamte Neurol Psychiatry 135:450–500, 1931

24. Guerrant J, Anderson WW, Fischer A, Weinstein MR, Jaros RM, Deskins A: Personality in Epilepsy. Springfield, Ill, Thomas, 1962

25. Hallen O: Das Oral-Petit mal. Beschreibung und Zergliederung der als uncinate-fit (Jackson) und psychomotor-fit (Lennox) bezeichneten epileptischen Äquivalente. Deutsch Z Nervenheilk 171:236–260, 1954

26. Hierons R, Saunders M: Impotence in patients with temporal lobe lesions. Lancet 2:761–764, 1966

27. Hoenig J, Hamilton C: Epilepsy and sexual orgasm. Acta Psychiat Neurol Scand 35:448–457, 1960

28. Hooshmand H, Brawley B: Temporal lobe seizures and exhibitionism. Neurology 19:1119–1124, 1969

29. Jackson JH: On a particular variety of epilepsy ("intellectual aura"), one case with symptoms of organic brain disease, in Taylor J (ed): Selected Writings of John Hughlings Jackson, vol 1. London, Staples Press, pp 404–405, 1958

30. Jackson JH: On temporary mental disorders after epileptic paroxysms, in Taylor J (ed): Selected Writings of John Hughlings Jackson, vol 1, London, Staples Press, p 121, 1958

31. James IP: Temporal lobectomy for psychomotor epilepsy. J Ment Sci 106:543–558, 1960

32. Janz D: Die Epilepsien. Stuttgart, G. Thieme, 1969

33. Kimura D: Right temporal lobe damage. Arch Neurol 8:264–271, 1963

34. Knox SJ: Epileptic automatism and violence. Med Sci Law 8:96–104, 1968

35. Landolt H: Serial electroencephalographic investigations during psychotic episodes in epileptic patients and during schizophrenic attacks. Folia Psychiat Neurol Neurochir Neerlandica Suppl 4:91–133, 1958

36. Levin S: Epileptic clouded states. J Nerv Ment Dis 116:215–225, 1952

37. Liddell DW: Observations on epileptic automatism in a mental hospital population. J Ment Sci 99:732–748, 1953

38. Milner B: Psychological defects produced by temporal-lobe excision. Res Publ Assoc Res Nerv Ment Dis 36:244–257, 1958

39. Milner B, Branch C, Rasmussen T: Study of short-term memory after intracarotid injection of sodium amytal. Trans Am Neurol Assoc 87:224–226, 1962

40. Milner B: Amnesia following operation on the temporal lobes, in Whitty CWM, Zangwill OL (eds): Amnesia. London, Butterworths, 1966

41. Milner B: Visual recognition and recall after right temporal-lobe excision in man. Neuropsychologia 6:191–209, 1969

42. Milner B: Further analysis of the hippocampal amnesic syndrome: 14-year follow-up study of H. M. Neuropsychologia 6:215–234, 1968

43. Mitchell W, Falconer MA, Hill D: Epilepsy with fetishism relieved by temporal lobectomy. Lancet 2:626–630, 1954

44. Nemiah JC: Hysterical amnesia, in Talland, GA, Waugh NC (eds): The Pathology of Memory. New York, Academic Press, 1969

45. Niedermeyer E, Khalifeh R: Petit-mal status ("spike-wave stupor"). Epilepsia 6:250–262, 1965

46. Niedermeyer E: The Generalized Epilepsies. Springfield, Ill, Thomas, 1972

47. Ounsted C, Lindsay J, Norman R: Biological Factors in Temporal Lobe Epilepsy. London, Heinemann, 1966

48. Penfield W, Jasper H: Epilepsy and the Functional Anatomy of the Human Brain. Boston Little, Brown, 1954

49.   Peters UH: Sexualstörungen bei psychomotorischer Epilepsie. J Neurovis Relat (Suppl 10):491–497, 1971
50.   Pond DA, Bidwell BH, Stein L: A survey of epilepsy in fourteen general practices. I. Demographic and medical data. Psychiat Neurol Neurochir 63:217, 1960
51.   Pond DA, Bidwell BH: A survey of epilepsy in fourteen general practices. II. Social and psychological aspects. Epilepsia 1:285, 1960
52.   Roger A, Dongier M: Corrélations électrocliniques chez 50 épileptiques internés. Rev Neurol 83:593–596, 1950
53.   Sano K, Malamud N: Clinical significance of sclerosis of the cornu ammonis. Arch Neurol Psychiatry 70:40–53, 1953
54.   Schmidt RP, Wilder BJ: Epilepsy, in Plum F, McDowell FH (eds). Contemporary Neurology Series. Philadelphia, Davis, 1968
55.   Serafetinides EA: Aggressiveness in temporal lobe epileptics and its relation to cerebral dysfunction and environmental factors. Epilepsia 6:33–42, 1965
56.   Serafetinides EA: Psychiatric aspects of temporal lobe epilepsy, in Niedermeyer E (ed): Epilepsy. Basel, Karger, 1970
57.   Slater E, Beard AW, Glithero E: The schizophrenia-like psychoses of epilepsy. Br J Psychiatry 109:95–150, 1963
58.   Slater E, Roth M: Clinical Psychiatry (ed 3). London, Baillière, Tindall, & Cassell, 1969
59.   Small JG, Milstein V, Stevens JR: Are psychomotor epileptics different? A controlled study. Arch Neurol 7:187–194, 1962
60.   Small JG, Small IF, Hayden MP: Further psychiatric investigations of patients with temporal and nontemporal lobe epilepsy. Am J Psychiatry 123:303–310, 1966
61.   Small JG, Small IF: A controlled study of mental disorders associated with epilepsy. Recent Adv Biol Psychiatry 9:171–181, 1966
62.   Stevens JR: Psychiatric implications of psychomotor epilepsy. Arch Gen Psychiatry 14:461–471, 1966
63.   Symonds C: Disorders of memory. Brain 89:625–644, 1966
64.   Szondi L: Triebpathologie. Bern, Huber, 1952
65.   Talland GA, Waugh NC (eds): The Pathology of Memory. New York, Academic Press, 1969
66.   Taylor DC: Sexual behavior and temporal lobe epilepsy. Arch Neurol 21:510–516, 1969
67.   Walker AE, Blumer D: Long-term effects of temporal lobe lesions on sexual behavior and aggressivity, in Fields WS, Sweet WH (eds): The Neurobiology of Violence. St. Louis, Warren H. Green, 1975
68.   Waxman SG, Geschwind N: Hypergraphia in temporal lobe epilepsy. Neurology 24:629–636, 1974
69.   Weingartner H: Verbal learning in patients with temporal lobe lesions. J Verb Learning Verb Behav. 7:520–526, 1968
70.   Whitty CWM, Zangwill OL (eds): Amnesia. London, Butterworths, 1966

Commentary

Epilepsy is a remarkably complex disorder, and the previous chapter has laid out some of the important interactions between neurologic and psychiatric symptomatology that are present. Many years ago it was stated that the study of epilepsy was a royal road to the understanding of the mind. There can be no doubt that the study of epilepsy does impinge on many of the interrelated portions of psychiatry and neurology. For example, symptoms such as dream-like states, illusions and hallucinations, terror, and elation are present in both epileptic and psychiatric disorders. Such symptoms are studied as intricate parts of a mental disorder by the psychiatrist, while the same symptoms are considered part of an aura indicating the specific portion of the cortex that is abnormal by the neurologist. The bridging of these two views should be helpful for understanding how the brain functions.

The following chapter presents another subject with both psychiatric and neurologic manifestations, which, at present, are rarely considered together. Despite the importance of sexually related matters to many psychiatric theories, there has been almost no interest in the neural basis of sexual arousal and response. The following chapter will present an overview of the neurologic basis of sex, particularly emphasizing the central nervous structures involved in sexual function, and outline the known clinico-anatomical correlates of sexual disorders.

Dietrich Blumer, M.D., and
A. Earl Walker, M.D.

11
The Neural Basis of Sexual Behavior

Although much has been written on various aspects of sexual function, no serious attempt has been made to bring together into a system the parts of the nervous system that contribute to sexuality. It now seems possible to describe a neural basis for sexual behavior.[69,70] The hypothalamo–hypophyseo-gonadal axis has generally been looked upon as the neuroendocrine basis of sexual behavior, and many animal studies support this view. Higher neuronal circuits must be involved in sexuality, at least in man, but there has been surprisingly little curiosity and little knowledge concerning these mechanisms.

The fact that many patients with certain forms of focal epilepsy have both ictal and interictal alterations of sexual behavior has been long overlooked. Two reasons for this failure can be enumerated. First, the future physician learns in medical school that he needs to undress his patient for full examination and soon overcomes a sense of shame; unfortunately, he is not similarly taught to explore the sex life of his patients. Second, there has been a stifling trend in research to investigate only what can be measured by objective methods. As a result, the systematic study of very private events in man, which to be valid requires a personal relationship of physician to patient, has been sorely neglected.

This essay will consider the neural factors participating in sexual behavior from the peripheral to the highest levels of the nervous system. Where gaps exist, hypotheses may be suggested or avenues of further investigation indicated.

PERIPHERAL NEURAL FACTORS

The sensibilities of the glans penis and, probably, the clitoris are quite unique in that they are subserved principally by protopathic systems. Both von Frey[18] and Head[23] clearly describe the protopathic and deep sensibilities. The glans is quite insensitive to stimulation with cotton, wool or tactile hairs, but 70–90 g/sq mm pain-hairs produce an unlocalized boring or stinging pain, much more uncomfortable than stimulation by the same hairs over the foreskin or shaft of the penis. The reaction to temperature is also peculiar. The corona of the glans is insensitive to heat, but objects colder than 21°C produce inconstant diffuse cold sensations. Stimulation by objects heated over 40°C may induce a diffuse, unpleasant, cold feeling. Between these temperatures, the responses are absent or inconstant. There is, however, a poorly localized touch sensation if pressure is applied to the glans, so that some vague localization of coronal sensation is possible.

The peripheral nerves mediating these sensibilities and the motor autonomic functions of the genitalia have been well described. The main parasympathetic supply to the male genital organs arise from the third and fourth sacral nerves and enter into the nervi erigentes. Stimulation of these nerves causes dilatation of the corpora cavernosa and penile erection. Prostatic secretions in the male and vaginal secretions in the female are increased.

Sympathetic innervation is by way of the pelvic plexus from the hypo-gastric plexus and the upper lumbar ganglia. Stimulation of these nerves in the male causes contraction of the seminal vesicles, ejaculatory ducts, and the vessels of the corpora cavernosa producing ejaculation. In the female, the effect is more complex depending on whether or not the uterus is gravid. In both sexes, the perineal muscles, innervated by the pudendal nerve, assist in orgasm. Sensory fibers are carried by both parasympathetic and sympathetic nerves as well as the pudendal nerve.

Sexual response remains possible despite major interferences with the peripheral sensory receptors. Thus, Money reports:[53] "In cases of extensive surgical resection of the genitals, erotic arousal may be initiated and carried to the completion of orgasm despite the loss of large zones of erotic sensory tissue, including the vulva or the penis itself."

SPINAL MECHANISMS

Erection appears to be purely a segmental reflex. The afferent arc arises from stimulation of the glans, passes by the internal pudic nerve to the second, third, and fourth sacral segments from where efferent fibers travel through the same segments to the parasympathetic nerves and pudendal nerve. The former dilates the arterioles of the penis, and the latter causes contraction of the periurethral muscles with compression of the draining channels from the penis.

This reflex is influenced by suprasegmental centers, although it may function independently. In spinal cord disease, particularly trauma, priapism spontaneously occurs to a greater or lesser degree, provided the lesion is in the thoracic or cervical cord. It may develop in partial interruptions but more commonly in complete cord transections. After trauma, it may outlast the period of spinal shock and recur in episodes lasting from minutes to hours. Erection is lost only if the trauma involves the sacral cord, the cauda equina or parasympathetic plexus.

What is the mechanism of these erections? Granted, some are purely reflex, but others occur without obvious stimulation and are probably due to abnormal neuronal activity in the spinal cord at or near the diseased segment. Pool[57] recorded spiky activity from the traumatized cord, which might account for the episodic priapism.

Ejaculation has a more complex mechanism that requires sympathetic activity mediated by the lower thoracic and upper lumbar, particularly the second, ganglia. After rehabilitation, Talbot[61] found that about one third of paraplegic men who had erections had successful intercourse and "gratification." In another study by Zeitlin et al.,[74] a somewhat smaller number of men reported orgasm and ejaculation. It is interesting to note that Retief[59] asserted that if the second lumbar ganglia on one or both sides are left intact, when a sympathectomy is done, ejaculation is not adversely affected.

After reaching the sacral cord, where do the fibers mediating the sexual responses go? The results of surgical cordotomies provide an answer to this question. After unilateral cordotomy in males, sexual function is variable. In general, the capacity for erection remains, but ejaculation may or may not be lost. There are, however, many reports of preservation of normal sexual enjoyment after the unilateral operation in both men and women. Following bilateral section of the antero–lateral tracts, both erection and ejaculation are apt to be absent in the male; with the passage of time, however, there may be a return of sexual desire and potentia. In the female, if the vulva and vagina are made analgesic by cordotomy, orgasm is lost. If some sensation persists in the female perineum, however, normal sexual satisfaction may be experienced according to White and Sweet.[72]

On the basis of these observations, it would seem that the afferent suprasegmental fibers carrying impulses—many protopathic—from the genitalia pass, in part or in whole, in the antero–lateral tracts of the spinal cord, probably in association with pain fibers. This localization in the spinothalamic tract apparently continues to the medullary level, since in Wallenberg's syndrome patients occasionally will describe a unilateral orgasmic response.

Chronic spinal cord injury, paraplegia or quadriplegia, produces a remarkable dichotomy in sexual response. In these patients genito–pelvic and cerebro–cognitive eroticism appear to function separately.[52] Stimulation of pelvic erotic zones will produce, by reflex action, erection and, much more rarely, ejaculation. Intercourse and even fertility have been reported in paraplegic males.[74] Paraplegia is less common in the female, but it is reported that menstruation continues unchanged and gestation has occurred.[61] Despite this appearance of normal sexual function, the patient with spinal cord transection is aware of what is happening in the genital area only by means of visual observation. These same patients, however, report sexual arousal from kissing, sex fantasies, and the occurrence of erotic dreams including the mental experience of orgasm. Thus, they can experience sexual responses from either genito–pelvic stimulation or on a purely cerebral basis, but the two responses remain disconnected.

BRAIN STEM ORGANIZATION

Although one might conjecture that the somesthetic fibers from the genitalia continue through the pons and mesencephalon intermingled with spinothalamic fibers, we know of no proof of this assumption. At the thalamic level, MacLean[42] reported that stimulation of the region in which the spinothalamic fibers terminate—basal ventrolateral and intralaminar nuclei—will produce, at times, erection and ejaculation. Details of the thalamic representation of the genitalia are not established, however. If the fibers from the glans follow the course of the spinothalamic fibers, one would expect that they would break into two bundles, one ending in the ventrobasal part of the thalamus, and the other in the intralaminar region. Despite the many thalamic stimulations carried out for localization by an exploring stereotaxic needle, and the multitude of thalamotomies performed, references to genital responses are lacking. Even Hess[25] in his extensive explorations of the diencephalon makes no mention of either erection or ejaculation.

LOCALIZATION OF SEX IN THE BRAIN

In order to trace the neural foundation of sex in the brain, review of a number of studies are necessary. For convenience, these have been subdivided into three major topics: animal studies, human evidence (including the effect of hormones) and the relationship of sex and epilepsy.

Evidence From Animal Studies

HYPOTHALAMIC CENTERS

Impressive evidence from animal studies supports the importance of the hypothalamus for overt expression of sexual behavior.[38-40] A hormone-dependent neuronal system initiating copulation has been localized in the preoptic hypothalamic region in almost all species studied. Implants of estrogen or testosterone propionate and electrical stimulation in this area elicit the copulatory response, while lesions decrease or eliminate sexual behavior, which is not restored by exogenous hormone treatment. A second center exists in the median eminence region that regulates gonadotropin release. Exogenous hormone replacement restores the mating ability in animals deprived by lesions in this second area.

Lisk[38] suggests that an inhibitory system regulating the level of sex drive is located in the region of the ventral border of diencephalon and mesencephalon. This is based on his findings of increased copulation following lesions involving the posterior hypothalamus and mammillary bodies in the male rat. The overt sexual behavior of both male and female, therefore, would depend on the balance of activity between a hormone-dependent integrative and facilitory system, probably located in the preoptic region, and a regulatory, inhibitory system located in the region of the mammillary bodies. Michael[49] showed specific uptake in certain regions of the brain, using systematically administered hexoestrol—H3. In the cat, localization of hormone in the brain was confined to a bilaterally symmetrical system involving the septal region, preoptic area, and hypothalamus. The primates showed an additional localization in the caudate nucleus.

HIGHER CENTERS AND PATHWAYS

In Rhesus monkeys and cats, hypersexuality has been described as a result of removal of both temporal lobes,[33] the amygdala and overlying piriform cortex,[60] or of small lesions in the piriform cortex.[21] Excitatory[66,73] as well as inhibitory[4,15] influences on the gonadotropin secretion are ascribed to the amygdala.

MacLean[41] found that electrical stimulation of the septum or caudal hippocampus in male cats induced after-discharges that resulted in enhanced pleasure and grooming reactions and sometimes penile erection. Similar effects were seen following local cholinergic stimulation of these structures.

MacLean's painstaking stereotaxic explorations for sexual responses in the squirrel monkey disclosed, in the brain stem above the level of the hypothalamus, two nodal regions that, when stimulated, elicited full penile erection.[46] One of these regions was located in the core of the medial dorsal nucleus of the thalamus from where the major pathway followed the inferior thalamic peduncle, then joined the median forebrain bundle. The other region was coextensive with the medial septopreoptic area, whose major efferent pathway was also traced to the medial forebrain bundle. Stimulation along the course of this bundle through the hypothalamus effectively elicited erection. At the level of the midbrain, the pathway was followed laterally into the substantia nigra, from which it descended through the ventrolateral pons and entered the medulla just lateral to the exit of the sixth nerve.[43] Stimulations at positive loci in the septum, anterior thalamus,[44,46] and the medial frontal cortex[14] recruited potentials in the hippocampus, leading in some instances to hippocampal afterdischarges. During these afterdischarges, the erection might throb, but despite this orgastic appearance, ejaculation was never observed. Seminal discharge, sometimes preceding erection, occurred only when stimulation involved loci that lie along the course of the spinothalamic pathway and its medial ramifications into the caudal intralaminar region of the thalamus.[45]

The significance of MacLean's findings for localization of sex in the brain is somewhat compromised by the squirrel monkey's habit of utilizing aggressively genital display in an attempt to dominate other males, or as a form of social greeting.[42] Analogous stereotaxic explorations in the female elicited no sexual responses whatsoever.

ROLE OF THE CORTEX: SEX DIFFERENCES

The cerebral cortex is judged relatively unimportant in the maintenance of mating behavior in most female mammals. Bard[3] removed increasingly larger portions of the cortex in the cat until all of the neocortex, most of the rhinencephalon, and a large part of the striatum and thalamus were destroyed, without eliminating estrous behavior in response to estrogen. That removal of the entire neocortex in the rat does not interfere with estrous cycle, mating, pregnancy, or delivery has repeatedly been confirmed. In contrast, the cortex has been found to be essential for the initiation of mating behavior in most male mammals. Beach[6] showed that while removal of 20 percent of the cortex in male rats did not reduce the percentage showing copulatory behavior, mo male mated if more than 60 percent of its cortex had been destroyed. Similarly, mounting behavior was lost in female rats after decortication, while their female patterns of activity were retained.[7] In these studies, the location of the cortical area removed was considered less important than the quantity, a conclusion that has since been clearly disproved.[35,36] For sexual response, the male mammal has a very complicated neuromuscular pattern to assume in contrast to the simple passive postural adjustment made by the female. The male response must include elements of recognition, orientation, mounting, pelvic thrusting, intromission, and ejaculation. It is obvious that many regions of the neural system must be involved in the performance of the complete copulatory response in the male.

The observation that the cortex may be superfluous for the maintenance of sexual behavior in female animals illustrates the vast gap between animal findings and the human condition.

Human Evidence

The continual sexuality of man contrasts sharply with the intermittent or seasonal sexuality of animals.[31] The male is constantly ready to engage in sexual behavior,[56] but sexual arousal in male animals tends to occur only in response to the cyclic female sexual behavior. The human female's sexual behavior is not connected to the estrous cycle, and the human male, therefore, is able to enjoy sex continually. In man, sexuality is intricately related to personality and general behavior, so that obviously the human cerebral cortex has a high degree of influence over sexual arousal and response.

SEXUAL ACTIVITY AND HORMONES

Sexual arousal in man is sometimes instantaneous and occurs independent of any change in the sex hormone levels in the cirulating blood. Migeon[50] has shown that during sexual intercourse the androgen level does not change, although an increase in corticosteroid levels can be documented. Threshold complements of androgen do need to be present, however, for normal sexual behavior in man. Castration, the application of antiandrogenic compounds such as progestogens, which are used for certain otherwise intractable sex deviations[12,54] or sectioning of the hypophyseal stalk (as practiced in cases of diabetic retinopathy), can abolish male sexual arousal by abnormally lowering the androgen level. Otherwise, sexual behavior in man is rather independent of hormonal mechanisms and depends largely on cerebral controls.

EFFECTS OF LESIONS AND STIMULATION

A number of clinical observations tend to confirm the importance for sexual behavior of those areas that were found involved in animal experiments.

1. Bauer[5] reviewed the findings in 60 autopsied cases of hypothalamic disease reported in the literature. Gonadal depression was associated predominantly with lesions in the inferior and more anterior region of the hypothalamus, whereas precocious puberty was associated frequently with disease in the posterior hypothalamus and often with disease in the mammillary bodies.
2. Heath[24] noted penile erection in three patients during electrical stimulation, and orgastic response in one female following chemical stimulation of the septal region. Conversely, Meyers[48] described loss of potency following lesions in the septo–fornico–hypothalamic region.

3. Poeck and Pilleri[58] described the case of a young woman who developed a gross hypersexuality following lethargic encephalitis. The autopsy showed lesions mainly in the mesodiencephalic border area (brain-stem limbic system).
4. Hypersexuality has been documented in cases with deep fronto–temporal tumors.[1,8,37,64,65] Rabies, a disease of the limbic system, reportedly has also resulted in hypersexual states.[20]

The frontal lobes may play a role in human sexual conduct according to Kleist.[32] He pointed out that orbital lesions appear to lead to the loss of moral–ethical restraints and gross sexual misconduct (without hypersexuality proper, that is, without increased frequency of sexual arousal). Lesions of the frontal convexity, on the other hand, are associated with a loss of general initiative, including sexuality, but the patient can still perform sexually if he is led step-by-step (see Chapter 9).

Meyer,[47] Walker,[67] and others have reported a decrease of sexual arousal and response after head injuries that tends to be global, affecting both libido and genital arousal. This emphasizes the significant vulnerability of sexual functions to cerebral injuries but does not specify localization.

Sexuality and Epilepsy

The most significant evidence of the higher neural basis for sexual behavior in man stems from observations in patients with focal epilepsy. The ancient Romans had an appropriate saying: "Coitus brevis epilepsia est." The mood of sexual desire is likened to the prodrome of an epileptic attack, the premonition of orgasm to the aura, and the sexual climax to the epileptic paroxysm. A refractory period, reduced tension, and sleep tend to follow both the sex act and the epileptic attack.[63] We must however, go beyond such loose analogies to a closer look at the relationship between sexual arousal and epilepsy.

Interictal sexuality: Of all forms of epilepsy, temporal lobe epilepsy is most clearly associated with abnormal sexual behavior. Table 11-1 lists the changes observed in 50 temporal lobe epileptics whose sexual behavior was carefully explored.[11] It is evident that sexual normality is the exception and a chronic disorder in the form of *global hyposexuality* is predominant. Hyposexuality in patients with minor seizures was originally observed a century ago by Griesinger,[22,55] then rediscovered and well documented by Gastaut and Collomb.[19] A marked decrease of both libido and genital arousal has been reported by a number of investigators. Hierons[26,27] described the deficit as impotence, since he was impressed by a continuing desire to perform sexually

Table 11-1

Changes of Sexual Behavior in 50 Temporal Lobe Epileptics (42 Operated)

Chronic global hyposexuality	29
Postoperative hypersexuality	2*
Hypersexuality induced by medication	1
Postictal sexual arousal	4†
Ictal sexual arousal	1
Homosexual behavior	2
Total	35 (70%)

*both patients were hyposexual, preoperatively.
†one patient also with homosexual behavior, another patient also with hypersexuality induced by medication (Mysoline).

despite inability to do so in late-onset temporal lobe epileptics. In contrast, Taylor[62,63] refers to a lack of appetence with continuing ability to perform sexually, which he calls a cerebral "fault of integration." Our own investigations[11,13] convince us that Gastaut's concept of a global hyposexuality is indeed correct. Patients with late-onset temporal lobe epilepsy who are married may complain of insufficiency, but on close scrutiny do not show any significant libido that cannot be satisfied. While complete sexual arousal can take place in a majority of temporal lobe epileptics, the frequency of arousal is drastically reduced. It is not unusual to find sexual arousal as rarely as once a year. Temporal lobe epileptics with onset of the illness prior to or at time of puberty may never or only rarely have sexual arousal.

The relationship of mesial temporal seizure discharges and sexual arousal is dramatically confirmed by findings in patients who were previously hyposexual but are completely free from any seizure activity after unilateral lobectomy. Normalization of sexual desire and ability is commonly observed, and, occasionally, a marked hypersexuality may present itself during the second postoperative month.[10,13] The hypersexuality is reversed if there is recurrence of temporal lobe seizures. In one case, we observed a hypersexual behavior that lasted 2 years following unilateral temporal lobectomy in a previously hyposexual woman. The hypersexuality gradually subsided without recurrence of seizures.

CASE 1

A boy developed normally until the age of 12 years, when he had an attack in which he became rigid with head retracted and eyes staring. In subsequent years, the episodes continued—sometimes occurring daily and again not for a week or so. The lad did well in school and at play. Although his secondary sexual characteristics developed normally, he developed no sexual arousal and throughout his 20s he had little interest or curiosity about women, with whom he had many associations in church work. The spells continued despite anticonvulsant medication and at age 30 his spiking right temporal lobe was removed. The attacks ceased completely. A few months after the operation, he began to notice how attractive women were. He took up dancing but he almost gave it up, when, for the first time in his life, he experienced an erection when he held a girl in his arms. This embarrassment heightened one evening 6 months after his operation, when at the age of 31 he had his first emission. He later married and at age 40 continued to consummate his marriage with great regularity.

The global hyposexuality is reversed not only by successful surgical treatment but, contrary to suspicion, anticonvulsants may reestablish sexual arousal if they suppress the seizure activity.[19,55]

Ictal sexual arousal: The hyposexuality of a majority of temporal lobe epileptics contrasts to the reputation of epileptics as suffering from deviant and/or excessive sexual arousal. Kraft–Ebbing[34] pointed out this paradox in the latter part of the last century. The excessive sexual excitement so vividly described in old psychiatric textbooks stems from strikingly abnormal sexual arousal in a few epileptics at the time of their seizures. Global hyposexuality, on the other hand, being a very silent condition, was overlooked despite its frequent occurrence. Our own observations indicate that sexual arousal may take place as a direct result of seizure discharges (ictal sexual arousal) or may *follow* the clinical seizure (postictal sexual arousal).

An understanding of the relationship between ictal events and sexual arousal in temporal lobe epilepsy, requires a clear understanding of the seizure pattern with differentiation of ictal and postictal phenomena (see Chapter 10). In most cases, an experienced observer can distinguish the ictal from the postictal phase of the attack and therefore identify a sexual arousal as ictal or postictal. Table 11-2 notes the types of ictal experiences that either precede or accompany the *ictal sexual arousal.* Fear is most often described and may be noted as a prepubertal phenomenon in seizures that assume a frankly sexual character after puberty. The aura associated with sexual seizures is frequently of the oro-alimentary kind. Sexual seizures are often triggered by sexual arousal in the form of intercourse or masturbation. By the same token, "nonsexual" seizures have been noted as a form of reflex epilepsy following sexual intercourse.[28] We believe that seizure phenomena may follow sexual stimulation more often than is generally assumed.

A clear example of the ictal attack was presented by a head-injured veteran of World War II who consulted one of us (A.E.W.) 10 years ago.

CASE 2

A 24-year-old man was having frequent spells and behavioral disturbances. In the course of the examination he had an attack. He stopped talking and stared into space,

Table 11-2
Symptomatology Associated With Psychomotor Ictal Sexual Arousal

---

Precipitating or triggering mechanisms
    Sexual intercourse or masturbation
    Erotically charged objects or events
    Hypnosis or suggestion
    Self-stimulation
Primictal
    Epigastric sensation
    Chest or anal sensation
    Abdominal pain
    Olfactory sensation
Ictal equivalents
    Fear (prepubertal)
    Paradoxical painful experience
    Urinary incontinence

---

a few twitchings occurred at the right corner of the mouth and he smacked his lips. At the same time, his hands began to move over his chest and abdomen, his right hand eventually moving about his pubis. For some minutes he mumbled incoherently and was unable to follow even simple commands. He gradually regained consciousness and was then able to reply coherently regarding his attack. He admitted that with the onset of the attack he always remembered experiencing a pleasant erotic sensation as if he were about to have an orgasm. Apparently, he would lose consciousness before it occurred.

Of particular interest is the case reported by Bancaud et al.[2]

CASE 3

    A girl, aged 20, had suffered from seizures since age 4, which, initially, consisted of a feeling of fear that prompted her to run to her mother. At age 8, the seizures changed; she would sit on the floor with her hands under her and turn around uttering incomprehensible words. Then she would lift her skirt, bite her cheeks, look around in a confused manner and urinate. She said these seizures were initiated by an epigastric pressure and undefinable fear. At age 11, she had her first spectacular and frankly sexual seizure: She called her mother, fell down with an expression of fear on her face and screamed loud and louder; then she made complex movements of her body and limbs while rubbing herself with closed fists in the pubic area and demanding silence. Abundant vaginal discharge took place with urination. She experienced as aura a sensation of diffuse oppression, then a contraction of thigh and pelvic muscles accompanied by a pleasurable feeling identical with the one she experienced with masturbation. The sexual pleasure replaced the fear she had experienced prior to age 11. Since that time, the seizures, usually provoked by masturbation but once brought on by heterosexual petting, remained about the same.

On examination the girl was mildly retarded. She had a left superior visual field defect. Neuroradiologic studies showed a right inferior temporal mass without misplacement of structures. An EEG showed sporadic right temporal spikes. During depth EEGs induced and spontaneous attacks were observed. The EEG analysis showed that participation of the right hippocampus was essential to the elaboration of the paroxysmal sexual manifestations. The amygdala, gyrus parahippocampi, and isocortex of the temporal lobe were secondarily involved while the contralateral limbic system was not implicated at all during the attacks. An astrocytoma, invading the amygdala as well as the anterior hippocampus, was found at operation and removed.

Although Freemon and Nevis[17] reported what they thought was the first case of sexual seizures, Bancaud and co-workers[2] summarized from the literature 26 cases of temporal lobe sexual seizures and ten cases of seizures with sexual manifestations due to involvement of the paracentral lobule. The French authors point out that *seizures due to lesions of the paracentral lobule* consist chiefly of lateralized genital paresthesias at the level of the penis or vagina, rectum, anus, abdomen, and sometimes the chest, which are experienced without sexual resonance; while with temporal lobe sexual seizures the entire pattern is integrated into the instinctive–affective content of dominating lust. This is in contrast to the impression given by Erickson's[16] well-known case with a hemangioma of the paracentral lobule, where his female patient's episodic genital sensation was probably misnamed "erotomania" or "nymphomania." Figure 11-1 depicts the involved structures: The paracentral lobule and hippocampus as well as the connection through the cingulate gyrus to the hippocampus. The role of the cingulate gyrus, however, is unclear.

The listing of sexual seizures by Bancaud and co-workers needs to be enlarged on the one hand but is somewhat uncertain on the other, because some of the authors quoted may have confused postictal with ictal sexual arousal.

Postictal sexual arousal is described in detail by Blumer.[10] It usually takes place in an appropriate setting with full recollection on the part of the patient and rarely seems engulfed in the phase of postictal amnesia. Reported cases of exhibitionism[29] may represent only confused undressing by a patient following a temporal lobe seizure, with or without sexual arousal. Postictal sexual arousal is not part of the immediate postictal phase and may be interpreted as a release phenomenon after excessive mesial temporal seizure discharges have terminated, not unlike the sexual arousal observed following successful temporal lobectomy. We have noted that it occurs in individuals who are not markedly hyposexual, while the belated sexual arousal manifested several weeks following unilateral temporal lobectomy typically occurs in patients who have been very hyposexual. We have never observed excessive sexual arousal following operation in patients who were not hyposexual prior to operation.

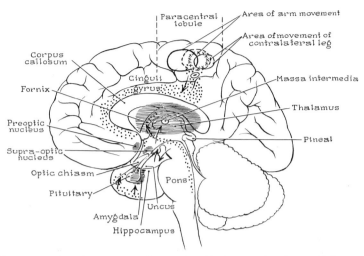

Fig. 11-1. Midsagittal section of the brain with the sexual pathways and centers indicated by dotted lines and areas. The brain stem tract passes to the base of the thalamus from whence fibers (not indicated in the sketch) project by way of the internal capsule to the paracentral lobule and also by way of the inferior thalamic peduncle to the amygdala. Fibers from the medial temporal structures pass to the cingulate gyrus and by the fornix to the hypothalamus which modulates the activity of the hypophysis. The paracentral area indicated by a dot in a circle is where Bates* obtained anal retraction upon electrical stimulation. The zones just above this area are the sites from which he elicited movements of the extremities (second motor area).

Sexual deviations and epilepsy: Homosexual, and in particular, trans-vestite and fetishistic deviations have been noted in a small number of temporal lobe epileptics.[9] A close relationship between perversion and temporal lobe abnormality is strongly suggested by two cases in the literature where the perversion was completely abolished following cure of the temporal lobe epilepsy by unilateral temporal lobectomy.[30,51] Unlike exhibitionism, which is most probably postictal, these sexual deviations apparently occur during the interictal phase. Two patients in our own series had homosexual behavior that disappeared following unilateral temporal lobectomy even though the seizures were not completely abolished.

It would appear that the role of the temporal lobe, especially the medial temporal structures, in the sexual system is more complicated and probably at a higher level than the paracentral center for the representation of the

*Bates, J.A.E.: Stimulation of the medial surface of the human cerebral hemisphere after hemi-spherectomy. Brain 76:405–447, 1953.

genitalia.[69,70] The temporal lobe is apparently concerned in the more global aspects of sexuality rather than in the primary integration of genital sensibility, and for this purpose, its wide connections to the hypothalamus, frontal lobe, thalamus, and cingulate gyrus are appropriate (Fig. 11-1).

COMMENTS

This discussion has emphasized the presence of centers in the hypothalamus, temporal lobe and paracentral cortex, which seem to modulate sexual activity in man and animals. To some extent, the influence is hormone-dependent.

The neural pathways involved are similar to other sensory systems. The paracentral representation seems to be the cortical representation of the perineal genital system akin to other somato–motor cortical receptor areas. The thalamic locus of this mechanism has not been defined. According to the charts of thalamic topography, it should lie in the basal lateral part of the ventral-thalamic nucleus, but stimulation of this area has not induced perineal or sexual hallucinations. Perhaps, future thalamic mappings may uncover the relay mechanisms. Theoretically, projections should be to the hypothalamus both anteriorly and posteriorly, and to the paracentral cortex. From the latter, fibers pass to the cingulate gyrus and hence to the amygdala and hippocampus and adjacent cortex. The efferent pathways probably involve direct fibers to the hypothalamus via the stria terminalis, anterior–thalamic peduncle, or anterior commissure. Thus, the neuronal basis for sexuality would seem to be related in part, at least, to the medial–temporal structures.

The complex changes resulting from interruption of one or more of these control systems is not easily understood. Not only are there secondary pathways that tend to restitute function, but the primary neuronal systems may undergo a hypersensitivity that modulates the activity of the complex system. The presence of both excitatory and inhibitory mechanisms manifest in sexual seizures on the one hand, and hyposexuality on the other allows for a delicate balance of the control of sexual arousal.

Let us assume that the chronic firing of an anterior temporal epileptic focus modifies the activity of diencephalic nuclei. Excision of the temporal structures not only eliminates the excitatory or inhibitory input to the hypothalamic neurons but by reason of denervation hypersensitivity makes them more susceptible to incoming impulses from other sources, especially frontal, which are likely to be excitatory. Multiple inputs from one or both sides of the brain to hypothalamic centers may account for the varied results of lobectomy. The delay in the onset of sexuality after anterior temporal lobectomy may be related to the gradual recovery of chronically depressed neurons, or to their slow development of hypersensitivity.[68]

We have described a neural basis utilizing phylogenetically old systems in the spinal cord and brain stem and newer structures in the telencephalon, which may subserve the genital as well as the libidinal arousal aspects of sex. This sexual system is analogous to other sensory–motor systems, and, in fact, in its more primitive course is integrated with certain parts of other systems. Its cortical representation is both in primary receptive areas (the paracentral region) and in associative and executive areas (the medial temporal lobe structures). The precise role played by the hippocampus, amygdala, hypothalamus, and connecting fiber bands is not clear, but, perhaps, this is not too important. The medial temporal structures often act as a unit,[71] and in epileptic discharge the functional limits of these structures are blurred. Probably the same is true for the regulation of sexual behavior, especially during sexual climax.

REFERENCES

1.   Anastasopoulos G: Hypersexualitaet, Wesensaenderung, Schlafstoerungen und Demenz bei einem Tumor des rechten Schlaefenlappens. Psychiatr Neurol 136:85–108, 1958
2.   Bancaud J, Favel P, Bonis A, Bordas-Ferrer M, Miraver J, Talairach J: Manifestations sexuelles paroxystiques et epilepsie temporale. Rev Neurol 123:217–230, 1970
3.   Bard, P: Central nervous mechanisms for emotional behavior patterns in animals. Res Publ Assoc Res Nervous Mental Disease (Proc.) 19:190–218, 1939
4.   Bar-Sela ME, Critchlow V: Delayed puberty following electrical stimulation of amygdala in female rats. Am J Physiol 211:1103–1107, 1966
5.   Bauer HG: Endocrine and metabolic conditions related to pathology in the hypothalamus. A review. J Nerv Ment Dis 128:323–338, 1959
6.   Beach FA: Effects of cortical lesions upon the copulatory behavior of male rats. J Comp Psychol 29:193–239, 1940
7.   Beach FA: Effects of injury to the cerebral cortex upon the display of masculine and feminine mating behavior by female rats. J Comp Psychol 36:169–199, 1943.
8.   Bente D, Kluge E: Sexuelle Reizzustaende im Rahmen des Uncinatus Syndroms. Arch Psychiat Z Neurol 190:357–376, 1953
9.   Blumer D: Transsexualism, sexual dysfunction, and temporal lobe disorder, in Green R, Money J (eds): Transsexualism and Sexual Reassignment. Baltimore, Johns Hopkins Press, 1969, pp213–219
10. Blumer D: Hypersexual episodes in temporal lobe epilepsy. Am J Psychiatry 126:1099–1106, 1970
11. Blumer D: Das Sexualverhalten der Schlaefenlappenepileptiker vor und nach chirurgischer Behandlung. J Neurovis Relat Suppl 10, 469–476, 1971
12. Blumer D, Migeon C: Hormone and hormonal agents in the treatment of aggression. J. Nerv Ment Dis 160:127–137, 1975

13. Blumer D, Walker AE: Sexual behavior in temporal lobe epilepsy. Arch Neurol 16:37–43, 1967

14. Dua S, MacLean PD: Localization for penile erection in medial frontal lobe. Am J Physiol 207:1425–1434, 1964·

15. Elwers M, Critchlow V: Precocious ovarian stimulation following hypothalamic and amygdaloid lesions in rats. Am J Physiol 198:381–385, 1960

16. Erickson T: Erotomania (nymphomania) as an expression of cortical epileptiform discharge. Arch Neurol Psychiatry 53:226–231, 1945

17. Freemon F, Nevis A: Temporal lobe sexual seizures. Neurology 19:87–90, 1969

18. von Frey M: Beitraege zur Sinnesfunction der Haut. Berichte ü.d. Verh. d. K. Saechs. Gesellsch Wissensch 2:166, 1895

19. Gastaut H, Collomb H: Etude du comportement sexuel chez les épileptiques psychomoteurs. Ann Med Psychol (Paris) 2:657–696, 1954

20. Gastaut H, Mileto G: Interprétation physiopathogenique des symptômes de la rage furieuse. Rev Neurol 92:5–25, 1955

21. Green JD, Clemente CD, de Groot J: Rhinencephalic lesions and behavior in cats. An analysis of the Klüver–Bucy syndrome with particular reference to normal and abnormal sexual behavior. J Comp Neurol 108:505–545, 1957

22. Griesinger W: Ueber einige epileptoide Zustaende. Arch Psychiat Nerv 1:329, 1868

23. Head H: Studies in Neurology, vol 1. London, Henry Frowde, Oxford University Press, Hodder and Stoughton, Ltd., 1920

24. Heath RG: Pleasure response of human subjects to direct stimulation of the brain: Physiologic and psychodynamic considerations, in Heath RG (ed): The Role of Pleasure in Behavior. New York, Harper & Row, 1964, pp 219–243

25. Hess WR: Das Zwischenhirn, Syndrome, Lokalisationen, Funktionen. Basel, B. Schwabe, 1949

26. Hierons R: Impotence in temporal lobe lesions. J Neurovis Relat Suppl. 10, 477–481, 1971

27. Hierons R, Saunders M: Impotence in patients with temporal lobe lesions. Lancet 2:761–764, 1966

28. Hoenig J, Hamilton C: Epilepsy and Sexual Orgasm. Acta Psychiatry Neurol Scand 35:448–457, 1960

29. Hooshmand H, Brawley B: Temporal lobe seizures and exhibitionism. Neurology 19:1119–1124, 1969

30. Hunter R, Logue V, McMenemy WH: Temporal lobe epilepsy supervening on long standing transvestism and fetishism. Epilepsia 4:60–65, 1963

31. Jensen GD: Human sexual behavior in primate perspective, in Zubin J, Money J (eds): Contemporary Sexual Behavior. Baltimore, The Johns Hopkins Univ Pr, 1973. pp 17–31

32. Kleist K: Gehirnpathologie. Leipzig, Barth, 1934

33. Klüver H, Bucy PC: "Psychic blindness" and other symptoms following bilateral temporal lobectomy in Rhesus monkeys. Am J Physiol 119:352–353, 1937

34. Krafft-Ebbing R: Psychopathia Sexualis (ed 12). London, Heinemann, 1931, p 469

35.   Larsson K: Mating behavior in male rats after cerebral cortex ablation. I. Effects of lesions on the dorsolateral and the median cortex. J Exp Zool 151:167–176, 1962

36.   Larsson K: Mating behavior in male rats after cerebral cortex ablation. II. Effects of lesions in the frontal lobes compared to lesions in the posterior half of the hemispheres. J Exp Zool 155:203–224, 1964

37.   Lechner H: Ein Beitrag zu den psychoorganischen Beziehungen der Sexualitaet. Wien Z Nerv 16:129–136, 1966

38.   Lisk R: Increased sexual behavior in the male rat following lesions in the mamillary region. J Exp Zool 161:129–136, 1966

39.   Lisk R: Sexual behavior: Hormonal control, in Martini L, Ganong WF (eds): Neuroendocrinology vol 2. New York, Academic Press, 1967, pp 197–239

40.   Lisk R: Neural localization for androgen activation of copulatory behavior in the male rat. Endocrinology 80:754–761, 1967

41.   MacLean PD: Chemical and electrical stimulation of hippocampus in unrestrained animals. Part II. Behavioral findings. Arch Neurol Psychiatr 78:128–142, 1957

42.   MacLean PD: New findings on brain function and sociosexual behavior, in Zubin J, Money J (eds): Contemporary Sexual Behavior. Baltimore, The Johns Hopkins Univ Pr, 1973, pp 53–74

43.   MacLean PD, Denniston RH, Dua S: Further studies on cerebral representation of penile erection: Caudal thalamus, midbrain, and pons. J Neurophysiol 26:273–293, 1963

44.   MacLean PD, Denniston RH, Dua S, Ploog DW: Hippocampal changes with brain stimulation eliciting penile erection, in Physiologie de l'hippocampe. Paris, Colloques Internationaux du Centre National de la Recherche Scientifique vol 107, 1962, pp 491–510

45.   MacLean PD, Dua S, Denniston RH: Cerebral localization for scratching and seminal discharge. Arch Neurol 9:485–497, 1963

46.   MacLean PD, Ploog DW: Cerebral representation of penile erection. J Neurophysiol 25:29–55, 1962

47.   Meyer JE: Die sexuellen Stoerungen der Hirnverletzten. Arch Psychiatr Z Neurol 193:449–469, 1955

48.   Meyers R: Central neural counterparts of penile potency and libido in humans and subhuman mammals. Cincinnati J Med 44:281–291, 1963

49.   Michael RP: The selective accumulation of estrogens in the neural and genital tissues of the cat, in Proceedings of First International Congress on Hormonal Steroids, vol 2. New York, Academic Press, 1962, pp 469–581

50.   Migeon C: Personal communication, 1972

51.   Mitchell W, Falconer MA, Hill D: Epilepsy with fetishism relieved by temporal lobectomy. Lancet 2:626–630, 1954

52.   Money J: Phantom orgasm in the dreams of paraplegic men and women. Arch Gen Psychiatr 3:373–382, 1960

53.   Money J: Components of eroticism in man. II. The orgasm and genital somesthesia. J Nerv Ment Dis 132:289–297, 1961

54.   Money J: Use of androgen-depleting hormone in the treatment of male sex

offenders. J Sex Res 6:165–172, 1970
55. Peters UH: Sexualstoerungen bei psychomotorischer Epilepsie. J Neurovis Relat Suppl. 10, 491–497, 1971
56. Phoenix CH, Goy RW, Young WC: Sexual behavior: General aspects, in Martini L, Ganong WF (eds): Neuroendocrinology, vol 2. New York, Academic Press, 1967, pp 163–196
57. Pool JL: Electrospinogram (ESG). Spinal cord action potentials recorded from a paraplegic patient. J Neurosurg 3:192–198, 1946
58. Poeck K, Pilleri G: Release of hypersexual behavior due to lesion in the limbic system. Acta Neurol 41:233–244, 1965
59. Retief PJM: Physiology of micturition and ejaculation. S Afr Med J 24:509, 1950
60. Schreiner L, Kling A: Effects of castration on hypersexual behavior induced by rhinencephalic injury in the cat. Arch Neurol Psychiatr 72:180–186, 1954
61. Talbot HS: Sexual function in paraplegics. J Urol 61:265, 1949
62. Taylor DC: Sexual behavior and temporal lobe epilepsy. Arch Neurol 21:510–516, 1969
63. Taylor, DC: Appetitive inadequacy in the sex behavior of temporal lobe epileptics. J Neurovis Relat Suppl. 10, 486–490, 1971
64. Torelli D, Bosna F: Alterazioni del'erotismo nell'epilessia e nei tumori cerebrali. Acta Neurol 23:154–165, 1958
65. Van Reeth PC, Dierkens J, Luminet D: L'hypersexualité dans l'épilepsie et les tumeurs du lobe temporal. Acta Neurol 58:194–218, 1958
66. Velasco ME: Opposite effects of platinum and stainless-steel lesions of the amygdala on gonadotropin secretion. Neuroendocrinology 10:301–308, 1972
67. Walker AE: A follow-up study of head wounds in World War II. VA Medical Monograph, Washington, DC, U.S. Government Printing Office, 1961
68. Walker AE: Man and his temporal lobes (John Hughlings Jackson Lecture). Surg Neurol 1:69–79, 1973
69. Walker AE, Blumer D: The localization of sex in the brain. Otfried Foerster Symposium on Cerebral Localization, Cologne, Sept. 20–22, 1973 (in press)
70. Walker AE, Blumer D: The sexual system. Inaugural Volume of the Columbian Neurological Institute, Bogota, Columbia (in press)
71. Walker AE, Mayanagi Y: Experimental temporal lobe epilepsy. Brain 97:423–446, 1974
72. White JC, Sweet WH: Pain, Its Mechanism and Surgical Control. Springfield, Ill, Thomas, 1955
73. Yamada T, Greer MA: The effect of bilateral ablation of the amygdala on endocrine function in the rat. Endocrinology 66:565–574, 1960
74. Zeitlin AB, Cottrell TL, Lloyd FA: Sexology of the paraplegic male. Fertil Steril 8:337, 1957

Commentary

With this presentation, the authors have demonstrated the localization of sexual functions in specific areas of the central nervous system. Particularly noteworthy is that many of the areas of the brain of significance for sexual function are also implicated in emotional behavior. The fact that sexual and emotional behavior are, at least in part, served by the same basic neuroanatomical structures accords with importance of sexual activities and fantasies in emotional life.

In the next chapter, the authors will discuss both the spontaneous and the drug-induced movement disorders that occur in psychiatric patients. For many years, the movement disorders occurring in schizophrenic patients have been of great interest. The introduction of the major tranquilizing drugs, in combination with more personal attention for the patient, has produced effective control of the acute catatonic symptomatology and this form of schizophrenic symptomatology has become rare. In its place, however, we now have a wealth of movement disorders that appear to be side effects of the drugs. The authors will discuss both the old and the new movement disorders of psychotic patients and will probe their relationship.

C. David Marsden, M. Sc., M.R.C.P.,
Daniel Tarsy, M.D., and
Ross J. Baldessarini, M.D.

12

Spontaneous and Drug-Induced Movement Disorders in Psychotic Patients

Abnormal movements have long been recognized as a frequent feature of both schizophrenia and the affective disorders. In certain cases, motor disturbances associated with psychosis bear a strong resemblance to abnormal movements appearing in neurologic disturbances of the extrapyramidal system. Kahlbaum was sufficiently impressed by the resemblance of the motor disorders of catatonia to disorders of movement occurring in neurologic disease that he believed they were symptomatic of underlying focal organic disease of the brain.[104] Kraepelin[165] and Bleuler[26,27] provided detailed descriptions of the various motor abnormalities associated with catatonic schizophrenia, and subsequent writers[102,103,159] have further subdivided catatonia according to these disturbances. The high incidence of stereotypy, mannerisms, tics, chorea, negativism, waxy flexibility, and akinesia in catatonic patients of that era seems remarkable, since catatonia is not frequent in contemporary clinical experience. There has probably been a decline in the incidence of catatonic schizophrenia,[230] and, in addition, it is likely that patients with organic neurologic disease were formerly included in populations of psychotic patients. The picture has been further complicated by the introduction of neuroleptic antipsychotic drug therapy, which itself results in extrapyramidal movement disorders.

Against this historical background, we will review movement disorders in psychotic patients under two headings: those occurring as part of the psychotic illness and those due to the drugs used to treat these conditions. There is also a third category comprised of patients with movement disorders due to neurologic disease who sometimes are referred for psychiatric evaluation and treatment. This occurs in cases of torsion dystonia (dystonia musculorum deformans), spasmodic torticollis, and blepharospasm, but such patients are usually considered to be suffering from structural or functional disorders of the motor system rather than primary psychiatric illness. Such conditions are extensively described in the neuropsychiatric literature[170] and will not be discussed further here.

MOVEMENT DISORDERS IN UNTREATED PSYCHOTIC PATIENTS

Schizophrenia

Stereotypies and mannerisms have most often been described in catatonic schizophrenia but occur in other forms of chronic schizophrenia as well.[143,144,249] According to traditional definitions,[26,27,104,165] *stereotypy* refers to isolated, purposeless movements carried out in a uniform and repetitive way. *Mannerism* is distinguished from stereotypy as an unusual or bizarre way of carrying out purposeful activity that results from the incorporation of stereotypy into goal-directed acts.[104] From a practical point of view, these two disorders usually occur together, making the distinction between them arbitrary. Stereotypy and mannerism may take the form of repetitive movements (hyperkinesia) or of persistent abnormal postures (hypokinesia). Although, in a broader sense, stereotypy and mannerism also refer to the recurrent use of certain words or phrases, the persistence of single thoughts or wishes, or oddities of dress and self-decoration,[165] the present discussion will be concerned only with abnormalities of movement and posture.

HYPERKINESIA

Stereotyped activity varies from simple tic-like movements of isolated portions of the body to complex patterns of behavior to which symbolic significance is sometimes attributed.[166,215,246] A variety of stereotyped movements were described by earlier writers[26,27,139,165] and are also mentioned in contemporary accounts.[143,144,249] The most elementary of these are listed in Table 12-1. A superficial resemblance of these stereotypies to oral-facial dyskinesias and choreiform activity of neurologic disorders is frequently apparent. The ritualistic incorporation of stereotyped movements into the performance of daily activities produces a caricature of purposeful activity known as manneristic behavior. Some examples of such behavior which have been described include unusual hand postures while writing, eating, or shaking hands, striking a plate before eating, tapping buttons before buttoning a coat, or circling a room before sitting.[27,165] Such motor activity is obviously more

Table 12-1
Stereotyped Movements Associated With Schizophrenia [19,29,88,119,141]

	Extremities
Eyes	*Manipulative*
Frowning	Picking
Opening wide	Pulling
Squeezing shut	Handling
Repetitive blinking	Twisting
Nose	Kneading
Wrinkling	Grasping
Sniffing	Tapping
Flaring nares	Rubbing
Mouth and Jaw	*Others*
Pouting	Intertwining fingers
Lipsmacking	Wringing hands
Grinning	Folding hands
Grimacing	Spreading fingers
Biting	Ballistic arm flinging
Chewing	
Tongue	Trunk and Whole Body
Protrusion	*Shoulder shrugging*
Licking	*Various contortionist movements*
Clicking	*Back-arching*
Others	*Rocking*
Wrinkling forehead	*Shuffling*
Facial twitching	*Hopping*
Head and Neck	*Turning*
Torsion movements	*Skipping*
Hyperextension	*Running*
Shaking	*Excessive leg lifting*
Nodding	

complex and purposeful in appearance than the hyperkinetic dyskinesias occurring in neurologic disorders. It was traditionally stated that over many years patients exhibiting manneristic behavior became increasingly awkward, clumsy, and ungraceful in nearly all of their activities.[27,103,165]

There are few reliable estimates of the incidence of these abnormalities in either the older or more contemporary psychiatric literature. In one recent study,[182] stereotypies were described in 24 percent, and mannerisms in 14 percent of 250 patients with catatonic schizophrenia among a total psychiatric population of 20,000 patients hospitalized over a 50-year period. According to classical descriptions,[27,165] stereotypies appear early in the course of schizophrenic illness, persist for many years and ultimately may dominate a patient's daily activity. A progressive degeneration of behavior from complex movements to more simplified fragments was also believed to occur,[9,27,165,215] although one recent study found no correlation between complexity of stereotypy and the age, length of illness, or duration of hospitalization.[143] There is little information concerning the influence of environmental factors on the severity of stereotypies, although they appear to be increased by interpersonal contacts and decreased during work, volitional movement of other portions of the body, or drowsiness.[143] Although it is uncertain whether or not stereotyped movements are partially attributable to the effect of chronic institutionalization, such behavior has been described in young schizophrenics with less than 2 years of hospitalization.[249] In this group of relatively drug-free patients, abnormal movements were associated with an earlier onset and poorer prognosis of schizophrenia than in an age-matched group of schizophrenic patients without such movements.[249]

Whether or not chorea or athetosis occurs in chronic schizophrenia uncomplicated by neurologic disease is presently difficult to determine. Kraepelin[165] described choreiform movements of the face and fingers in schizophrenic patients, which he called "athetoid ataxia." A virtually identical disturbance referred to as "parakinesia," a term introduced by Wernicke,[139] was also commonly compared with chorea.[103,104,159] This was characterized by continuous, irregular motor activity, whereby patients grimaced, twitched, and jerked continuously. Volitional motor activity was said to become fragmented, stiff, and jerky with loss of the normal, smooth transition between movements.[103,159] Involvement of facial musculature in continuous grimacing and bizarre distortions of facial expression were especially prominent. Speech was often disjointed and characterized by short, sharp bursts, clicking and snorting noises, or utterances of meaningless syllables or words.[102] Bleuler, on the other hand, stated that he had never seen chorea in schizophrenia and attributed the high incidence described by other observers to differences in definition of the term.[26] It is likely that many choreoathetotic signs described in the older literature[208] occurred as a result of organic neurologic disease. More recent studies[144,178] indicate that true chorea or athetosis is extremely rare in chronic psychiatric populations and, when present, is nearly always associated with organic neurologic disease.

Although several of the facial movements listed in Table 12-1 certainly resemble oral–facial dyskinesias of neurologic diseases, the vast majority are best regarded as tic-like disturbances whose repetitive, stereotyped quality differentiates them from chorea, athetosis or dystonia. By contrast with chorea or athetosis, motor activity of the extremities in psychosis usually consists of handling of body parts or external objects, involves the hands more than the feet and toes, and often resembles ordinary volitional activity. Indeed, the presence of typical chorea or dystonia in a psychotic patient should raise the possibility that the illness is symptomatic of an organic extrapyramidal disorder, such as drug-induced dyskinesia, Huntington's chorea, or familial torsion dystonia (dystonia musculorum deformans).

HYPOKINESIA

As with the hyperkinetic disorders, abnormal hypokinetic states most frequently have been described in catatonic schizophrenia. Stereotyped postures refer to awkward and sometimes bizarre body positions that are maintained for long periods of time.[104] Examples include lying in bed with the head elevated as if on a ''psychological pillow,'' lying with knees drawn up to the chin, or sitting with the upper and lower portion of the body twisted at right angles. Manneristic postures, by contrast, are said to be less rigidly maintained and usually are caricatured exaggerations of more normal positions.[104]

The most striking catatonic hypokinetic disorders are those exemplifying states of *automatic obedience* and *negativism*.[104] Automatic obedience is characterized by an abnormal degree of compliance and is manifested by a variety of abnormal postures, the best known of which is ''waxy flexibility'' or *catalepsy,* a relatively uncommon disturbance in which an individual allows himself to be placed in awkward positions that are maintained for prolonged periods. Variations of this unusual disturbance include *mitgehen,* in which a body part continues to move in a given direction in response to light pressure applied by the examiner, or *cooperation,* in which a displaced body part springs back to its original position when released.[104]

Negativism encompasses a broad category of disordered behavior characterized by the failure to do what is suggested, leading to varying states of akinesia. In its most severe form, catatonic stupor, the patient sits or lies motionless with fixed, expressionless facies and resists all efforts at communication or mobilization. Muscle tone is quite variable and, although often increased, the clenched fist or fixed jaw and head position frequently described[104,139,165,215] differs considerably from the more generalized rigidity of extrapyramidal disease. Muscle tone in the limbs or trunk is actually quite inconstant[230] and may increase only in response to attempts to manipulate the patient. Occasionally tone may be extremely flaccid.[139] Hypokinetic and hyperkinetic disturbances sometimes occur in the same patient, either simultaneously or alternately.[103,182] Transient akinetic episodes, often called *blocking,*[230] may occur suddenly and intermittently in the midst of hyperkinetic or normal motor activity or speech, while sudden bursts of hyperkinetic activity may interrupt prolonged periods of akinesia.

The akinetic features of catatonic schizophrenia often closely resemble akinetic disorders of the extrapramidal system. Lack of spontaneity, expressionless facies, fixed postures, transient bursts of activity in akinetic patients, sudden blocking, and frequent hypertonia all have their counterparts in

Parkinson's syndrome. The similarities that have been emphasized,[141,159] however, appear to be limited to external appearances, while the disordered thought processes and extreme degree of negativism characterizing catatonic patients almost never have a counterpart in Parkinson's disease.[139]

Manic-Depressive Illness

Isolated hyperkinetic movement disorders are rarely associated with manic-depressive illness. In manic excitement, a state of generalized psychomotor hyperactivity characterized by well-coordinated motor activity, exaggerated expressions of affect, and pressure of speech often occur but bear little resemblance to any extrapyramidal disorder. The psychomotor retardation associated with severe depression, on the other hand, may so closely resemble Parkinsonian akinesia that practical difficulties in differential diagnosis may arise.[169] Patients perform all movements slowly, speak softly in monotone, and exhibit fixed, unchanging facial expressions. In Parkinson's disease uncomplicated by significant depression, however, the mood, mental content, and facial expression are rarely characterized by the quality of sadness and despair seen in retarded psychotic depression.

Mechanisms of Psychiatric Motor Disorders

There have been attempts on both neurologic and psychologic levels to suggest mechanisms for disorders of movement associated with schizophrenia. Early neurologic approaches (see Bleuler[26]) were strongly influenced by the organic views of Kahlbaum and Wernicke and assumed that focal cerebral pathology would account for these disturbances. Consistent with Hughlings Jackson's hierarchical conception of brain function, it was suggested that because of presumed cortical dysfunction, disinhibited subcortical levels of nervous system function were expressed as catatonic motor activity.[9,192,215] Other examples of presumed release of subcortical mechanisms, such as the behavior of "idiots"[165] and the awkward and repetitive motility of children,[114,215] were offered as supporting evidence. According to Kleist,[159] both hyperkinetic and hypokinetic movement disorders were identical in origin with the motor manifestations of neurologic disease and were due to focal cerebral pathology within cortical and subcortical structures. Other writers, who were strongly influenced by the similarities between postencephalitic Parkinsonism and the motor manifestation of catatonia (see Jeliffe[141]), have also proposed an organic basis for the psychologic and motor disturbances of catatonia.

Psychodynamic interpretations have also been suggested. Kraepelin and Bleuler laid the basis for this approach by attributing them to underlying disturbances of will, thought content, and emotion. Psychoanalytic explanations of catatonic motor disorders[246] provided symbolic explanations of complex stereotypies in which motor behavior was viewed as an external representation of delusional thought content. Although dynamic relationships may occasionally be inferred, relevant delusional thought content is usually undetectable,[143] and even when apparent, is unlikely to be causally related to stereotyped behavior in schizophrenia.[230] A possible contribution of chronic institutionalization and social isolation in stereotyped behavior is suggested by the finding that isolation of non-human primates leads to an increase in stereotyped behavioral patterns that can then be reduced by environmental stimulation.[24] The observation that stereotyped behavior has become less prevalent among chronic schizophrenics in recent years[230] with decreased reliance on prolonged hospitalization also suggests that chronic institutional neglect and social isolation may contribute to the development and maintenance of stereotyped behaviors in chronic psychosis.

Most writers[104,139,141,215,230,236] have recognized the limitation of purely neurologic or psychologic approaches to psychotic motor disturbances and suggested instead that they be referred to as "psychomotor" phenomena.[139,230,236] Implicit in this terminology is the assumption that superficial similarity of appearance does not necessarily indicate a common etiology or pathophysiology for movement disorders in psychiatric and neurologic syndromes. One suggestion has been that abnormal movements may appear either when abnormal regulatory mechanisms of the extrapyramidal system alter output from the motor cortex (the dyskinesias of neurologic disease) or when abnormal influences of other cortical or limbic structures alter the function of the voluntary motor system (the "psychomotor" stereotypies of psychosis).[15]

BIOCHEMICAL MECHANISMS

Recently, "neuropsychopharmacologic" studies have had considerable impact on research and theories directed to an understanding of the phenomena of psychosis. One important observation has been that chronic abuse of amphetamine may produce a paranoid psychosis virtually indistinguishable from paranoid schizophrenia,[56,89] and associated with striking stereotyped behaviors.[211] The psychologic characteristics of this syndrome include paranoid ideation, auditory hallucinations, euphoria, and, in later states, withdrawal and apathy. Although the classical schizophrenic disorder of thought associations and flattening of affect are characteristically absent, amphetamine psychosis is a useful model of acute paranoid schizophrenia.[231] The stereotyped behavior associated with amphetamine psychosis, referred to in Scandanavia as "punding,"[211] closely resembles the motor disturbances of catatonic schizophrenia. Individuals spend hours repetitively handling objects or body parts, dismantling and assembling mechanical equipment, tidying up, applying cosmetics, or pacing in circles. In addition to these complex patterns, simpler manifestations including twisting movements of the trunk and extremities, grimacing, and chewing or bruxism[89,211] have been described. True chorea and athetosis are uncommon but have occasionally occurred in patients with preexisting choreoathetosis or organic brain damage.[173] It is also clear that stimulants such as L-dopa, amphetamine, and methylphenidate can produce transient exacerbations of idiopathic schizophrenia.[7,69]

When given to animals in high doses, amphetamine produces a distinctive motor syndrome characterized by repetitive stereotyped behavior that becomes increasingly variable and complex in higher animals. Rodents continuously sniff, lick, and chew; cats show continuous head movements; dogs persistently run in circles; and monkeys show various movements of the eyes, head, trunk, and extremities or other repetitive behavioral patterns.[206]

The behavioral effects of amphetamine are generally believed to be mediated by the endogenous catecholamines, dopamine and norepinephrine, which act as synaptic neurotransmitters in the central nervous system.[16,207] Amphetamines probably act primarily indirectly through release of catecholamines into the synaptic cleft, blockade of their inactivation by reuptake into the presynaptic nerve terminals, and weak antagonism of monoamine oxidase (MAO).[16] These actions presumably increase the amount of catecholamine available at the postsynaptic receptor site. The weight of evidence strongly indicates that in animals the production of stereotyped behavior by amphetamine is due to activation of dopaminergic mechanisms in the striatum and limbic system.[107,207] Other drugs with dopaminergic activity such as apomorphine, L-dopa, trivastal, and methylphenidate also produce stereotyped behavior in animals identical to that produced by amphetamine.[58,207] Study of the distribution of monoamine containing neurons in both the animal and human brain by fluorescence histochemical methods[5,186] has identified at least two ascending dopaminergic systems important in the mediation of motor activity. A nigrostriatal system which originates in the zona compacta of the midbrain substantia nigra and terminates primarily in the caudate nucleus and putamen (neostriatum), and a mesolimbic system which originates in regions surrounding the interpeduncular nucleus of the ventral tegmentum in midbrain and terminates in the nucleus accumbens, nucleus of the stria terminalis, and the olfactory tubercle—all believed to be elements of the limbic forebrain. Recent studies of the effects of intracerebral injection of dopamine agonists or antagonists, or of lesions within these two pathways,[57,107] indicate that stereotyped behavior is mediated by both systems.

Since the occurrence of stereotyped behavior in animals treated with stimulant drugs is apparently universal and increases in complexity as one ascends the phylogenetic scale, it is reasonable to assume that human stereotyped behavior associated with amphetamine psychosis is an analogous although more complex phenomenon. Nevertheless, the metabolic basis for hyperkinetic motor disorders in schizophrenia remains conjectural. A direct test of the dopamine hypothesis by clinical studies of cerebrospinal fluid or cerebrovascular monoamine metabolites such as homovanillic acid (HVA) have not been done in large numbers of psychotic patients with prominent movement disorders. Nevertheless, the hypothesis that stereotyped motor behavior in schizophrenic psychosis results from functional overactivity of a central dopaminergic system forms a useful starting point for clinical pharmacologic investigations. In support of the idea, cocaine, which has pharmacologic properties similar to amphetamine, was reported by Bleuler to produce a psychotic behavioral syndrome that included "a preoccupation with various tasks that leads to nothing."[27] L-dopa, when given to patients with Parkinson's disease, occasionally produces psychotic agitation as well as stereotyped motor behavior in addition to the more common choreiform dyskinesias induced by this drug. The observation that amphetamines produce stereotyped motor behavior more frequently than extrapyramidal dyskinesias, while the reverse is true for L-dopa, may be due partly to the fact that these drugs are taken by very dissimilar populations of patients. Angrist et al[7] administered a short oral course of L-dopa to schizophrenic patients; although psychosis was exacerbated in each case, motor stereotypies and involuntary facial movements appeared only rarely. It has additionally been observed that pimozide, an antipsychotic drug that appears to act primarily through dopaminergic blockade, abolishes schizophrenic stereotypies.[183]

Even less is known about the biochemical basis for the various hypokinetic manifestations of psychotic illness. Their superficial resemblance to some aspects of Parkinsonism has been commented on, but firm metabolic data to support or refute the hypothesis that either catatonic or depressive stupor is associated with a functional deficiency of dopamine are not available. De Jong[73] demonstrated that a state of akinesia characterized by marked catalepsy could be produced in animals by bulbocapnine, a substance that may interfere with striatal dopamine neurotransmission.[90] Cataleptic behavior in animals appears to have little specific relationship with schizophrenic catatonia, however, and may be produced experimentally by a variety of unrelated compounds, anoxia, electric shock, hepatic failure,[73] and by virtually all of the antipsychotic drugs used in the treatment of schizophrenia.[28] It is also worth noting the general resemblance of the various "amine hypotheses" of affective disorders[18,216] to the concepts of dopamine deficiency that are now well established for Parkinson's disease.

EXTRAPYRAMIDAL SYNDROMES ASSOCIATED
WITH ANTIPSYCHOTIC DRUGS

The antipsychotic drugs are a group of compounds that are effective primarily in schizophrenic psychosis, produce characteristic extrapyramidal syndromes in man, and profoundly affect the motor behavior of laboratory animals. Their effect on motor behavior, which accounts for their designation as "neuroleptic" drugs,[74] is an important feature distinguishing them from the antidepressants, sedative-hypnotics, and minor tranquilizers. Several classes of antipsychotic drugs have been developed since the introduction of psychopharmacologic therapy. These include reserpine and its derivatives, phenothiazines and thioxanthines, butyrophenones, and dibenzodiazepines, a new series of drugs structurally related to the tricyclic antidepressants.[14] All produce distinctive extrapyramidal syndromes, although reserpine has been associated with a more limited variety of neurologic effects,[109,115] and clozapine, a dibenzodiazepine, has a particularly low incidence of such effects.[6,14,20] Antidepressant drugs and lithium salts used in the treatment of manic-depressive illness have rarely been associated with extrapyramidal syndromes and will be discussed only briefly. Inhibitors of monamine oxidase, particularly in toxic doses or combined with tricyclic antidepressants, produce states of extreme restlessness and agitation. The tricyclic antidepressant drugs, such as imipramine, have central anticholinergic effects and accordingly are rarely associated with Parkinsonian effects and can even exert therapeutic effects in Parkinson's disease.[226] A persistent, fine, and rapid tremor of the upper extremities occurs in 10 percent of patients treated with imipramine[160] and may be similar to the physiologic tremor commonly produced by drugs potentiating peripheral adrenergic activity. Severe tremor with ataxia[160] and chorea[39] have occurred following ingestion of toxic amounts of tricyclic antidepressants, but do not appear during routine clinical use. Lithium salts often produce tremor and their toxic effects include myoclonus, but these effects are not necessarily of central origin and are not accompanied by unequivocal extrapyramidal disturbances.

The neuroleptic antipsychotic drugs include a large number of agents with similar pharmacologic action that differ widely in potency and capacity for producing extrapyramidal syndromes. Among the phenothiazines, the relationship between modification of the three-ringed nucleus or the side-chain and pharmacologic activity has been described in detail.[80,82] Modifications of the side-chain produce major changes in potency for both antipsychotic and extrapyramidal effects among the aliphatic (for example, chlorpromazine), piperidine (for example, thioridizine) and piperazine (for example, trifluoperazine) phenothiazines. The piperazine compounds are approximately 10–30 times as potent per milligram as the other classes of phenothiazines for both effects, while the piperidine compounds are relatively low in therapeutic potency (but not in efficacy) and are associated with the lowest incidence of extrapyramidal effects. The side-chain terminal nitrogen-diethyl-substituted analogue of chlorpromazine (diethylperazine) is strongly anticholinergic and is therefore useful as an antiparkinson agent. Modification of the phenothiazine nucleus has led to the development of the antipsychotic thioxanthenes (for example, chlorprothixene). Substitution in the side-chains of the thioxanthenes produces effects similar to the phenothiazines, although there are conflicting reports concerning the relative incidence of extrapyramidal effects during treatment with these drugs.[80,167] The replacement of the sulfur atom of the central ring with an ethylene group resulted in the nonplanar tricyclic antidepressant drugs that are characterized by central adrenergic and anticholinergic effects. Somewhat surprisingly, analogs of imipramine include the new dibenzodiazepines (for example, clozapine), which appear to be effective antipsychotic agents, although they are said to be virtually free of extrapyramidal side effects.[14,20,229]

The butyrophenones (for example, haloperidol) have evolved from normeperidine, have an entirely different chemical structure from the tricyclic antipsychotic agents, and appear to be comparable to the piperazine class of phenothiazines with regard to potency for antipsychotic and extrapyramidal effects.[13] A group of agents closely related to the butyrophenones, the diphenylbutylpiperidines (for example, pimozide) are also highly potent antipsychotic drugs.[235]

Parkinsonism

Each of the cardinal neurologic signs of Parkinson's disease, including akinesia, rigidity, postural abnormalities, and tremor may be associated with antipsychotic drugs so that this syndrome, although sometimes referred to as "pseudoparkinsonism,"[85] in fact closely resembles the major spontaneous forms of Parkinson's disease: paralysis agitans and postencephalitic Parkinsonism.

Bradykinesia ("akinesia") is the earliest, most common, and frequently the only manifestation of drug-induced Parkinsonism[12,85,121] and accounts for the expressionless facies, loss of associated movements, slow initiation of motor activity, soft and monotonous speech, and slow, micrographic handwriting, that are so common in drug-treated psychiatric patients. Alterations in handwriting,[121] reduction in facial expression,[74] and reduced arm-swing[123] are important early signs of akinesia and may be accompanied by subjective symptoms such as muscle fatigue or weakness. Although often difficult, it is important to distinguish these features of drug-induced akinesia from the psychomotor retardation commonly associated with underlying psychiatric illness such as depression or catatonia. Rigidity of the extremities, neck or trunk, usually without a "cogwheel" phenomenon, appears from days to weeks *after* the onset of akinesia. Characteristic Parkinsonian postural abnormalities are also frequent, including flexed posture, impairment of righting responses, and a propulsive or retropulsive gait.

The characteristic 4–6 Hz alternating "pill-rolling" tremor of Parkinson's disease, present at rest and disappearing with action, occurs still later in the course of drug-induced Parkinsonism and is relatively uncommon.[217] As in Parkinson's disease, the tremor is often variable, occurring at higher frequencies and during movement as well as at rest. A fine, perioral tremor, referred to as the "rabbit syndrome," has also been described.[244] A fine distal tremor sometimes occurs acutely following the administration of piperazine phenothiazines,[74,77] but is entirely unlike Parkinsonian tremor and probably represents a toxic exaggeration of physiologic tremor.

Signs of Parkinsonism may begin within a few days of drug treatment with a gradual increase in incidence so that 50–75 percent of cases appear by 1 month and 90 percent of cases within 3 months.[12,109] Following piperazine phenothiazines, the progression of signs is often telescoped so that acute akinesia with mutism may appear within 48 hours followed within days by rigidity and a resultant "akinetic-hypertonic" syndrome.[74] After discontinuation of the neuroleptic drugs, the majority of patients are free of extrapyramidal signs within a few weeks, but in some cases these signs persist for several months[123,126,195] and rarely for as long as a year. Although it is often stated that tolerance develops for the Parkinsonian effects of antipsychotic drugs, few prospective clinical studies have adequately dealt with this phenomenon. Observations that withdrawal of coadministered anticholinergic drugs after several months of administration leads to the appearance of a relatively small incidence of Parkinsonism[81,161] presently provide the only clinical basis for this assumption, although "tolerance" and even "cross-tolerance" to the neuroleptic actions of antipsychotic drugs in animals have been amply demonstrated.[10,181]

Parkinsonism occurs following the use of reserpine, phenothiazines, thioxanthenes, and the butyrophenones. The incidence of Parkinsonism following reserpine given in high doses (usually 5–10 mg/day) as an antipsychotic drug has ranged from 5 to 29 percent.[19,109,115] Following phenothiazines or butyrophenones, incidence has varied between 5 and 60 percent,[109,110,115,221] although incidence in routine psychiatric practice is about 10–15 percent.[12,45]

The reported incidences of drug-induced Parkinsonism appear primarily to have been determined by the potency of antipsychotic drugs studied and the sensitivity of clinical examination. Studies using the potent piperazine phenothiazines[77] or the butyrophenones,[55] and those using sensitive methods for the detection of Parkinsonism,[121,205] have frequently yielded an incidence of greater than 90 percent.

In spite of this nearly universal susceptibility, individual predisposition appears to play a significant role. Attempts to correlate total drug dosage with incidence of Parkinsonism have usually failed to show a clear relationship.[109,115,123,227] In one study,[227] the total doses of trifluoperazine required to produce a similar degree of Parkinsonism ranged from 20 to 480 mg. Dramatic examples of severe Parkinsonism appearing within several days of treatment with small doses of antipsychotic drugs are not uncommon.

There are few clues as to the basis of individual susceptibility to extrapyramidal effects of antipsychotic drugs. In large studies, the age distribution of drug-induced Parkinsonism has closely paralleled that of Parkinson's disease with a sharp rise in incidence after the age of 40.[12] However, some young adults are also affected and occasional cases are reported in children[85] and even in neonates.[127,237] A female-to-male preponderance of 2:1 has been reported,[12,109] but the rates of treatment and dosage of antipsychotic drugs used in females and males are frequently not equivalent.[72,85] One report indicated a higher incidence of drug-induced Parkinsonism in premenopausal than postmenopausal women and found that administration of estrogen hormones to patients being treated with phenothiazines precipitated Parkinsonism within 24–48 hours.[116] In another study,[130] the incidence of Parkinsonism in chronic schizophrenics with previous lobotomy was somewhat higher than in a matched control group given the same phenothiazine. The possibility that increased susceptibility to drug-induced extrapyramidal reactions may be related to subclinical Parkinson's disease has also been raised,[74] but only isolated case reports document such an occurrence.[109,131] The increased prevalence of Parkinson's disease reported to occur in the families of patients with drug-induced Parkinsonism[184] is relatively small and has not been confirmed.[121] The recent finding that drug-induced extrapyramidal syndromes occur with increased incidence in patients with systemic lupus erythematosus treated with steroids[29] is of interest but diffiuclt to interpret.

Acute Dyskinesia (Acute Dystonia)

The acute dyskinesias occur soon after treatment with neuroleptic antipsychotic drugs is started and consist primarily of intermittent or sustained muscular spasms and abnormal postures. Involvement of the muscles of the eyes, face, neck, and throat includes oculogyric crises or other aversive eye movements, blepharospasm, trismus, forced jaw-opening, grimacing, protrusion or twisting of the tongue, distortions of the lips, and glossopharyngeal contractions. Dysarthria, dysphagia, jaw dislocation, and respiratory stridor with cyanosis all may result. When the neck is affected, there may be spasmodic torticollis or retrocollis. The trunk is more prominently affected in children, who may show opisthotonus, scoliosis, lordosis, trunk-flexion, writhing movements, or tortipelvis with a characteristic dystonic gait. Continuous slow writhing movements of the extremities with exaggerated postures of hyperpronation and adduction complete the clinical picture. Acute dyskinesias of lower amplitude unaccompanied by severe muscle spasm also occur,[66] including tongue-protrusion, lip-smacking, blinking, athetosis of the fingers and toes, shoulder-shrugging, and a variety of myoclonic muscle contractions of the face, neck, and extremities.[74,77,213] Subtle forms of these disturbances, such as muscular cramps or tightness of the jaw and tongue with difficulty in chewing or speaking, may occur by themselves or precede the more obvious manifestations.

The acute dyskinesias are very disturbing, frequently painful, and often frightening to affected patients. When severe, they have often been confused with status epilepticus, tetanus, encephalitis, meningitis, rabies, or intracerebral hemorrhage. In addition, because signs may spontaneously remit and exacerbate, and may respond to a broad variety of drugs and sometimes even to suggestion, they may be mistaken as hysterical reactions.[8]

Acute dyskinesias are the earliest drug-induced syndrome to appear and may begin within hours of a single dose of a neuroleptic agent. As a rough generalization, 50 percent occur within 48 hours and perhaps 90 percent within 5 days of drug treatment.[12,78] They may either remit or fluctuate spontaneously over several hours or days but often reappear on reintroduction of other drugs of equal potency.[228] Long-acting phenothiazines given by injection, such as fluphenazine decanoate, may produce acute dyskinesias within 72 hours of each administration.[142] Persistent dyskinesia does not occur following acute exposure to ordinary doses of antipsychotic drugs. Although recently a concept of "side-effect breakthrough" has been discussed in relation to an apparently lower incidence of both acute dyskinesias and Parkinsonism when extremely large doses of the drugs are used in young patients,[209] this intriguing observation requires further documentation. There appear to be no well-documented cases of acute dyskinesias following the use of reserpine or its analogs. Following routine clinical use of neuroleptic agents, the overall incidence of acute dystonic reactions is approximately 2 1/2 to 5 percent,[12,45] and is therefore the least frequent drug-induced extrapyramidal syndrome. As in the case of Parkinsonism, however, the more potent agents, including the piperazine phenothiazines and the butyrophenones, are particularly likely to produce acute dyskinesias and, in some series, are reported to account for dystonic reactions in 50 percent or more of cases.[78,177]

Few factors contributing to increased susceptibility to these reactions have been uncovered. Incidence rates that are twice as high in men than women and also higher in young adults and children[12,120] have been reported for the acute drug-induced dyskinesias. Children under 15 years of age frequently show more severe and generalized involvement of the trunk and extremities, while older individuals tend to show more restricted involvement of the neck, face, tongue, and upper extremities.[12] There is one report of several patients with untreated hypoparathyroidism and hypocalcemia who suffered severe acute dystonia within hours of the administration of small doses of a phenothiazine.[214] Treatment of hypocalcemia and removal of the antipsychotic drug resulted in disappearance of this reaction and the failure to provoke it by further challenges with the drug. Whether this reaction was due to increased peripheral neuromuscular excitability or the presence of occult extrapyramidal disease, which occasionally accompanies hypoparathyroidism, is uncertain. There is reportedly a relatively high incidence of drug-induced acute dystonia in the relatives of patients with torsion dystonia,[88] and occasionally other families with striking susceptibility to drug-induced dyskinesias are reported.[11]

Akathisia

Akathisia is a state of motor restlessness that occurs following administration of all antipsychotic drugs. Because of its occurrence in postencephalitic and idiopathic Parkinson's disease and its occasional response to antiparkinsonian medications, it is often assumed to be an extrapyramidal disturbance, although there is little compelling evidence to support this assumption. There is usually a striking complaint of tension, being driven to move, pulling or drawing sensations in the legs, and an inability to tolerate inactivity.[213] The objective manifestations include a variety of patterns of restless motor activity. When mild, these may be confined to shuffling or tapping movements of the feet while sitting and continuous shifting of weight and rocking of the trunk while standing. In more severe cases, patients appear agitated, are unable to sit, stand or lie still and pace or run incessantly. Earlier writers referred to these are ''paradoxical behavioral reactions''[213] or ''turbulent reactions.''[19] Since this syndrome may be confused with psychotic agitation or anxiety, it must be differentiated from states of restlessness determined psychologically or by other causes.[213,247]

Akathisia may begin within several days following the start of drug-treatment but usually does not occur within the first 48 hours. Unlike acute dyskinesias, the incidence of akathisia continues to increase with time so that about 50 percent of such reactions occur within a month and 90 percent within 2 or 3 months of the start of exposure to a neuroleptic drug.[12] The duration of akathisia is extremely variable, and symptoms may spontaneously appear and disappear. If the offending drug is continued, akathisia may subside within several days or weeks but frequently persists without change. Although drug withdrawal usually results in improvement, the symptoms may persist unchanged for several months or may even worsen.[126,166] The fact that akathisia often occurs simultaneously with other extrapyramidal syndromes has complicated its clinical description. Its frequent association with akinesia and rigidity, for example, may result in the paradoxical and striking appearance of incessant walking in patients frozen in fixed postures.[77,93] Although chewing movements of the tongue and jaw and lip-smacking are included in some descriptions of akathisia,[12,217] they probably represent coexistent acute or chronic dyskinesias which should be considered separately.

Akathisia is probably the most common reaction to antipsychotic drugs and occurs following administration of reserpine,[19,109,115] the phenothiazines,[12] and the butyrophenones.[13] The incidence of akathisia following reserpine has ranged between 0.5 and 8 percent.[109,115] As in the other drug-induced syndromes, the reported incidence among the phenothiazines varies primarily with the potency of the drug being studied. Following the potent piperazine phenothiazines incidences between 5 and 50 percent have been reported,[77,110,115] although in routine clinical use the incidence is about 20 percent.[12]

Factors that might account for differences in individual susceptibility are not known. Akathisia has been reported to be more common in women than men[12] but this finding is inconstant and, as in Parkinsonism, such data may be influenced by the tendency for women to receive somewhat higher doses of antipsychotic drugs. Unlike the other drug-induced syndromes, no specific age predisposition has been noted so that incidence is fairly uniform between the ages of 12 and 65 years.[12]

Tardive dyskinesia

Tardive dyskinesia (late or persistent dyskinesia) is a hyperkinetic movement disorder which occurs following prolonged exposure to phenothiazines or butyrophenones and may be chronic or irreversible.[137] It is characterized by a remarkable variety of diverse involuntary movements which include oralfacial dyskinesia, chorea, athetosis, dystonia, hemiballismus, tics, and other abnormal postures. Tremor, however, does not occur as a part of this syndrome.

Oralfacial dyskinesia, also known as the buccolinguomasticatory syndrome,[99,223] is the most characteristic and well-known feature of tardive dyskinesia. Restricted vermicular movements of the tongue on the floor of the mouth are said to be a particularly early sign of oral dyskinesia.[66] Protruding, twisting, and curling tongue movements combined with pouting, sucking, and twisting lip movements, bulging of the cheeks, and various chewing jaw movements are characteristic in fully developed cases. In contrast with acute dyskinesia, upper portions of the face are often relatively spared,[70] although frequent blinking, blepharospasm, and brief upward deviation of the eyes[66] may also occur. In elderly individuals, oralfacial dyskinesia is often the earliest and most prominent feature but this usually becomes associated with restless, choreiform movements of the extremities and distal athetosis, consisting of twisting, flexion-extension, and spreading movements of the fingers, tapping motions of the feet, and dorsiflexion of the toes. Abduction postures and ballistic movements of the arms are additional features. Abnormalities of gait and trunk-posture are frequent and include lordosis, rocking and swaying, shifting of weight, shoulder shrugging, and rotatory pelvic movements. Although some of these movements resemble akathisia, they differ in being unaccompanied by a strong subjective need to move or walk incessantly.[66] Myoclonic jerks, grunting vocalizations, and disturbances or respiratory rhythm form additional features of the syndrome.[135]

In adults, cases in which severe axial dystonia dominate the clinical picture have been relatively uncommon and, interestingly, in reported cases, have usually affected individuals below the age of 50 years.[49,64,83,137,149] In children a syndrome resembling tardive dyskinesia has been reported[1,174,200] which is characterized predominantly by chorea of the extremities, athetosis, myoclonus, and hemiballismus. In contrast to the adult syndrome, involvement of the mouth and face is rare in children.[1,200] To date, all reported pediatric cases have appeared for the first time following the discontinuation of a phenothiazine and have resolved completely within one year of stopping the drug.

As in other choreoathetotic disorders, movements increase with emotional stress and decrease with drowsiness or sedation. Repetitive voluntary activity using other parts of the body,[70,223] concentration on motor tasks,[70] or attempts at voluntary inhibition of one portion of the dyskinesia[83] usually enhance the dyskinesia. Although extreme oralfacial dyskinesia may interfere with speech, eating, or respiration and occasionally produce oral ulcerations, reports of significant disability are exceptional.[135] Institutionalized patients characteristically seem unaware of and undisturbed by their movement, although this is not universal,[242] as some patients are quite troubled and embarrassed by them.

Tardive dyskinesia begins following a minimum of 3–6 months of exposure to antipsychotic drugs, though the majority of cases have been reported after at least 2 years of treatment.[64,99] Although onset within the first 6 months is occasionally reported,[72,99,223] it is possible that the early hypokinetic effects of antipsychotic drugs mask the signs of tardive dyskinesias and delay their diagnosis.[72,97] The dyskinesia usually appears while patients are still taking an antipsychotic drug,[70] but characteristically it increases or even makes its initial appearance following the reduction of dose or complete withdrawal of the drug.[72] According to one review,[64] 5–40 percent of asymptomatic patients develop dyskinesia upon discontinuation of prolonged treatment with neuroleptic agents.

Irreversibility of dyskinesia following discontinuation of antipsychotic drugs is the most distinctive and disturbing feature of the syndrome. Despite earlier statements to the contrary,[162] the fact that dyskinesia may persist for years following discontinuation of antipsychotic drugs or be irreversible is now well-documented[64] and widely accepted.[1] Although short-term studies of the effects of drug-withdrawal have frequently found an increase of dyskinesia in a large proportion of patients,[66,70,86] long-term studies indicate that once dyskinesia appears, it is not progressive and either remains unchanged or shows gradual improvement on discontinuation of treatment.[64]

The prognosis with regard to recovery has been difficult to assess. Some patients show what appears to be a "withdrawal" dyskinesia which is limited to a period of several weeks following reduction or discontinuation of antipsychotic drugs.[137,201] During one 7–10 month follow-up study of 273 patients with tardive dyskinesia whose antipsychotic medications were discontinued, dyskinesias disappeared in 19 percent, were reduced in 19 percent, and remained unchanged in 50 percent.[70] In another study, all signs of dyskinesia regressed more or less completely within 3 years of discontinuation of antipsychotic drugs.[122] Complete recovery is said to be more likely in young adults[70,137] and, to date, has been universal in children.[1,174] The course of dyskinesias in patients who continue to receive antipsychotic drugs is presently unclear. In one study[125] approximately 40 percent of patients became free of symptoms after 15 months of unchanged drug treatment. In other studies, however, assessment of patients 6–18 months following therapeutic trials of phenothiazines used to suppress dyskinesia have indicated either no change[51] or worsening[62] of dyskinesia.

Tardive dyskinesia has been reported in patients exposed to virtually all phenothiazines as well as butyrophenones[137] but has only rarely been associated with reserpine.[70,242,248] Piperazine phenothiazines are reported to produce the syndrome earlier and more frequently..[99,242] Evaluation of incidence following specific drugs, however, is complicated by the fact that most patients have been exposed to multiple drugs by the time of its appearance.

Evidence of an etiologic role of antipsychotic drugs in tardive dyskinesia is mainly epidemiologic but at this time seems to be thoroughly convincing.[17,64,65] Comparative studies of treated and untreated patients within the same institution,[99,205] and in institutions where drugs are used freely compared with those in which they have been avoided,[61,72] have disclosed, with few exceptions,[75] a significantly higher incidence of chronic dyskinesia in drug-treated patients. Attempts to determine the amount of drug-exposure necessary to produce the disorder have been inconclusive.[64] Although some studies have found an association with duration of drug treatment,[67,205] or drug dosage,[62] others have not confirmed this point.[34,72,151] Nevertheless, most patients who develop tardive dyskinesia while being treated with antipsychotic drugs have received large quantities of drugs by the time the dyskinesia is observed. They have usually been exposed to several antipsychotic drugs and antiparkinson agents.

The reported prevalence of tardive dyskinesia in chronic, institutionalized patients has varied between 0.5 and 40 percent.[17,64] Differences in definitions of the syndrome, patient populations, methods of case-ascertainment, and neurologic assessment have made an accurate determination of incidence impossible,[64] but it is currently estimated that 3–6 percent of patients in mental hospitals and approximately 20 percent of elderly, chronically institutionalized patients exhibit drug-induced tardive dyskinesia.[1] Although tardive dyskinesia is relatively uncommon among outpatients or in acute psychiatric units, cases have been reported in this group as well.[92,137]

Factors predisposing to tardive dyskinesia have been widely discussed. There is no evidence that the specific underlying psychiatric disorder plays any role in predisposition. Although the point has not been studied formally, there is no evidence that pre-existing hyperkinetic movement disorders associated with chronic psychoses have any relationship to subsequent appearance of tardive dyskinesia. The majority of cases have been reported in patients with chronic schizophrenia, affective illness and a variety of dementias,[34,72,99] reflecting the fact that these patients are most often chronically treated with antipsychotic-neuroleptic drugs. Importantly, however, tardive dyskinesia also occurs in patients treated with neuroleptics for psychoneurosis, gastrointestinal disturbances, chronic pain syndromes, and personality disorders.[72,83,92,99,155] Although prospective studies have not been done, there is no evidence that tardive dyskinesia occurs with a higher incidence in patients previously manifesting acute dyskinesia. On the other hand, a history of drug-induced Parkinsonism does occur with increased frequency in patients who subsequently develop tardive dyskinesia, although cases frequently occur without antecedent Parkinsonism.

Although early reports[83,99,135,162] emphasized a relationship with organic brain disease, with rare exception[86] subsequent studies seriously question an association of tardive dyskinesia with preceding organic brain damage, electroconvulsive therapy,[34,72,75] or leukotomy. Other reports have claimed an association with advanced age[34,99] and female sex.[135,151] However, studies taking into account the characteristics of patient populations at risk have suggested that advanced age[151,205] and female sex[62,72,99] are not correlated with the development of tardive dyskenesia. In view of the complex characteristics of chronically treated patient populations, the precise contribution of brain damage and advanced age to individual susceptibility remains problematical.

Comparison of Drug-induced Syndromes
With Spontaneous Movement Disorders

In general, the extrapyramidal syndromes induced by antipsychotic drugs bear close resemblance to well-known spontaneous movement disorders. From a practical point of view, the similarity is usually so great that clinical differentiation depends on the history of drug exposure; nevertheless, certain distinctive clinical features can be pointed out.

In drug-induced Parkinsonism, the sequence of appearance, topographic pattern, and relative frequency of signs typically show important differences when compared with paralysis agitans or post encephalitic Parkinsonism. While a rhythmic resting tremor, frequently restricted to one extremity, is a common early feature of paralysis agitans, it occurs infrequently and late in the course of drug-induced Parkinsonism. On the other hand, postural or action tremors of higher frequency seem to be more common following drugs that in Parkinson's disease. Drug-induced Parkinsonism nearly always produces symmetrical akinesia and rigidity from the time of onset, while paralysis agitans and postencephalitic Parkinsonism, especially in early stages, are characteristically asymmetrical in distribution. It should be emphasized, however, that variability also exists among patients with spontaneous forms of Parkinson's disease. Despite the fact that drug-induced Parkinsonism, postencephalitic Parkinsonism, and idiopathic forms of paralysis agitans all differ in the frequency of certain physical signs, it is often impossible to differentiate individual cases solely on the basis of clinical appearance.

Drug-induced acute dystonia closely resembles dystonia as it occurs in a number of toxic, metabolic, infectious, traumatic, or degenerative diseases of the basal ganglia. By contrast with disorders in which dystonia represents only one of several neurologic deficits, torsion dystonia (dystonia musculorum deformans) is manifested exclusively by dystonic postures and movements and, as a result, often strongly resembles the drug-induced syndrome. The broad spectrum of severity, which in torsion dystonia ranges from restricted involvement of one extremity to generalized dystonia, is reproduced in the broad range of signs occurring acutely following antipsychotic drugs. Interestingly, age appears to influence the distribution of dystonia similarly in both conditions. Children under 15 years frequently manifest generalized dystonia following drugs, which resembles the distribution of childhood torsion dystonia, while adults more commonly manifest localized involvement of the neck, face, and upper extremities similar to the more restricted distribution of adult torsion dystonia.[12] Additionally, in both disorders, dystonia may increase or remit in response to emotional stress or verbal suggestion, respectively, leading to the misdiagnosis of hysteria.[8,88]

The akathisia associated with antipsychotic drugs is indistinguishable from that which occasionally occurs in Parkinson's disease. In Parkinson's disease, however, akathisia is relatively uncommon and rarely dominates the clinical picture as it often does following antipsychotic drugs.[217] Although drug-induced akathisia has also been referred to as a "restless legs syndrome," its relationship to those uncommon disorders of unknown etiology[87,233] characterized by leg pain and isolated continuous movements of the lower extremities and toes, is obscure.

Individually considered, the manifestations of tardive dyskinesia are quite similar to those characterizing a number of spontaneous extrapyramidal diseases. The choreiform movements of the extremities closely resemble those of Huntington's chorea; the oralfacial movements are indistinguishable from those of spontaneous oralfacial dyskinesia, and the dystonic postures may be identical to those of familial torsion dystonia. As in drug-induced acute dyskinesia and familial torsion dystonia, age may determine the topographical distribution of tardive dyskinesia. Young adults[70] and children[174,200] tend to have greater involvement of the extremities and trunk while older individuals tend to show more restricted involvement of the oral region. The possible resemblance of tardive dyskinesia to other spontaneous disorders of the extrapyramidal system has been widely considered. One issue is whether tardive dyskinesia is distinct from the oral dyskinesias that occur spontaneously in the chronically institutionalized patients likely to be exposed chronically to treatment with antipsychotic drugs. Oralfacial dyskinesias in such patients are often associated with advanced age, cerebral arteriosclerotic disease, and the edentulous state and may be indistinguishable in appearance from those of tardive dyskinesia. As a rule however, the fact that such dyskinesias are characteristically restricted to the mouth is the principal feature which differentiates them from the more generalized choreoathetosis usually evident in tardive dyskinesia. Because of its generalized distribution, tardive dyskinesia is commonly compared with Huntington's chorea. The resemblance in many cases is strong, although distinguishing features have been pointed out.[34] In contrast to Huntington's chorea, tardive dyskinesia is characterized by more extreme involvement of oral structures, relative sparing of the upper face, and a less prominent disturbance of gait. As in drug-induced Parkinsonism, however, differences of this type are frequently not helpful in the identification of individual cases.

Taken as a group, it is striking how closely the drug-induced extrapyramidal syndromes resemble the various neurologic syndromes that were associated with encephalitis lethargica. Virtually identical syndromes characterized by akinesia, rigidity, dystonia, dyskinesia, akathisia, chorea, tic, and autonomic disturbances have been described in both conditions.[77,213] The similarities are so strong that some classifications of the antipsychotic drug-induced syndromes have used terminology identical to that of original descriptions of encephalitis lethargica and the post encephalitic states.[74,77,78] A feature particularly common to both conditions is the frequency with which hysteria has been suspected in patients with isolated extrapyramidal signs. In addition, certain individual signs such as the oculogyric crisis have been virtually unique for these two conditions, while others, such as the "fly-catcher tongue" described in both acute[213] and tardive[135] dyskinesia occur in such high frequency that they have been regarded as characteristic features of each syndrome.

MECHANISMS OF EXTRAPYRAMIDAL SYNDROMES INDUCED BY ANTIPSYCHOTIC DRUGS

Current information concerning putative neurotransmitters in the central nervous system and the action of antipsychotic drugs, although far from complete, allows tentative neuropharmacologic explanations of some features of the drug-induced syndromes. Dopamine, acetylcholine, gamma-aminobutyric acid (GABA) and serotonin all occur in relatively high concentrations in the basal ganglia—structures that form much of the anatomical substrate of the extrapyramidal system. A reciprocal balance between dopaminergic and cholinergic activity in the neostriatum (caudate nucleus and putamen) has been proposed as an important basis for normal extrapyramidal function. This concept derives from numerous experimental and clinical observations in animals and man.[2,21,84,107,154,176,177] The most compelling clinical example of this balance occurs in Parkinson's disease in which a deficiency of dopamine in the neostriatum results in a state of apparent relative cholinergic sensitivity. Thus, physostigmine, a centrally active anticholinesterase which increases the striatal concentration of acetylcholine, dramatically worsens Parkinsonism, while anticholinergic drugs improve Parkinsonism.[84] All of the currently available antipsychotic drugs produce extrapyramidal syndromes and also interfere with dopaminergic mechanisms within the brain. For the Parkinsonism and tardive dyskinesia induced by antipsychotic drugs, a reciprocal "dopaminergic:cholinergic balance" also appears to exist. This conclusion is supported by the pattern of responses of these syndromes to a variety of drugs which are known to act on the metabolism or receptors of dopamine and acetylcholine (Table 12-2). Recent studies of the effects of some agonists (L-dopa, apomorphine, amphetamine, trivastal) and antagonists of dopamine (phenothiazines and butyrophenones) suggest a more specific hypothesis concerning the balance between dopamine and acetylcholine than has heretofore

Table 12-2

Dopaminergic–Cholinergic Effects on Drug-induced Extrapyramidal Syndromes

	Dopamine Effects		Acetylcholine Effects	
	*Increased**	*Decreased*	*Increased†*	*Decreased††*
Parkinsonism				
Phenothiazine-induced	No change (L-dopa)[106,251] Improved (L-dopa)[36]	—	Worse [2,112]	Improved [177,221,224]
Reserpine-induced	Improved (L-dopa)[71]	—	—	—
Acute dyskinesia	Improved [95,113] (apomorphine, methylphenidate)	—	No change[212]	Improved
Akathisia	Improved[42] methylphenidate	—	No change[2]	Little change
Tardive dyskinesia	Worse [45,112,128] (L-dopa)	Improved [45,147] (antipsychotic drugs; α-methyl-p-tyrosine)	No change [112,240] Slight improvement[158]	Worse[112]

*Drugs used indicated in parentheses.

†Physostigmine used in all cases.

††Anticholinergic drugs.

241

been proposed. Thus, the phenothiazines and butyrophenones increase the rate of synthesis[220,241] and the neuronal release[234] of acetylcholine in the striatum, while dopamine agonists have the opposite effects.[220,234] These findings provide evidence for the hypothesis that there may be inhibitory dopamine-receptors located on striatal cholinergic neurones that can modulate cholinergic activity. Hence, at the neuronal level, dopamine antagonists, as a consequence of their interference with striatal dopaminergic neurotransmission, appear to increase the activity of striatal cholinergic neurones.[220,234,241] Such an effect would readily account for the reciprocal dopaminergic-cholinergic relationship in behavioral and motor activity which has been observed. Although a possible role of other neurotransmitters in the actions of antipsychotic drugs has not been excluded, at the present time, their consideration does not further clarify the mechanism of drug-induced extrapyramidal syndromes.

Striatal-nigral Feedback Mechanisms

The phenothiazines and butyrophenones appear to exert their pharmacologic action by interfering with the synaptic functions of catecholamines, particularly of dopamine, in the brain. They may act in this way by inhibiting the presynaptic release of dopamine[218] and by blocking postsynaptic dopamine receptors. The concept that phenothiazines interact with dopamine receptors is supported by the similarity of the three-dimensional molecular structures of chlorpromazine and dopamine.[132] By the use of cell fractionation techniques it has been shown that, similar to peripheral adrenergic receptor blocking agents such as phenoxybenzamine or propranolol, neuroleptic drugs have a high binding-affinity for nerve-ending membranes.[79,219] There is evidence for the blockade of peripheral adrenergic receptors by neuroleptic drugs,[35,252] and recently electrophysiologic[38,253] and biochemical[53,146,148] studies have provided evidence that they block central dopamine receptors as well.

It has been suggested that the synthesis and release of dopamine in the nigrostriatal system are enhanced in response to the blockade of dopamine receptors by the effects of neuronally mediated feedback mechanisms involving descending striatal-nigral pathways.[21] Blockade of dopamine neurotransmission by antipsychotic drugs results in what has been interpreted as removal of feedback inhibition, and hence an increased firing rate of nigrostriatal neurones[38] and activation of the synthesis and release of dopamine, as if to overcome the more primary antidopaminergic actions of the drugs.[50] L-dopa, apomorphine, and trivastal, on the other hand, are agonists of dopamine receptors and seem to induce increased feedback inhibition, as evidenced by decreased firing in nigrostriatal neurones[37] and reduced metabolic turnover of dopamine in the neostriatum.[187] The neuronally mediated control of the turnover of dopamine is distinct from other mechanisms of feedback inhibition that have been described, including biochemical end-product inhibition of tyrosine hydroxylase by catechols[140] and poorly characterized local "perisynaptic" receptor-mediated feedback mechanisms,[150] and may be abolished by a lesion in the ascending nigrostriatal tract.[189] Nevertheless, L-dopa (and its product, dopamine) and apomorphine are catechols and even trivastal produces catecholic metabolites and so may partly alter the metabolism of dopamine by inhibiting striatal tyrosine hydroxylase directly.

Since anticholinergic drugs prevent the enhancement of dopamine-turnover by phenothiazines,[31] it has been suggested that striatal-nigral feedback may be at least partially mediated by cholinergic neurones.[21] Although there is histochemical evidence for a cholinergic striatal-nigral pathway based on relatively nonspecific techniques,[190] interruption of these putative cholinergic striatal-nigral connections does not alter the increased turnover of dopamine in the nigrostriatal neurons.[22] Moreover, such lesions fail to lower nigral levels of acetylcholine or the activity of the enzyme that synthesizes it, choline acetyltransferase;[175] moreover, there are no physiologic data to indicate the existence of a descending cholinergic striatal-nigral connection. It is therefore likely that any cholinergic role in the regulation of dopamine turnover by feedback is limited to intrastriatal neurones or to local cholinergic neurones in the midbrain.

Recent evidence suggests that a striatal-nigral pathway for feedback inhibition may be mediated by GABA neurones.[100,124,204] Electrical stimulation in the caudate nucleus inhibits the firing of neurones of the substantia nigra; this effect is blocked by putative blockers of GABA receptors and is thought to be mediated through a descending striatonigral projection using GABA as a neurotransmitter.[204] Midbrain neurones in the zona compacta of the substantia nigra inhibited by stimulation at the caudate nucleus are also strongly depressed by microiontophoretic application of GABA but not acetylcholine, glycine, or dopamine.[100] The facts that the substantia nigra contains the highest concentration of GABA and its synthesizing enzyme (glutamic acid decarboxylase) in the brain,[93] and furthermore that lesions of the caudate nucleus or its efferent projections lead to depletion of nigral GABA and loss of glutamic acid decarboxylase activity,[152] provide additional support for a functionally important striatonigral GABA-mediated pathway.

One method commonly used for estimating the metabolic turnover of dopamine is to determine brain concentrations of homovanillic acid (HVA), the principal metabolite of dopamine.[21] A transient rise in cerebral ventricular HVA levels, a reasonably accurate reflection of striatal HVA, has also been demonstrated following the acute administration of antipsychotic drugs in several species.[119,171] Studies of the effect of phenothiazines and butyrophenones on concentrations of HVA in the lumbar cerebrospinal fluid of humans indicate that a similar mechanism is identifiable in man. Thus, Persson and Roos[198] found levels of cerebrospinal fluid HVA to be higher in chronic schizophrenics treated with antipsychotic drugs than in normal controls; they also reported an increase in the levels of HVA within hours following intravenous administration of haloperidol to two chronic schizophrenic patients.[197] Moreover, Bowers[30] found a rise in HVA concentrations after treatment of psychotic patients with antipsychotic drugs when the cerebrospinal fluid was obtained following probenecid, a drug that blocks reabsorption of acidic metabolites of monoamines from the cerebrospinal fluid into blood. Chase and his colleagues[48] studied this phenomenon in relation to drug-induced extrapyramidal syndromes and measured cerebrospinal fluid HVA in 20 chronic schizophrenic patients. Some of the patients manifested Parkinsonism, tardive dyskinesia, or a combination of the two syndromes, and had significantly lower levels of HVA than patients without neurologic signs while receiving antipsychotic drugs. It was therefore suggested that drug-induced extrapyramidal syndromes may preferentially appear in patients in whom compensatory acceleration of monoamine formation in response to antipsychotic drugs is impaired.

Further clinical investigations of the relationship between extrapyramidal syndromes and the activation of monoamine-turnover by antipsychotic drugs may, by identifying patients with abnormal cerebral metabolic responses to antipsychotic drugs, help to predict an increased susceptibility to drug-induced extrapyramidal syndromes. Since the actions of phenothiazines and butyrophenones appear to include competition with dopamine at striatal dopamine receptor sites,[53] a compensatory increase in the synthesis and release of dopamine in patients treated with antipsychotic drugs may be of some functional importance. Increased turnover of dopamine as measured by the probenecid-induced accumulation of cerebrospinal fluid HVA before and after haloperidol treatment has been demonstrated in patients with various spontaneous extrapyramidal disorders,[46] and is currently being studied in patients with drug-induced syndromes as well.[47]

Parkinsonism

A variety of anatomical[5,186] and physiologic studies[245] have demonstrated an ascending dopaminergic nigrostriatal pathway, and its functional importance in relation to Parkinson's syndrome has been reviewed extensively.[133] Reserpine depletes brain dopamine, norepinephrine, and serotonin by interfering with presynaptic vesicular storage mechanisms, thereby permitting increased degradation by monoamine oxidase. Reserpine and tetrabenazine, a synthetic analog of reserpine with a similar mechanism of action, can produce Parkinsonism.[45] In animals, reserpine induces a state of catalepsy characterized by profound akinesia and rigidity that is dramatically reversed by L-dopa.[41] The phenothiazines, thioxanthenes, and butyrophenones appear to produce a state of functional deficiency of dopamine by their antagonistic actions at synapses that utilize dopamine. In laboratory animals, these drugs induce catalepsy and antagonize the behavioral effects of the dopamine agonists L-dopa, apomorphine, and amphetamine.[28] When used clinically, α-methyl-p-tyrosine, a drug that prevents the synthesis of catecholamines by inhibition of tyrosine hydroxylase, also produces Parkinsonism.[45] Although a significant role for norepinephrine blockade has not been entirely excluded by these observations, the weight of evidence indicates that drug-induced Parkinsonism is primarily due to interference with extrapyramidal dopaminergic mechanisms.[133]

The effects of drugs used to treat drug-induced Parkinsonism are generally consistent with this neuropharmacologic mechanism. L-dopa reverses the motor inhibitory effects of reserpine in animals[41] and man,[71] presumably by replacement of depleted catecholamines. In cases of Parkinsonism induced by neuroleptic drugs, oral L-dopa has been ineffective,[106,251] presumably because of persistent blockade of postsynaptic dopamine-receptors due to continued use of the offending drugs; nevertheless, in one study,[36] intravenous L-dopa produced a transient improvement of Parkinsonism induced by chlorpromazine or haloperidol. In general, L-dopa cannot be used in the management of neurologic syndromes of patients who are also psychotic because of the risk of agitation and worsening of their mental status.[250]

If drug-induced Parkinsonism is due to a functional deficiency of dopamine, then, as in Parkinson's disease, cholinergic sensitivity should be demonstrable. In two studies, physostigmine was found to exacerbate phenothiazine-induced Parkinsonism.[2,112] The effect of anticholinergic drugs is less clear, however. The failure of many investigators to distinguish between acute dyskinesias, in which anticholinergic drugs are known to be dramatically effective, and Parkinsonism has obscured the question somewhat. When given after the appearance of Parkinsonian signs, anticholinergic drugs are usually of some benefit, [177,221,224] although, in one study, no effect was observed following intravenous administration.[224] When given prophylactically, the frequency of Parkinsonism may not be affected,[81] although the severity of signs is probably reduced. Recent studies in which anticholinergic drugs have been withdrawn during the course of chronic antipsychotic drug therapy have estimated the incidence of Parkinsonism during treatment with antipsychotic drugs to be between 9 and 30 percent.[81,161,191] There is some indication that the rate of appearance of Parkinsonism is higher when anticholinergics are discontinued within 3 months of the start of therapy than at later times.[81,161] These findings suggest that "tolerance" to extrapyramidal effects of neuroleptic agents develops within 3 months; they have important parallels in animal experiments in which tolerance, and even cross-tolerance among dissimilar agents to the dopamine-receptor blocking and dopamine-turnover increasing actions of the drugs, have been reported recently.[10,181] The differences in extrapyramidal effects of antipsychotic drugs have been attributed to their potency as anticholinergic agents.[179,232] Thus, the fact that drugs with relatively strong anticholinergic properties, such as thioridazine or clozapine, are associated with a lower incidence of Parkinsonism provides additional evidence that cholinergic mechanisms influence this syndrome.

Akathisia

The pathophysiology of motor restlessness or akathisia following neuroleptic drugs is unknown at the present time. Like Parkinsonism, it is commonly associated with treatment with reserpine, phenothiazines, and butyrophenones, although a form of motor restlessness has also been associated with the use of barbiturates.[43] Akathisia is relatively resistent to treatment with anticholinergic and antihistaminic drugs and shows no response to physostigmine.[2] A possible animal model of akathisia is suggested by the observation that very small doses of haloperidol, but not higher doses, stimulate locomotor activity in rats.[60] Amphetamines reportedly ameliorate akathisia in man,[42] suggesting that akathisia may be related to interference with catecholamine mechanisms. More convincing evidence to support a specific relationship between akathisia and the effects of antipsychotic drugs on catecholamine transmission is lacking, however. Furthermore, although akathisia's occurrence in Parkinson's disease has led to its commonly assumed extrapyramidal origin, the existence of a similar syndrome that occurs in the absence of evident extrapyramidal disease[87] raises the possibility that an entirely different and perhaps even peripheral mechanism may be responsible.

Acute Dyskinesia (Acute Dystonia)

Biochemical and neurophysiologic mechanisms underlying the acute dyskinesias associated with neuroleptic drugs are presently as obscure as the spontaneously occurring dystonic syndromes. Animal models are not available, since acute dystonia evidently does not occur following phenothiazines in lower laboratory animals, and it has only occasionally been observed in monkeys.[91] The fact that acute dystonia may follow relatively small doses of phenothiazines or butyrophenones but does not occur following even large doses of reserpine suggests that the unique effect of the phenothiazines and butyrophenones on neuronal membranes in general and at dopaminergic synapses in particular may be responsible, but little additional evidence supports this assumption. The immediate reversal of these reactions by anticholinergic drugs suggests, by analogy to Parkinsonism, that an acute functional deficiency of dopamine may play a role. Reports of reversing acute dyskinesias by drugs with dopaminergic effects such as apomorphine and methylphenidate[95,113] provide additional evidence along these lines. However, a number of other drugs with various actions have also been reported to reverse acute dyskinesia, including barbiturates,[111] caffeine,[213] diazepam,[164] and meperidine.[196] Physostigmine has apparently not been given during acute dyskinesia, although in one study its repeated administration early in the course of treatment to patients receiving fluphenazine did not increase the frequency of acute dyskinesias.[212]

The resemblance of many acute dyskinesias to those produced by L-dopa in patients with Parkinson's disease suggests the alternative possibility that the acute extrapyramidal effects of the antipsychotic drugs may be related to dopaminergic hyperactivity rather than deficiency. A systematic test of this hypothesis by the administration of even higher acute parenteral doses of the offending neuroleptic agents in search of a paradoxical beneficial effect has apparently not been reported. The capacity of the phenothiazines and butyrophenones to accelerate acutely the synthesis and turnover of dopamine may be relevant for such a mechanism. Possibly, in susceptible individuals, increased availability of dopamine successfully competes with or outlasts the dopamine-antagonistic effects of the precipitating drug. A related hypothesis suggests that the release of dopamine may be activated in branches of nigro-striatal neurones at whose terminals the effects of neuroleptic drugs are incomplete.[172] The capacity of phenothiazines to block presynaptic reuptake of dopamine[136] and theoretically to potentiate its effect in this manner is relatively minor and unlikely to be relevant to their clinical effects.

Finally, it is quite possible that acute dyskinesias arise by mechanisms entirely separate from dopaminergic blockade in the nigrostriatal system. The fact that metoclopramide, a nonphenothiazine antiemetic drug, occasionally produces acute dyskinesia[44] but has not been reported to produce Parkinsonism or to worsen spontaneously occurring Parkinson's disease suggests that alternative mechanisms should be explored.

Tardive Dyskinesia

The prolonged and frequently irreversible course of tardive dyskinesia strongly suggests that permanent structural alterations are responsible for this disorder. However, neuropathologic studies following acute or chronic administration of antipsychotic drugs in laboratory animals have not demonstrated specific or localized pathologic changes in the brain beyond those secondarily produced by the diverse systemic effects of these drugs.[145,210] A recent report[193] of reduced neuronal cell counts in the basal ganglia of rats receiving chronic phenothiazine treatment is interesting but, since associated degenerative changes or gliosis were not present, it is of uncertain significance.

Neuropathologic changes following chronic phenothiazine treatment in patients without extrapyramidal syndromes have usually consisted of scattered areas of neuronal degeneration and gliosis without convincing localization.[108,210] Individual patients with drug-induced Parkinsonism or tardive dyskinesia have been reported to have postmortem changes in the globus pallidus and putamen,[202] caudate nucleus and substantia nigra,[117] and inferior olive.[118] Hunter et al[134] reported no significant neuropathologic abnormality in three patients with tardive dyskinesia, although two of these showed, among other lesions, neuronal degeneration in the substantia nigra believed to be consistent with their advanced age. Christensen et al.[52] reported the presence of neuronal degeneration and gliosis of the substantia nigra in 27 of 28 brains from patients with chronic oral dyskinesias, 21 of which were attributed to antipsychotic drugs, while only 7 of 28 control brains matched for age and psychiatric diagnosis showed similar changes. Although this finding may represent a toxic effect of the drugs, its occurrence in some elderly individuals without tardive dyskinesia raised the possibility that it is an accompaniment of aging which predisposes in some poorly understood manner to the subsequent appearance of tardive dyskinesia.

Several clinical observations have indicated that this syndrome is associated with a state of relative dopaminergic overactivity or hypersensitivity. It tends to worsen on withdrawal of the dopamine-antagonistic neuroleptic drugs. Furthermore, tardive dyskinesia closely resembles the dyskinesias produced by L-dopa in patients with Parkinson's disease and administration of L-dopa exacerbates tardive dyskinesia.[45,112,128] The fact that tardive dyskinesia may be suppressed by treatment with drugs that deplete or block the action of dopamine, such as tetrabenazine, reserpine, phenothiazines, and butyrophenones[147] as well as α-methyl-p-tyrosin[45,112] provides additional support for a state of relative dopaminergic hypersensitivity. Since improvement after such antiadrenergic agents is often quite prompt and usually occurs without the appearance of significant Parkinsonism,[147] it is unlikely that the benefits are due solely to the superimposition of a hypokinetic state. The observation that anticholinergic drugs worsen tardive dyskinesia,[112,135,158] similar to their worsening effect in Huntington's chorea[157] and ability to induce dyskinesias in Parkinson's disease,[94] is also consistent with a state of dopaminergic overactivity or hypersensitivity. The anticholinesterase agent, physostigmine, by potentiating central cholinergic mechanisms, would be expected to improve tardive dyskinesia, but has been associated variously with mild improvement,[112,158] little change, or even worsening.[240]

There have been few studies of monoamine metabolites in the cerebrospinal fluid during tardive dyskinesia. In one study, the lumbar cerebrospinal fluid concentration of homovanillic acid (HVA) measured after probenicid was normal,[199] while other findings indicate that the turnover of dopamine may be diminished in patients with tardive dyskinesia.[47] Although conclusions would be premature, it has been suggested that such changes may reflect structural alterations in dopamine neurones or a functional response to a change in sensitivity of dopamine receptors.[47]

The accelerated turnover of dopamine produced by neuroleptic drugs is a transient effect[10] that is unlikely to explain the persistence of dyskinesia for months to years after withdrawal. An alternative mechanism to account for overactivity or hypersensitivity to dopamine is the development of denervation—or disuse supersensitivity—of dopamine receptors.[40,153,154,238,239] Since the drugs responsible for tardive dyskinesia appear to produce pharmacologic blockade of transmission at dopamine-mediated synapses, disuse supersensitivity produced by alteration of receptors may be a long-term consequence of their use.[153,239] Evidence of phenomena presumably related to synaptic supersensitivity in the central nervous system has been obtained in numerous experiments.[239] Destruction of dopamine-containing neurones of the nigrocaudate pathway of cats with intraventricular 6-hydroxydopamine produced a significant increase in the sensitivity of caudate neurones to microiontophoretically applied dopamine.[101] Following unilateral destruction of the nigrostriatal tract in rats, L-dopa or low doses of apomorphine produced contralateral turning behavior consistent with enhanced sensitivity of the denervated striatum.[243] Intraventricular administration of 6-hydroxydopamine to newborn rats resulted in the appearance of stereotyped behavior following doses of apomorphine which had been ineffective 3 months previously.[68] The unilateral destruction of the nigrostriatal tract of the rat has recently been reported to induce an increased responsiveness of dopamine-sensitive adenylate cyclase in tissue prepared from the ipsilateral neostriatum; this biochemical change may reflect supersensitivity of dopamine receptors.[180] Furthermore, the administration of L-dopa or apomorphine to monkeys pretreated with intraventricular or intracaudate 6-hydroxydopamine resulted in the appearance of abnormal lip and tongue movements, chorea, dystonia, and hemiballismus, which did not appear in animals not given 6-hydroxydopamine.[185] Recent behavioral evidence accumulated in several animal species[105,156,238] suggests that chronic administration of antipsychotic or other antiadrenergic[239] drugs may also produce a state of denervation supersensitivity lasting for several weeks after they are discontinued.

If tardive dyskinesia results from prolonged blockade of dopamine receptors, it might be expected to appear predominantly in patients previously exhibiting significant drug-induced Parkinsonism. Although one controlled study suggests that this may be true,[63] tardive dyskinesia may also occur in patients without previous Parkinsonism. Microiontophoretic studies of the caudate nucleus have disclosed the presence of two populations of neurones, respectively inhibited or facilitated by dopamine.[177] In order to explain the appearance of tardive dyskinesia without previous Parkinsonism, Klawans[153,154] has proposed that these two receptors may not be equally susceptible to blockade with antipsychotic drugs. The fact that these two populations of dopamine-sensitive neurones have been shown to be blocked equally well by microiontophoretically applied chlorpromazine[253] would argue against this theory, however.

Although denervation or disuse supersensitivity may be produced experimentally, it remains unproven that this mechanism is responsible for the development of tardive dyskinesia. The usually prolonged and frequently irreversible course of the syndrome would be inconsistent with a purely pharmacologic state of denervation supersensitivity and suggests instead that significant structural or other neurotoxic changes have taken place, possibly related to the other effects of phenothiazines, for example, on cell membranes or cellular respiratory mechanisms.[98] It has alternatively been suggested that increased sensitivity to dopamine in tardive dyskinesia may be due to impaired presynaptic reuptake and inactivation of dopamine due to preexisting subclinical disease of the nigrostriatal system insufficient to produce Parkinson's disease but sufficient to interfere with reuptake mechanisms.[163] According to this hypothesis, however, oralfacial dyskinesias would be expected early in the course of spontaneous Parkinson's disease but, in fact, do not occur.

The possibility of changes in neuronal systems mediated by other putative neurotransmitters has not been widely studied. Administration of L-tryptophan to patients with tardive dyskinesia on the basis of a proposed defect in serotonin mechanisms does not produce a lasting effect.[203] If centrally effective agonists of α-amino-butyric acid (GABA) become available for clinical use, they may be worthy of trail in various dyskinetic disorders.

The attempts to reproduce tardive dyskinesia in animals have been generally disappointing. Oral dyskinesias have been produced in monkeys by chronic administration of antipsychotic drugs.[76,194] In 5 out of 15 monkeys fed chlorpromazine (30 mg/kg) daily for 3 to 9 months, buccolingual dyskinesias, biting behavior, and self-destructive acts occurred that were maximal several hours after each dose but ceased when chlorpromazine was discontinued.[194] Possibly similar to tardive dyskinesia, discontinuation of chronic chlorpromazine has been associated with the appearance of at least transient dyskinetic or hyperkinetic behavior in animals.[33,194] Although in one study, chronic administration of haloperidol did not produce dyskinesia,[194] there is another report of choreoathetosis and oral dyskinesias in monkeys during 6 months of treatment with haloperidol.[23] These dyskinesias were not long-lasting, and, because of their appearance in some instances following each dose of a neuroleptic agent[194] and their response to an anticholinergic drug,[76] they more closely resemble the acute dyskinesias seen in humans, or the acute "withdrawal" dyskinesias reported to occur on discontinuation of large or prolonged doses of neuroleptic drugs in adults[137] or of ordinary doses in children.[174] The fact that chronic exposure appears to be necessary for their appearance in animals, however, may make these reactions relevant to understanding clinical tardive dyskinesia, and worthy of further pharmacologic and pathologic study.

Relationship of Antipsychotic and Extrapyramidal Effects

A widely discussed aspect of the actions of antipsychotic drugs is the relationship of their antipsychotic effects to their capacity to produce extrapyramidal syndromes.[28] The high incidence of extrapyramidal syndromes in patients treated with these drugs led some early investigators to conclude that they were necessary for the achievement of antipsychotic effects.[77,78] It was soon established, however, that antipsychotic effects could be achieved without prominent extrapyramidal reactions,[25,54] although a minimal degree of akinesia did appear to correlate highly with clinical effectivness.[121,225] Although it has become clear that extrapyramidal effects have no direct role in antipsychotic efficacy, an extremely high correlation appears to exist between these two pharmacologic properties. Behavioral[138] and metabolic[4, 146] studies of large numbers of antipsychotic drugs have shown that they may be classified according to their relative ability to block receptors for dopamine and norepinephrine. Some drugs such as chlorpromazine, thioridazine, and chlorprothixene block these receptors approximately equally; others, such as piperazine phenothiazines and thioxanthenes as well as most butyrophenones, block dopamine receptors more effectively than norepinephrine receptors; a third group, the diphenylbutylpiperidines, including pimozide, which is structurally related to the butyrophenones, appear to be virtually pure dopamine receptor antagonists.[4] It is believed that antipsychotic effects correlate best with effects on dopaminergic mechanisms, while blockade of norepinephrine receptors correlates more highly with sedative properties.[4,188] There is some recent evidence that clozapine, which is relatively free of extrapyramidal effects, produces more striking effects on dopamine turnover in the limbic forebrain than in the basal ganglia.[6]

Two other important effects of the antipsychotic drugs, their antiemetic and extrapyramidal actions, also appear to be related to the blockade of dopamine receptors in the brain. Antiemetic effects are probably related to effects on dopamine-receptive neurones in the "chemoreceptor trigger zone" of the area postrema.[195] Some phenothiazines, such as promethazine, appear to be relatively active on this system, but are devoid of neurologic and antipsychotic effects. There is also some evidence that antipsychotic drugs may interfere with the actions of dopamine in the hypothalamus, and thus lead to changes in pituitary function, such as decreased release of growth hormone[222] and increased output of prolactin.[168] According to recent biochemical studies in animals, tolerance to the dopamine-antagonistic effects of antipsychotic drugs occurs in the caudate nucleus[10,32] but does not occur in limbic or hypothalamic regions.[32] This regional selectivity suggests that the effects of chronic neuroleptic agents on hypothalamic-pituitary function are more closely similar to antipsychotic effects to which there is also no tolerance, than to extrapyramidal effects to which tolerance probably occurs.

It is possible that extrapyramidal and antipsychotic effects may similarly be separable and that drugs with exclusively antipsychotic effects can be developed. The lack of availability of such selective antipsychotic agents is in no small measure due to the screening of potential new agents by seeking neuroleptic (neurological) effects in animals to predict possible antipsychotic efficacy. The anatomical substrate for this hoped-for separability of effects may parallel the separation of nigro-neostriatal and mesolimbic dopaminergic systems demonstrated in both animals and man.[5,28,186] The recently described projections of dopamine-containing neurones to cerebral cortical portions of the limbic system[129] may also be important in psychosis. There is evidence that the antipsychotic drugs in current use block dopamine synaptic transmission in both mesolimbic centers and the neostriatum.[3] Recent approaches to this problem have attempted to determine which effects in animals correlate with antipsychotic activity and which correlate with extrapyramidal effects in order to select drugs with predominantly antipsychotic effects.[28,59] Since clozapine has been reported to possess antipsychotic effects without producing catalepsy in rats or extrapyramidal disorders in man,[20,229] it is likely that extrapyramidal and antipsychotic effects may ultimately prove to be separable pharmacologic phenomena.

In summary, it is clear that modern neuroanatomical, physiologic, metabolic, and pharmacologic studies are having a profound impact on the theory and clinical management of chronic psychosis and the disorders of the extrapyramidal motor system. It is also clear that psychiatry and neurology have an increasing area of common interest, notably including the topics that we have discussed.

REFERENCES

1. American College of Neuropsychopharmacology-Food and Drug Administration Task Force: Neurologic syndromes associated with antipsychotic drug use. N Engl J Med 289:20, 1973
2. Ambani LH, Van Woert MH, Bowers MB Jr: Physostigmine effects on phenothiazine-induced extrapyramidal reactions. Arch Neurol 29:444, 1973

3. Andén N-E: Dopamine turnover in the corpus striatum and the limbic system after treatment with neuroleptic and anti-acetylcholine drugs. J Pharm Pharmacol 24:905, 1972
4. Andén N-E, Butcher SG, Corrodi H, Fuxe K, Ungerstedt U: Receptor activity and turnover of dopamine and noradrenaline after neuroleptics. Eur J Pharmacol 11:303, 1970
5. Andén N-E, Dahlstrom K, Fuxe K, Larsson K, Olson L, Ungerstedt U: Ascending monoamine neurons to the telencephalon and diencephalon. Acta Physiol Scand 67:313, 1966
6. Andén N-E, Stock G: Effect of clozapine on the turnover of dopamine in the corpus striatum and in the limbic system. J Pharm Pharmacol 25:346, 1973
7. Angrist B, Sathanamthan G, Gershon S: Behavioral effects of L-dopa in schizophrenic patients. Psychopharmacologia(Berl.) 31:1, 1973
8. Angus JWS, Simpson GM: Hysteria and drug-induced dystonia. Acta Psychiatr Scand (Suppl 212):52, 1970
9. Arieti S: Primitive habits and perceptual alterations in the terminal stage of schizophrenia. Arch Neurol Psychiatry 53:378, 1945
10. Asper H, Baggiolini M, Burki HR, Lauener H, Ruch W, Stille G: Tolerance phenomena with neuroleptics. Eur J Pharmacol 22:287, 1973
11. Ayd FJ Jr: Drug-induced extrapyramidal reactions: Their clinical manifestations and treatment with Akineton. Psychosomatics 1:143, 1960
12. Ayd FJ Jr: A survey of drug-induced extrapyramidal reactions. JAMA 175:102, 1961
13. Ayd FJ Jr: Haloperidol: Fifteen years of clinical experience. Dis Nerv Syst 33:459, 1972
14. Ayd FJ Jr: Clozapine: A unique new neuroleptic. Internat Drug Therapy Newsletter 9:5, 1974
15. Baker AB: Discussion In Crane GE, Gardner R Jr (eds): Psychotropic Drugs and Dysfunctions of the Basal Ganglia. Washington, U.S. Public Health Service, Publ. No. 1938, p 60
16. Baldessarini RJ: Pharmacology of the amphetamines. Pediatrics 49:694, 1972
17. Baldessarini RJ: Tardive dyskinesia: An evaluation of the etiologic association with neuroleptic therapy. J Can Psychiat Assoc, 1974 (in press)
18. Baldessarini RJ: Amine hypotheses in the affective disorders, in Flach F, Draghi S (eds): The Nature and Treatment of Depression. New York, Wiley, 1975 (in press)
19. Barsa JA, Kline NS: Use of reserpine in disturbed psychotic patients. Am J Psychiatry 112:684, 1956
20. Bartholini G, Haefely W, Jalfre M, Keller HH, Pletscher A: Effects of clozapine on cerebral catecholaminergic neurone systems. Br J Pharmacol 46:736, 1972
21. Bartholini G, Stadler H, Lloyd KG: Cholinergic-dopaminergic interactions in the extrapyramidal system. In Calne DB (ed): Progress in the Treatment of Parkinsonism. New York, Raven, 1973, p 233–241
22. Bédard P, LaRochelle L: Effect of section on the strionigral fibers on dopamine turnover in the forebrain of the rat. Exp Neurol 41:314, 1973

23. Bédard P, LaRochelle L, De Léan J, Lafleur J: Dykinesias induced by long term administration of haloperidol in the monkey. The Physiologist 15:836, 1972

24. Berkson G, Mason WA, Saxon SU: Situation and stimulus effects on stereotyped behaviors of chimpanzees. J Comp Physiol Psychol 56:786, 1963

25. Bishop MP, Gallant DM, Sykes TF: Extrapyramidal side effects and therapeutic response. Arch Gen Psychiatry 13:155, 1965

26. Bleuler EP: Dementia Praecox or the Group of Schizophrenias. New York, International Universities, 1950, pp 180–205, 445–449

27. Bleuler EP: Textbook of psychiatry. New York, Dover, 1951, pp 142–156, 359, 400–413

28. Bobon DP, Janssen PAJ, Bobon J: Modern Problems of Pharmacopsychiatry. Vol 5, The Neuroleptics. Basel, Karger, 1970

29. Boston Collaborative Drug Surveillance Program: Drug-induced extrapyramidal symptoms. JAMA 224:889, 1973

30. Bowers MB Jr: 5-Hydroxyindoleacetic acid (5 HIAA) and homovanillic acid (HVA) following probenecid in acute psychotic patients treated with phenothiazines. Psychopharmacologia (Berl.) 28:309, 1973

31. Bowers MB Jr, Roth RH: Interaction of atropine-like drugs with dopamine-containing neurones in rat brain. Br J Pharmacol 44:301, 1972

32. Bowers MB Jr, Rozitis A: Regional differences in homovanillic acid concentrations after acute and chronic administration of antipsychotic drugs. J Pharm Pharmacol 26:743, 1974

33. Boyd EM: Chlorpromazine tolerance and physical dependence. J Pharmacol Exp Ther 128:75, 1960

34. Brandon S, McClelland HA, Protheroe C: A study of facial dyskinesia in a mental hospital population. Br J Psychiatry 118:171, 1971

35. Brotzu G: Inhibition by chlorpromazine of the effects of dopamine on the dog kidney. J Pharm Pharmacol 22:664, 1970

36. Bruno A, Bruno SC: Effects of L-dopa on pharmacological parkinsonism. Acta Psychiatr Scand 42:264, 1966

37. Bunney BS, Aghajanian GK, Roth RH: Comparison of effects of L-dopa, amphetamine and apomorphine on firing rate of rat dopaminergic neurones. Nature New Biol 245:123, 1973

38. Bunney BS, Walters JR, Roth RH, Aghajanian GK: Dopaminergic neurons: Effect of antipsychotic drugs and amphetamine on single cell activity. J Pharmacol Exp Ther 185:560, 1973

39. Burks J, Walker J, Ott JE, Rumack B: Chorea associated with imipramine poisoning: Reversal by physostigmine. Neurology (Minneap.)23:393, 1973

40. Carlsson A: Biochemical implications of dopa-induced actions on the central nervous system, with particular reference to abnormal movements, in Barbeau A. McDowell FH (ed): L-dopa and Parkinsonism. Philadelphia, Davis, 1970, p 205

41. Carlsson A, Lindqvist M, Magnusson T: 3,4-Dihydroxyphenylalanine and 5-hydroxytryptophan as reserpine antagonists. Nature 180:1200, 1957

42. Carman JS: Methylphenidate in akathisia. Lancet 2:1093, 1972
43. Casey JF, Lasky JJ, Klett CJ, Hollister LE: Treatment of schizophrenic reactions with phenothiazine derivatives. Am J Psychiatry 117:97, 1960
44. Casteels-Van Daele M, Jaeken J, Van Der Schueren P, Zimmerman A, Van Den Bon P: Dystonic reactions in children caused by metoclopramide. Arch Dis Child 45:130, 1970
45. Chase TN: Drug-induced extrapyramidal disorders. Res Publ Ass Nerv Ment Dis 50:448, 1972
46. Chase TN: Central monoamine metabolism in man. Arch Neurol 29:349, 1973
47. Chase TN: Catecholamine metabolism and neurologic disease, in Usdin E, Snyder SM (eds): Frontiers in Catecholamine Research. New York, Pergamon Press, 1974, pp 941–945
48. Chase TN, Schnur JA, Gordon EK: Cerebrospinal fluid monoamine catabolites in drug-induced extrapyramidal disorders. Neuropharmacology 9:265, 1970
49. Chateau R, Fau R, Groslambert R, Perret J: A propos d'un cas de torticolis spasmodique irreversible, survenu au cours d'un traitement par neuroleptiques. Rev Neurol 114:65, 1966
50. Cheramy A, Besson MJ, Glowinski J: Increased release of dopamine from striatal dopaminergic terminals in the rat after treatment with a neuroleptic: Thioproperazine. Eur J Pharmacol 10:206, 1970
51. Chien C-P, Cole JO: Eighteen-months follow-up of tardive dyskinesia treated with various catecholamine-related agents. Psychopharm Bull 9:38, 1973
52. Christensen E, Møller, JØ, Faurbye A: Neuropathological investigation of 28 brains from patients with dyskinesia. Acta Psychiatr Scand 46:14, 1970
53. Clement-Cormier YC, Kebabian JW, Petzgold GL, Greengard P: Dopamine-sensitive adenylate cyclase in mammalian brain: A possible site of action of antipsychotic drugs. Proc Nat Acad Sci USA 71:1113, 1974
54. Cole JO, Clyde DJ: Extrapyramidal side effects and clinical response to the phenothiazines. Rev Can Biol 20:565, 1961
55. Collard J: Psychopharmacologie comparée du haloperidol et de ses dérivés (tripéridol, methylpéride et R 1647). Rev Can Biol 20:456, 1961
56. Connell PH: Amphetamine Psychosis. London, Chapman and Hall, 1958
57. Costall B, Naylor RJ: The role of telencephalic dopaminergic systems in the mediation of apomorphine-stereotyped behavior. Eur J Pharmacol 24:8, 1973
58. Costall B, Naylor RJ: The site and mode of action of ET 495 for the mediation of stereotyped behavior in the rat. Naunyn-Schmiedeberg's Arch Pharm (Weinheim)278:117, 1973
59. Costall B, Naylor RJ: Is there a relationship between the involvement of extrapyramidal and mesolimbic brain areas with the cataleptic action of neuroleptic agents and their clinical antipsychotic effect? Psychopharmacologia (Berl.) 32:161, 1973
60. Costall B, Naylor RJ, Olley JE: On the involvement of the caudate-putamen, globus pallidus and substantia nigra with neuroleptic and cholinergic modification of locomotor activity. Neuropharmacology 11:317, 1972

61. Crane GE: Dyskinesia and neuroleptics. Arch Gen Psychiatry 19:700, 1968
62. Crane GE: High doses of trifluoperazine and tardive dyskinesia. Arch Neurol 22:176, 1970
63. Crane GE: Pseudoparkinsonism and tardive dyskinesia. Arch Neurol 27:426, 1972
64. Crane GE: Persistent dyskinesia. Br J Psychiatry 122:395, 1973
65. Crane GE: Clinical psychopharmacology in its 20th year. Science 181:124, 1973
66. Crane GE, Naranjo ER: Motor disorders induced by neuroleptics. Arch Gen Psychiatry 24:179, 1971
67. Crane GE, Smeets RA: Tardive dyskinesia and drug therapy in geriatric patients. Arch Gen Psychiatry 30:341, 1974
68. Creese I, Iversen S: Blockage of amphetamine-induced motor stimulation and stereotypy in the adult rat following neonatal treatment with 6-hydroxydopamine. Brain Res 55:369, 1973
69. Davis JM, Janowsky DS: Amphetamine and methylphenidate psychosis, in Usdin E, Snyder SH (eds): Frontiers in Catecholamine Research. Oxford, Pergamon, 1973, pp 977–981
70. Degkwitz R: Extrapyramidal motor disorders following long-term treatment with neuroleptic drugs, in Crane GE, Gardner RJ Jr (eds): Psychotropic Drugs and Dysfunctions of the Basal Ganglia. Washington, U.S. Public Health Service Publication No. 1938, 1969, pp 22–32
71. Degkwitz R, Frowein R, Kulenkamff C, Mohs U: Über die Wirkungen des L-DOPA bein Menschen und deren Beeinflussung durch Reserpin, Chlorpromazin, Iproniazid und Vitamin B6. Klin Wochenschr 38:120, 1960
72. Degkwitz R, Wenzel W: Persistent extrapyramidal side effects after long-term application of neuroleptics, in Brill H (ed): Neuropsychopharmacology (International Congress Series No. 129). Amsterdam, Excerpta Medica, 1967, pp 608–615
73. De Jong HH: Experimental Catatonia. Baltimore, Williams & Wilkins, 1945
74. Delay J, Deniker P: Drug-induced extrapyramidal syndromes, in Vinken PJ, Bruyn GW (eds): Handbook of Clinical Neurology, vol 6, Diseases of the Basal Ganglia. Amsterdam, North-Holland, 1968, pp 248–266
75. Demars JCA: Neuromuscular effects of long-term phenothiazine medication, electroconvulsive therapy, and leucotomy. J Nerv Ment Dis 143:73, 1966
76. Deneau GA, Crane GE: Dyskinesia in rhesus monkeys tested with high doses of chlorpromazine, in Crane GE, Gardner R Jr (eds): Psychotropic Drugs and Dysfunctions of the Basal Ganglia. Washington, U.S. Public Health Service Publication No. 1938, 1969, pp 12–13
77. Denham J, Carrick DJ: Therapeutic value of thioproperazine and the importance of the associated neurological disturbances. J Ment Sci 107:326, 1961
78. Deniker P: Experimental neurological syndromes and the new drug therapies in psychiatry. Compr Psychiatry 1:92, 1960
79. De Robertis E: Molecular biology of synaptic receptors. Science 171:963, 1971
80. Di Mascio A: Classification and overview of psychotropic drugs, in Di Mascio

A, Shader RI (eds): Clinical Handbook of Psychopharmacology. New York, Academic Press, 1970, pp 3–15

81. Di Mascio A, Demirgian E: Antiparkinson drug overuse. Psychosomatics 11:596, 1970

82. Domino EE: Substituted phenothiazine antipsychotics, in Efron D (ed): Psychopharmacology: A Review of Progress 1957–1967. Washington, U.S. Public Health Service Publication No. 1836, 1968, pp 1045–1056

83. Druckman R, Seelinger D, Thulin B: Chronic involuntary movements induced by phenothiazines. J Nerv Ment Dis 135:69, 1962

84. Duvoisin RC: Cholinergic-anticholinergic antagonism in parkinsonism. Arch Neurol 17:124, 1967

85. Duvoism RC: Neurological reactions to psychotropic drugs, in Efron D (ed): Psychopharmacology: A Review of Progress 1957–1967. Washington, U.S. Public Health Service Publication No. 1836, 1968, pp 561–573

86. Edwards H: The significance of brain damage in persistent oral dyskinesia. Br J Psychiatry 116:271, 1970

87. Ekbom KA: Restless legs syndrome. Neurology (Minneap)10:868, 1960

88. Eldridge R: The torsion dystonias: Literature review and genetic and clinical studies. Neurology (Minneap)20(Part 2):1, 1970

89. Ellinwood EH Jr: Amphetamine psychosis: I. Description of the individuals and process. J Nerv Ment Dis 144:273, 1967

90. Ernst AM: Experiments with an O-methylated product of dopamine on cats. Acta Physiol Pharmacol Neerl 11:48, 1962

91. Essig CF, Carter WW: Convulsions and bizarre behavior in monkeys receiving chlorpromazine. Proc Soc Exp Biol Med 95:726, 1957

92. Evans JH: Persistent oral dyskinesia in treatment with phenothiazine derivatives. Lancet 1:458, 1965

93. Fahn S, Côté LJ: Regional distribution of gamma-aminobutyric acid (GABA) in brain of the Rhesus monkey. J Neurochem 15:209, 1968

94. Fahn S, David E: Oral-facial-lingual dyskinesia due to anticholinergic medication. Trans Am Neurol Assoc 97:277, 1972

95. Fann WE: Use of methylphenidate to counteract acute dystonic effects of phenothiazines. Am J Psychiatry 122:1293, 1966

96. Fann WE, Davis JM, Janowsky DS: The prevalence of tardive dyskinesias in mental hospital patients. Dis Nerv Syst 37:182, 1972

97. Fann WE, Lake CR: On the coexistence of parkinsonism and tardive dyskinesia. Dis Nerv Syst 35:324, 1974

98. Faurbye A: The structural and biochemical basis of movement disorders in treatment with neuroleptic drugs and in extrapyramidal diseases. Compr Psychiatry 11:205, 1970

99. Faurbye A, Rasch PJ, Peterson PB, Brandborg G, Pakkenberg H: Neurological symptoms in pharmacotherapy of psychoses. Acta Psychiat Scand 40:10, 1964

100. Feltz P: γ-Aminobutyric acid and a caudal-nigral inhibition. Can J Physiol Pharmacol 49:1113, 1971

101. Feltz P, De Champlain J: Enhanced sensitivity of caudate neurones for mic-

roiontophoretic injections of dopamine in 6-hydroxydopamine-treated cats. Brain Res 43:601, 1972

102.   Fish FJ: The classification of schizophrenia. J Ment Sci 103:433, 1957
103.   Fish FJ: Leonhard's classification of schizophrenia. J Ment Sci 104:943, 1958
104.   Fish FJ: Clinical Psychopathology. Bristol, Wright, 1967, pp 84–106
105.   Fjalland B, Møller-Nielsen I: Enhancement of methylphenidate-induced stereotypies by repeated administration of neuroleptics. Psychopharmacologia (Berl.) 34:105, 1974
106.   Fleming P, Makar H, Hunter KR: Levodopa in drug-induced extrapyramidal disorders. Lancet 2:1186, 1970
107.   Fog R: On stereotypy and catalepsy: Studies on the effect of amphetamines and neuroleptics in rats. Acta Neurol Scand 48(Suppl 50):1–66, 1972
108.   Forrest FM, Forrest IS, Roizin L: Clinical, biochemical and postmortem studies on a patient treated with chlorpromazine. Agressologie 4:259, 1973
109.   Freyhan FA: Psychomotility and parkinsonism in treatment with neuroleptic drugs. Arch Neurol Psychiatry 76:56, 1957
110.   Freyhan FA: Therapeutic implications of differential effects of new phenothiazine compounds. Am J Psychiatry 115:577, 1959
111.   Gailitis J, Knowles RR, Longobardi A: Alarming neuromuscular reactions due to prochlorperazine. Ann Intern Med 52:538, 1960
112.   Gerlach J, Reisby N, Randrup A: Dopaminergic hypersensitivity and cholinergic hypofunction in the pathophysiology of tardive dyskinesia. Psychopharmacologia (Berl.) 34:21, 1974
113.   Gessa R, Tagliamonte A, Gessa GL: Blockade by apomorphine of haloperidol-induced dyskinesia in schizophrenic patients. Lancet 2:981, 1972
114.   Glynn A: The nature of schizophrenia and its early diagnosis. Acta Psychiat Neurol Scand 28:123, 1953
115.   Goldman D: Parkinsonism and related phenomena from administration of drugs: Their production and control under clinical conditions and possible relation to therapeutic effect. Rev Can Biol 20:549, 1961
116.   Gratton L: Neuroleptiques, parkinsonnisme et schizophrenie. Union Med Can 89:679, 1960
117.   Gross H, Kaltenbäck E: Hirnbetunde nach neuroleptischer Langzeittherapie. Zentralbl Gesamte Neurol 188:400, 1967
118.   Grünthal VE, Walther-Buel H: Über Schädigung der Oliva Inferior durch Chlorperphenazine (Trilafon). Psychiat Neurol 140:249, 1960
119.   Guldberg HC, Yates CM: Some studies of the effects of chlorpromazine, reserpine and dihydroxyphenylalanine on the concentrations of homovanillic acid, 3,4-dihydroxyphenylacetic acid and 5-hydroxyindole-3-ylacetic acid in ventricular cerebrospinal fluid of the dog using the technique of serial sampling of the cerebrospinal fluid. Br J Pharmacol Chemother 33:457, 1968
120.   Gupta JM, Lovejoy FH Jr: Acute phenothiazine toxicity in childhood: A five-year survey. Pediatrics 39:771, 1967
121.   Haase HJ, Janssen PAH: The Action of Neuroleptic Drugs. Amsterdam, North-Holland, 1965

122. Haddenbrock S: Zur wirkungsweise und zur frage zentralorganischer spatschaden der neuroleptischen dauergehandlung, Nervenarzt 20:199, 1966

123. Hall RA, Jackson RB, Swain JM: Neurotoxic reactions resulting from chlorpromazine administration. JAMA 161:214, 1956

124. Harris JE, Baldessarini RJ: Amphetamine-induced inhibition of tyrosine hydroxylation in homogenates of the rat corpus striatum. J Pharm Pharmacol 25:755, 1973

125. Heinrich K, Wegener I, Bender HJ: Späte extrapyramydalen hyperkinesen bei neuroleptischer Langzeit-therapie. Pharmakopsychiat Neuropsychopharmacol 1:169, 1968

126. Hershon HI, Kennedy PF, McGuire RJ: Persistence of extrapyramidal disorders and psychiatric relapse after withdrawal of long-term phenothiazine therapy. Br J Psychiatry 120:41, 1972

127. Hill RM, Desmond MM, Kay JL: Extrapyramidal dysfunction in an infant of a schizophrenic mother. J Pediatr 69:589, 1966

128. Hippius H, Lange J: Zur Problematik der späten extrapyramydalen Hyperkinesen nach langfristiger neuroleptischer Therapie. Arzneim Forsch 20:888, 1970

129. Hökfelt T, Ljungdahl Å, Fuxe K, Johansson O: Dopamine nerve terminals in the rat limbic cortex: aspects of the dopamine hypothesis of schizophrenia. Science 184:177, 1974

130. Holden JMC, Itil TM, Keskiner A: The treatment of lobotomized schizophrenic patients with butaperazine. Curr Ther Res 11:418, 1969

131. Hollister LE, Glazener FS: Concurrent paralysis agitans and schizophrenia. Dis Nerv Syst 22:187, 1961

132. Horn AS, Snyder SH: Chlorpromazine and dopamine: Conformational similarities that correlate with the antischizophrenic activity of phenothiazine drugs. Proc Natl Acad Sci USA 68:2325, 1971

133. Hornykiewicz O: Dopamine in the basal ganglia. Br Med Bull 29:172, 1973

134. Hunter R, Blackwood W, Smith MC, Cumings JN: Neuropathological findings in three cases of persistent dyskinesia following phenothiazine medication. J Neurol Sci 7:263, 1968

135. Hunter R, Earl CJ, Thornicroft S: An apparently irreversible syndrome of abnormal movements following phenothiazine medication. Proc R Soc Med 57:758, 1964

136. Iversen LI: Catecholamine uptake processes. Br Med Bull 29:130, 1973

137. Jacobson G, Baldessarini RJ, Manschreck T: Tardive dyskinesia associated with haloperidol. Am J Psychiatry 131:910, 1974

138. Janssen PAJ, Niemegeers CJE, Schellekens KHL, Lenaerts FM: Is it possible to predict the clinical effects of neuroleptic drugs (major tranquilizers) from animal data? Arzneim Forsch 17:841, 1967

139. Jaspers K: General Psychopathology. Manchester, Manchester University Press, 1963, pp 179–185

140. Javoy F, Agid Y, Bouvet D, Glowinski J: Feedback control of dopamine synthesis in dopaminergic terminals of the cat striatum. J Pharmacol Exp Ther 182:454, 1972

141. Jelliffe SE: The mental pictures in schizophrenia and in epidemic encephalitis. Res Publ Assoc Nerv Ment Dis 5:204, 1928

142. Johnson DAW: The side-effects of fluphenazine decanoate. Br J Psychiatry 123:519, 1973

143. Jones IH: Observations on schizophrenic stereotypies. Compr Psychiatry 6:323, 1965

144. Jones M, Hunter R: Abnormal movements in patients with chronic psychiatric illness, in Crane GE, Gardner R Jr (eds): Psychotropic Drugs and Dysfunctions of the Basal Ganglia. Washington, U.S. Public Health Service Publication No. 1938, 1969, pp 53–65

145. Julou L, Ducrot R, Ganter P, Maral R, Populaire P, Durel J, et al.: Chronic toxicity, side effects and metabolism of neuroleptics of the phenothiazine group, in Proceedings of the European Society for Study of Drug Toxicity, vol. 9, Toxicity and Side Effects of Psychotropic Drugs. Amsterdam, Excerpta Medica, International Congress Series No. 145, 1968, pp 36–51

146. Karobath M, Leitich H: Antipsychotic drugs and dopamine-stimulated adenylate cyclase prepared from corpus striatum of rat brain. Proc Natl Acad Sci USA 71:2915, 1974

147. Kazamatsuri H, Chien C-P, Cole JO: Therapeutic approaches to tardive dyskinesia. Arch Gen Psychiatry 27:491, 1972

148. Kebabian JW, Petzold GL, Greengard P: Dopamine-sensitive adenylate cyclase in the caudate nucleus of rat brain and its similarity to the "dopamine receptor." Proc Natl Acad Sci USA 61:2145, 1972

149. Keegan DL, Rajput AH: Drug-induced dystonia tarda: Treatment with L-Dopa. Dis Nerv Syst 38:167, 1973

150. Kehr W, Carlsson A, Lindqvist M, Magnusson T, Atack CV: Evidence for a receptor-mediated feedback control of striatal tyrosine hydroxylase activity. J Pharm Pharmacol 24:744, 1972

151. Kennedy PF, Hershon HI, McGuire RJ: Extrapyramidal disorders after prolonged phenothiazine therapy. Br J Psychiatry 118:509, 1971

152. Kim JS, Bak IJ, Hassler R, Okada Y: Role of γ-aminobutyric acid (GABA) in the extrapyramidal motor system. II. Some evidence for the existence of a type of GABA-rich strionigral neurons. Exp Brain Res 14:95, 1971

153. Klawans HL Jr: The pharmacology of tardive dyskinesias. Am J Psychiatry 130:82, 1973

154. Klawans HL Jr: The Pharmacology of Extrapyramidal Movement Disorders. Basel, Karger, 1973, pp 7–47, 64–70

155. Klawans HL Jr, Bergen D, Bruyn GW, Paulsen GW: Neuroleptic-induced tardive dyskinesias in nonpsychotic patients. Arch Neurol 30:338, 1974

156. Klawans HL Jr, Rubovits R: An experimental model of tardive dyskinesia. J Neural Transmission 33:235, 1972

157. Klawans HL Jr, Rubovits R: Central cholinergic-anticholinergic antagonism in Huntington's chorea. Neurology (Minneap)22:107, 1972

158. Klawans HL Jr, Rubovits R: Effect of cholinergic and anticholinergic agents on tardive dyskinesia. J Neurol Neurosurg Psychiatry 27:941, 1974

159. Kleist K: Schizophrenic symptoms and cerebral pathology. J Ment Sci 106:246, 1960
160. Klerman GL, Cole JO: Clinical pharmacology of imipramine and related antidepressant compounds. Pharmacol Rev 17:101, 1965
161. Klett CJ, Caffey E Jr: Evaluating the long-term need for antiparkinson drugs by chronic schizophrenics. Arch Gen Psychiatry 26:374, 1972
162. Kline NS: On the rarity of "irreversible" oral dyskinesias following phenothiazines. Am J Psychiatry 124(Suppl):48, 1968
163. Korczyn AD: Pathophysiology of drug-induced dyskinesias. Neuropharmacology 11:601, 1972
164. Korczyn AD, Goldberg GJ: Intravenous diazepam in drug-induced dystonic reactions. Br J Psychiatry 121:75, 1972
165. Kraepelin E: Dementia Praecox and Paraphrenia. Edinburgh, Livingstone, 1919
166. Kruse W: Persistent muscular restlessness after phenothiazine treatment: Report of 3 cases. Am J Psychiatry 117:152, 1960
167. Lader MH: Drug-induced extrapyramidal syndromes. J R Coll Physicians (London)5:87, 1970
168. Lu K-H, Amenomori Y, Chen D-L, Meites J: Effects of central acting drugs on serum and pituitary prolactin levels in rats. Endocrinology 87:667, 1970
169. Mandell AJ, Markham CH, Tallman FF, Mandell MP: Motivation and ability to move. Am J Psychiatry 119:544, 1962
170. Marsden CD, Parkes JD: Abnormal movement disorders. Br J Hosp Med 10:428, 1973
171. Matthysse S: Antipsychotic drug actions: Clue to the neuropathology of schizophrenia? Fed Proc 32:200, 1973
172. Matthysse S: Implications of feedback control in catecholamine neuronal systems, in Usdin E, Snyder SH (eds): Frontiers in Catecholamine Research. Elmsford, New York, Pergamon Press, 1974, pp 1139–1142
173. Mattson RH, Calverly JR: Dextroamphetamine-sulfate-induced dyskinesias. JAMA 204:400, 1968
174. McAndrew JB: Effects of prolonged phenothiazine intake on psychotic and other hospitalized children. J Autism Child Schizo 2:75, 1972
175. McGeer PL, Boulding JE, Gibson WC, Foulkes RG: Drug-induced extrapyramidal reactions. JAMA 177:665, 1961
176. McGeer EG, Fibiger HC, McGeer PL, Brooke S: Temporal changes in amine synthesizing enzymes of rat extrapyramidal structures after hemitransections or 6-hydroxydopamine administration. Brain Res 52:289, 1973
177. McLennan H, York DH: The action of dopamine on neurones of the caudate nucleus. J Physiol 189:393, 1967
178. Mettler FA, Crandell A: Neurologic disorders in psychiatric institutions. J Nerv Ment Dis 128:148, 1959
179. Miller RJ, Hiley CR: Antimuscarinic properties of neuroleptics and drug-induced parkinsonism. Nature 248:596, 1974
180. Mishra RK, Gardner EL, Katzman R, Makman MH: Enhancement of

dopamine-stimulated adenylate cyclase activity in rat caudate after lesions in substantia nigra: evidence for denervation supersensitivity. Proc Natl Acad Sci USA 71:3883, 1974

181. Møller-Nielsen I, Fjalland B, Pedersen V, Nymark M: Pharmacology of neuroleptics upon repeated administration. Psychopharmacologia (Berl.) 34:95, 1974

182. Morrison JR: Catatonia. Retarded and excited types. Arch Gen Psychiatry 28:39, 1973

183. Munkvad I, Hein G, Herskin B: The treatment of chronic schizophrenics with pimozide. Clin Trials J (Lond) 8 (Suppl 2):67, 1971

184. Myrianthopolous NC, Kurland AA, Kurland LT: Hereditary predisposition in drug-induced parkinsonism. Arch Neurol 6:5, 1962

185. Ng LKY, Gelhard RE, Chase TN, MacLean PD: Drug-induced dyskinesia in monkeys. A pharmacologic model employing 6-hydroxydopamine, in Barbeau A, Chase TN, Paulson GW (eds): Huntington's Chorea, 1872–1972. New York, Raven, 1973, pp 651–655

186. Nobin A, Björkland A: Topography of the monamine neuron systems in the human brain as revealed in fetuses. Acta Physiol Scand 88(Suppl 388):1, 1973

187. Nybäck H, Schubert J, Sedvall G: Effect of apomorphine and pimozide on synthesis and turnover of labeled catecholamines in mouse brain. J Pharm Pharmacol 22:622, 1970

188. Nybäck H, Sedvall G: Further studies on the accumulation and disappearance of catecholamines formed from tyrosine-^{14}C in mouse brain. Effect of some phenothiazine analogues. Eur J Pharmacol 10:193, 1970

189. Nybäck H, Sedvall G: Effect of nigral lesion on chlorpromazine-induced acceleration of dopamine synthesis from (^{14}C)-tyrosine. J Pharm Pharmacol 23:322, 1971

190. Olivier A, Parent A, Simard H, Poirier LJ: Cholinesterasic striatopallidal and striatonigral efferents in the cat and the monkey. Brain Res 18:273, 1970

191. Orlov P, Kasparian G, Di Mascio A, Cole JO: Withdrawal of antiparkinson drugs. Arch Gen Psychiatry 25:410, 1971

192. Orton ST: Some neurologic concepts applied to catatonia. Arch Neurol Psychiatry 23:114, 1930

193. Pakkenberg H, Fog R, Nilakantan B: The long-term effect of perphenazine enanthate on the rat brain. Psychopharmacologia (Berl.) 29:329, 1973

194. Paulson GW: Dyskinesias in Rhesus monkeys. Trans Am Neurol Assoc 97:109, 1973

195. Peng MT: Locus of emetic action of epinephrine and dopa in dogs. J Pharmacol Exp Ther 139:345, 1963

196. Perez LM: Treatment of extrapyramidal symptoms. N Engl J Med 264:1269, 1961

197. Persson T, Roos B-E: Clinical and pharmacological effects of monoamine precursors or haloperidol in chronic schizophrenia. Nature (Lond)217:854, 1968

198. Persson T, Roos B-E: Acid metabolites from monoamines in cerebrospinal fluid of chronic schizophrenics. Br J Psychiatry 115:95, 1969

199. Pind K, Faurbye A: Concentration of homovanillic acid and 5-hydroxyindoleacetic acid in the cerebrospinal fluid after treatment with probenecid in patients with drug-induced tardive dyskinesia. Acta Psychiat Scand 46:323, 1970

200. Polizos P, Engelhardt DM, Hoffman SP: CNS consequences of psychotropic drug withdrawal in schizophrenic children. Psychopharmacol Bull 9:34, 1973

201. Polvan N: Fluphenazine hydrochloride and enanthate in the management of chronic psychosis. Dis Nerv Syst 31 (Suppl 9):48, 1970

202. Poursines Y, Alliez J, Toga M: Syndrome parkinsonien consécutif á la prise prolongée de chlorpromazine avec ictus mortel intercurrent. Rev Neurol 100:745, 1959

203. Prange AJ Jr, Wilson IC, Morris CE, Hall CD: Preliminary experience with tryptophan and lithium in the treatment of tardive dyskinesia. Psychopharmacol Bull 9:36, 1973

204. Precht W, Yoshida M: Blockage of caudate-evoked inhibition of neurons in the substantia nigra by picrotoxin. Brain Res 32:229, 1971

205. Pryce IG, Edwards H: Persistent oral dyskinesia in female mental hospital patients. Br J Psychiatry 112:983, 1966

206. Randrup A, Munkvad I: Stereotyped activities produced by amphetamine in several species and man. Psychopharmacologia (Berl.) 11:300, 1967

207. Randrup A, Munkvad I: Biochemical, anatomical and psychological investigations of stereotyped behavior induced by amphetamine, in Costa E, Garattini S (eds): Amphetamines and Related Compounds. New York, Raven, 1970, pp 695–713

208. Reiter PJ: Extrapyramidal motor disturbances in dementia praecox. Acta Psychiat Neurol Scand 1:287, 1926

209. Rifkin A, Quifkin F, Carillo C, Klein DF: Very high dosage fluphenazine for nonchronic treatment-refractory patients. Arch Gen Psychiatry 25:398, 1971

210. Roisin L, True C, Knight M: Structural effects of tranquilizers. Res Publ Assoc Nerv Ment Dis 37:285, 1959

211. Rylander G: Psychoses and the punding and choreiform syndromes in addiction to central stimulant drugs. Psychiat Neurol Neurochir 75:203, 1972

212. Safer DJ, Allen RP: The effect of fluphenazine in psychologically normal volunteers: Some temporal, performance and biochemical relationships. Biol Psychiatry 3:237, 1971

213. Sarwer-Foner GJ: Recognition and management of drug-induced extrapyramidal reactions and "paradoxical" behavioral reactions in psychiatry. Can Med Assoc J 83:312, 1960

214. Schaar M, Payne CA: Dystonic reactions to prochlorperazine in hypoparathyroidism. N Engl J Med 275:991, 1966

215. Schilder P: Brain and Personality: Studies in the Psychological Aspects of Cerebral Neuropathy and the Neuropsychiatric Aspects of the Motility of Schizophrenia. A Nervous and Mental Disease Monograph 53. Washington, The Nervous and Mental Disease Publication Co., 1931, pp 92–135

216. Schildkraut JJ: Neuropsychopharmacology and the affective disorders. N Engl J Med 281:197, 1969

217. Schwab RS, England AC: Parkinson syndromes due to various causes, in Vinken PJ, Bruyn GW (eds): Handbook of Clinical Neurology, vol. 6, Diseases of the Basal Ganglia. Amsterdam, North-Holland, 1968, pp 227–247
218. Seeman P, Lee T: Antipsychotic drugs: Direct correlation between clinical potency and presynaptic action on dopamine neurones. Science, 1974 (in press)
219. Seeman P, Wong M, Lee T: Dopamine receptor-block and nigral impulse-blockade by major tranquilizers. Fed Proc 33:246, 1974
220. Sethy VM, Van Woert MH: Modification of striatal acetylcholine concentration by dopamine receptor agonists and antagonists. Res Comm Chem Path Pharm 8:13, 1974
221. Sheppard C, Merlis S: Drug-induced extrapyramidal symptoms: Their incidence and treatment. Am J Psychiatry 123:886, 1967
222. Sherman L, Kim S, Benjamin F, Kolodny HD: Effect of chlorpromazine on serum growth-hormone concentration in man. N Engl J Med 284:72, 1971
223. Sigwald J, Bouttier D, Raymondeaud C, Piot C: Quatre cas de dyskinesie facio-bucco-linguo-masticatrice à évolution prolongée secondaire á un traitement par les neuroleptiques. Rev Neurol 100:751, 1959
224. Simpson GM: Controlled studies of antiparkinsonism agents in the treatment of drug-induced extrapyramidal symptoms. Acta Psychiatr Scand (Suppl 212):44, 1970
225. Simpson GM, Amuso D, Blair JH, Farkas T: Phenothiazine-produced extrapyramidal system disturbance. Arch Gen Psychiatry 10:199, 1964
226. Simpson GM, Krakov L, Kunz-Bartholini E: A controlled trial of combined medications on behavioral and extrapyramidal effects. Acta Psychiatr Scand (Suppl 212):20, 1970
227. Simpson GM, Kunz-Bartholini E: Relationship of individual tolerance, behavior and phenothiazine produced extrapyramidal system disturbance. Dis Nerv Syst 29:269, 1968
228. Simpson GM, Laska E: Sensitivity to a phenothiazine (butaperazine). Can Psychiatr Assoc J 13:499, 1968
229. Singer K, Lam CM: Evaluation of Leponex (clozapine) in schizophrenia with acute symptomatology. J Internat Med Res 1:627, 1973
230. Slater E, Roth M: Clinical Psychiatry (ed 3). London, Bailliére, Tindall and Cassell, 1969, pp 271–287
231. Snyder SH: Amphetamine psychosis: A "model" schizophrenia mediated by catecholamines. Am J Psychiatry 130:61, 1973
232. Snyder SH, Greenberg D, Yamamura HI: Antischizophrenic drugs and brain cholinergic receptors. Arch Gen Psychiatry 31:58, 1974
233. Spillane JD, Nathan PW, Kelly RE: Marsden CD: Painful legs and moving toes. Brain 94:541, 1971
234. Stadler H, Lloyd KG, Gadea-Ciria M, Bartholini G: Enhanced striatal acetylcholine release by chlorpromazine and its reversal by apomorphine. Brain Res 55:476, 1973
235. Sterkmans P, Brugmans J, Gevers F: The clinical efficacy of pimozide in chronic psychotic patients. Clin Trials J (Lond)5:1107, 1968

236. Straus EW, Griffith RM: Pseudoreversibility of catatonic stupor. Am J Psychiatry 111:680, 1955

237. Tamer A, McKey R, Arias D, Worley L, Fogel BJ: Phenothiazine-induced extrapyramidal dysfunction in the neonate. J Pediatr 75:479, 1969

238. Tarsy D, Baldessarini R: Pharmacologically induced behavioral supersensitivity to apomorphine. Nature [New Biol] 245:262, 1973

239. Tarsy D, Baldessarini RJ: Behavioral supersensitivity to apomorphine following chronic administration of drugs which interfere with the synaptic function of catecholamines. Neuropharmacology 13:927, 1974

240. Tarsy D, Leopold N, Sax DS: Physostigmine in choreiform movement disorders. Neurology (Minneap)24:28, 1974

241. Trabucchi M, Cheney D, Racagni G, Costa E: Involvement of brain cholinergic mechanisms in the action of chlorpromazine. Nature 249:644, 1974

242. Uhrbrand L, Faurbye A: Reversible and irreversible dyskinesia after treatment with perphenazine, chlorpromazine, reserpine, and electroconvulsive therapy. Psychopharmacologia (Berl.) 1:408, 1960

243. Ungerstedt U: Postsynaptic supersensitivity after 6-hydroxydopamine induced degeneration of the nigrostriatal dopamine system. Acta Physiol Scand 82(Suppl 367):69, 1971

244. Villeneuve A: The rabbit syndrome, a peculiar extrapyramidal reaction. Can Psychiat Assoc J 17:SS69, 1972

245. Vogt M: Functional aspects of the role of catecholamines in the central nervous system. Br Med Bull 29:168, 1973

246. Weiner H: Diagnosis and symptomatology in Bellak L (ed): Schizophrenia: A Review of the Syndrome. New York, Logos Press, 1958, p 143

247. Windelman NW: The interrelationship between the physiological and psychological etiologies of akathisia, in Bordeleau JM (ed): Extrapyramidal System and Neuroleptics. Montreal, Editions Psychiatriques, 1961, pp 563–568

248. Wolf SM: Reserpine: Cause and treatment of oral-facial dyskinesia. Bull Los Angeles Neurol Soc 38:80, 1973

249. Yarden PE, Discipio WJ: Abnormal movements and prognosis in schizophrenia. Am J Psychiatry 128:317, 1971

250. Yaryura-Tobias JA, Diamond B, Merlis S: The action of L-Dopa on schizophrenic patients. Curr Ther Res 12:528, 1970

251. Yaryura-Tobias JA, Wolpert A, Dana L, Merlis S: Action of L-Dopa in drug-induced extrapyramidalism. Dis Nerv Syst 31:60, 1970

252. Yeh BK, McKay JL, Goldberg LI: Attenuation of dopamine renal and mesenteric vasodilation by haloperidol: Evidence for a specific dopamine receptor. J Pharmacol Exp Ther 168:303, 1969

253. York DH: Dopamine receptor blockade—a central action of chlorpromazine on striatal neurones. Brain Res 37:91, 1972

Commentary

The authors have provided a great deal of clinical information and a useful foundation for the understanding of future drug problems. While many points in this chapter deserve emphasis, the editors particularly want to point out that many of the movement disorders described in this chapter were known to occur in psychiatric patients, particularly in schizophrenics, prior to the introduction of the major tranquilizing drugs. This would suggest that the drugs may facilitate certain CNS metabolic abnormalities already present in schizophrenic patients. Study of the pharmacology of the antipsychotic agents and drug-induced movement disorders should represent an important means of studying the pathophysiology of psychiatric disorders.

The following chapter presents a neuropsychiatric study of the natural course of a single disease, Huntington's chorea. In outlining the full course of this disease, the authors touch on most of the major neuropsychiatric problems previously presented in this volume. In simplified form, the initial "functional" symptomatology seen in Huntington's chorea disappears with emergence of a major personality disorder, which, in turn, degenerates into dementia.

Paul R. McHugh, M.D., and
Marshal F. Folstein, M.D.

13

Psychiatric Syndromes of Huntington's Chorea: A Clinical and Phenomenologic Study

We report our detailed observations on the psychologic symptoms of eight patients with Huntington's chorea. The symptoms cluster into two clearly recognizable syndromes: (1) a progressive dementia syndrome afflicting all the patients and (2) an intermittent affective disorder afflicting a majority of the patients. A few schizophrenic-like symptoms occur in Huntington's chorea. One patient of ours had an hallucinatory–delusionary state that was most like schizophrenia. It could have been instead an atypical affective change. The issues of paranoid features and personality change are discussed and exemplified in our patients. The possibility that Huntington's chorea may represent degeneration of one of the ascending, transmitter-specific pathways is suggested and briefly discussed in the light of the particular psychiatric symptoms found in this disorder.

In his original description of Huntington's chorea,[10] George Huntington made "insanity with a tendency to suicide" one of three distinguishing characteristics of the illness, along with the facts that it is hereditary and that it first appears in adulthood. Subsequent students of the disease have confirmed Huntington's observation but noted that several different mental disturbances occur in these patients; a dementia syndrome,[8] psychotic symptoms variously labeled schizoid, paranoid, or depressive,[2, 3,6] and personality changes.[4,17,27] The clinical descriptions of these disturbances, however, are usually brief,

Supported by Grant MH11000-06 from the National Institutes of Health, Department of Health, Education and Welfare, and by Grant MR06710-15, from the National Institute of Mental Health, Department of Health, Education and Welfare.

perhaps because little enthusiasm could be kindled for the drawing of subtle psychiatric distinctions from among the manifestations of a rare, idiopathic disorder with an intractable course.

But now we know that some pathologic disruption of the neural paths with specific chemical transmitters may explain several extrapyramidal disorders. These concepts resting on a new neuroanatomy have led to a new treatment—L-Dopa—in Parkinsonism and to a new interest in all the extrapyramidal disorders including Huntington's chorea. Although the choreic movements and the motoric disability in Huntington's chorea attract most attention, these new concepts may provide an appreciation of mechanisms behind the mental disturbances in this disease and even for the mental illnesses that it can mimic. Therefore, we are encouraged to describe the psychiatric symptoms in Huntington's chorea and to consider their resemblance to symptoms in other disorders by a renewed sense of purpose.

SAMPLE

It was important that all of our patients were seen at a psychiatric hospital, the New York Hospital, Westchester Division, since patients gathered from a neurologic or medical setting might have less prominent psychologic symptomatology. All eight patients were personally studied, and had a psychiatric history obtained from relatives and friends. These eight patients are listed in Table 13-1 with pertinent demographic and clinical features. Two are related, L.M. and K.M., being father and daughter, respectively.

All patients had family histories of Huntington's chorea and were themselves certain examples of the disorder. One developed her illness in adolescence and showed the rigidity that characterizes the juvenile form of Huntington's chorea.

The patients were studied for the first time at varying periods in their illnesses. Four of them, K.M., B.U., B.B., and A.S., were seen prior to the advent of their neurologic symptoms and were referred for evaluation of psychologic disturbance. Eventually, choreic movements or rigidity did develop, but these patients demonstrated that the very first symptoms of the condition may be of a psychologic nature. The others were seen after chorea had appeared and been diagnosed but were referred because of psychologic complications.

THE DEMENTIA SYNDROME

The mental disorder most consistently suffered by patients with Huntington's chorea is a dementia syndrome, eventually seen in nearly all

Table 13-1
Eight Patients from New York Hospital, Westchester Division.

Patient	Age	Sex	Duration of Illness on admission	WAIS I.Q. Full Score	Verbal Performance	Memory Difficulty	Suicidal Attempts	Other Diagnoses Entertained
K.M.	18	F	1 year	71	78 65	No	No	Schizophrenia Paranoid type
L.M.	49	M	3 years	—	—	Yes	Yes	Manic–depressive Alzheimer's disease
J.M.	40	F	5 years	94	102 84	Yes	No	—
B.U.	41	F	1 year	111	127 95	No	No	Manic–depressive
E.Z.	60	F	7 years	72	80 65	Yes	No	Manic–depressive
B.B.	39	F	1 year	80	88 71	No	Yes	Manic–depressive
A.S.	51	F	1 year	107	118 91	Yes	No	Schizophrenia Paranoid type
H.P.	45	M	8 years	91	105 74	Yes	No	—

examples. Reports of its frequency vary from 50 to 100 percent, perhaps depending on the vigor with which it was sought.[2,6, 21] All of our patients manifested a dementia syndrome, the severity of which depended on the duration of the illness, but the characteristics were always the same: They were those of a syndrome in which impaired cognitive function was combined with a progressive mental apathy. These two features of the syndrome will be separately described for purposes of clarity, even though they appear and advance together.

Impaired Cognitive Functions

Although the symptoms of the dementia syndrome are usually obvious when the choreic movements are clearly established, they can precede the abnormal movements and then present diagnostic problems, as they did in four of our patients, L.M., H.P., K.M., and A.S. The earliest symptoms of this syndrome are hard to describe with confidence, since they are easily disregarded and explained as expression of fatigue, distraction, or emotional disturbance. They usually appear, however, as a change in the capacity of the patient to think through problems at home or at work with his accustomed efficiency. Problems that had been easy for him to solve now seem more difficult. He is less able to appreciate situations and to recall information for his purposes. This can be obvious in patients with professional occupations. H.P.'s first symptom was difficulty in organizing simple programs of digitalis therapy for his patients, even though he was a recognized cardiologist.

Although these difficulties may be vague, insidious in their onset and progression, and unaccompanied by clear signs on bedside mental testing, formal psychologic testing of cognitive functions will usually document the problem, particularly by a decline in the performance scores of the Wechsler Adult Intelligence Scale (WAIS) (see table 13-1). In our patients, the average discrepancy between verbal and performance scores was 21 points when the patient was first seen.

With the onset of the dementia syndrome, and usually contemporaneous with the appearance of the choreic symptoms, the impaired capacity to think becomes apparent in everyday situations. Now the patient is seen to have difficulty in following the gist of a conversation, to become vague and uncertain in speech, and to fail to appreciate humor or subtle distinctions of meaning. Patient A.S. was observed by her husband to speak vaguely and off the point, to be repetitious, and difficult to follow in her conversation, a notable change for this college graduate. L.M. had a similar loss of coherence and was thought by his family to have ''aged very remarkably'' in a few months.

Also at this stage, patients themselves will often complain of difficulties in memory, with inability to learn or to recall important events. Five of our eight patients clearly had trouble with memory, which will be discussed in more detail below.

At this time, the patient's judgments are often poor. Liable to misinterpret situations and the meanings of other people's actions, they may react inappropriately and emotionally. Patient A.S., in fact, developed a morbid jealousy after observing her husband talk to a young woman. H.P. refused to surrender his aviator's license, even though his motor incoordination was obvious and he admitted to difficulty following the directions for navigating his aircraft.

Bedside mental examination now clearly documents the disability in thinking. Although patients are usually oriented to time and place, tasks that require attention and concentration, like the serial sevens, are particularly badly performed. Similarly, they misunderstand complex commands and make mistakes in the tests of memory. Patient L.M. is a good example. He was able to count and do simple arithmetic but could not subtract 7 from 100, nor do any "carryover" subtractions. He was unable to repeat any of the parts of the cowboy story nor to interpret it. He could repeat only three digits forwards and none backwards and was unable to remember any of the word pairs of the paired associate learning test. The impression gained on bedside examination is not of a specific deficit in any particular cognitive function, such as memory, but rather a general loss of efficiency in all aspects of thinking including memory functions.

Psychologic tests show a worsening of the overall I.Q. with lowering of both verbal and performance scores. Patient H.P. has been followed for 8 years. His initial WAIS, given 2 years after the onset of his illness, already reflected a verbal-performance difference with full I.Q., 109, verbal score, 126, performance, 87. These scores fell in the next 6 years to a full I.Q. of 91, with verbal, 105, and performance, 74. A 78 on the Raven's Progressive Matrices, a test given at the same time as the WAIS that does not require movement to complete, demonstrated that the low performance score was not due to motor disability.

The absolutely terminal stage of the dementia syndrome in Huntington's chorea has not been observed in our eight patients, as they are all still alive. Patients with Huntington's chorea live on the average of 16 years after the onset of their illness but can live as much as 25–30 years.[21] Thus, the natural history of this dementia is different from that in other degenerative diseases impairing cognitive powers, particularly Alzheimer's disease.[25] In Alzheimer's disease, 3–4 years after the first symptoms are seen, a severe dementia syndrome is present and by 6–8 years, the patient has died in an amentia. Most patients with Huntington's chorea who survive long despite the progressive motor incapacity and cachexia will show a very severe cognitive loss with disorientation, memory loss, and a total collapse of verbal and performance scores.

When the disabilities of the dementia syndrome are prominent, the patient usually has other symptoms that interfere with his thinking capacities. Most distressing and dramatic are the appearance of typical catastrophic reactions. These are not different from the catastrophic reactions seen in patients whose dementia syndromes rest on other pathology. They are transient, explosive, emotional collapses of the capacity to think, judge, and behave appearing in situations that are taxing to the patient's diminished abilities. These reactions may appear during formal testing or when the patient's cooperation is needed in disagreeable circumstances and may then lead to behaviors for which the patient is often remorseful on recovery of his composure. Patient J.M. would have such a reaction during each home visit. On appreciating that she was returning to the hospital, she would cry, curse, and strike out at her husband and children. Even though she was repentant after these outbursts and recognized that they jeopardized her visiting privileges, she never seemed able to control them.

There are several aspects of cognitive function that are always spared in Huntington's chorea. These preserved functions help define the dementia syndrome here and differentiate it from dementia syndromes seen with some other brain diseases. The most important is that Huntington's chorea patients do not develop aphasia. They may have impaired word-finding and some difficulty in abstract communication, but these difficulties are reflections of their problems in the preconditions for language, such as capacity to attend, to understand, to interpret, and to respond. Specifically, the patient with Huntington's chorea never develops jargon aphasia that is so characteristic of patients whose dementia syndromes rest primarily on cortical degeneration, such as Alzheimer's disease[25] and Jakob–Creutzfeldt disorder.[22] The list of mental symptoms not seen in Huntington's chorea can be enlarged to include cortical blindness and unilateral neglect. Bruyn[3] reports that Shternberg[23] has made similar observations and adds the absence of alexia, apraxia, and agnosia to the list of symptoms seen in other dementias but not in Huntington's chorea.

The issue of memory disorder in Huntington's chorea is also of interest and slightly controversial, some textbooks reporting that memory is spared[26] and others that memory is affected early and considerably in Huntington's chorea.[30] It is our experience that patients with Huntington's chorea do have a memory disorder. Two of them, patients H.P. and L.M., complained of trouble with memory when they were first examined. As shown in Table 13-1, five of our eight patients had a memory disorder manifested by impaired recall of recent events, by difficulty in remembering items on bedside testing, and by low scores on formal psychologic tests, such as the Wechsler Memory Scale. Patient J.M. with a performance I.Q. of 84 scored a Wechsler M.Q. of 65. Table 13-1 also reveals that the memory disorder is an aspect of advancing illness. Of the four patients in the first year of the illness, only one had a disturbance of memory; the other four patients with a longer duration of illness all had demonstrable difficulties with memory.

The memory impairment is not, however, disproportionate to other difficulties in cognitive function, such as attention and interpretation. The Huntington patient does not have the memory disorder called Korsakov's syndrome, in which the patient, disoriented to time and place, and without the capacities to recall recent events or to learn new things, has retained many other cognitive functions such as powers of abstraction and reasoning.

These clinical impressions could be improved with data specifically comparing the psychologic performance of Huntington patients with other syndromes such as the Korsakov. We and others are doing such studies.[19] Our present view is that memory is disturbed in Huntington's chorea but can be described as a quantitative impairment in learning new things that is proportional to other cognitive deficits and can be at least partially overcome by attention, repetition, and practice, whereas the memory problem of the Korsakov syndrome is a qualitative defect that interferes absolutely and specifically with learning in a fashion not susceptible to improvement by compensatory efforts. Further empirical work is needed to confirm or deny this view.

Mental Apathy

Right from the onset of the difficulties in thinking and with their progressive manifestation, a feature often described as a change in personality is developing that is an integral part of the dementia syndrome in this disorder. This change both worsens the cognitive disturbances and makes them harder to measure accurately. It is the appearance of an apathetic state affecting the intellectual vitality, physical energy, and curiosity of the patient and usually first recognized by a lessening interest in work, appearance, current affairs, or even in the progress of the illness. This apathy, or loss of initiative, can result in a much poorer performance in daily affairs than would be thought likely from the modest difficulties found on formal intellectual assessment in the earliest stage of the syndrome. An excellent example of this symptom is K.M., who over 6 months and prior to any other symptom, stopped caring about her dress and make-up, lost her job, and changed from an active and effective young person to one who would prefer to stay home watching television or resting in bed.

In the late stages of Huntington's chorea, there is marked progression of apathy and inertia to the point of profound self-neglect, double incontinence, and mutism. This state in which the patient is inaccessible to examination resembles the akinetic mute syndrome. Curran[5] reported an excellent example of this symptom, and our patient K.M. progressively manifested it until she was bedridden and mute. As with typical examples of akinetic mutism, sometimes spontaneously and sometimes in response to a stimulus, K.M. would speak giving evidence that some capacities to remember and appreciate her situation, were present but masked by her apathy, inertia, and mutism.

Although in the full course of the illness this apathetic feature steadily worsens, it can be transiently interrupted by periods of restlessness and irritation lasting minutes to days and occasionally leading to assaults on the family and attendants. At these times, the patient's judgment is poor, his intentions vague and uncertain, and his actions impulsive and unpredictable. The more short-lived attacks probably represent examples of the catastrophic reactions described above. Others that extend over days are not likely to represent the same kind of disturbance. These longer periods of overactivity can usually be recognized as responses of a person with impaired cognitive powers to misindentifications, mood changes, or delusions. These precipitating mental changes are described in more detail below. But H.P. was an excellent example of how they can lead to rather long periods of restless irritability. He was usually apathetic and disinterested but intermittently his mood changed to one of elation and overactivity as he simultaneously developed the belief that he was the inventor of a new gyroscope. He then wanted to buy bicycles to test out his invention and, when discouraged in these plans, became angry and aggressive. He would stay in this angry overactive state for several weeks until the mood of elation and the false belief subsided. He would then return to his customary apathetic condition.

Summary

To summarize these observations, thère are three distinctive features of the dementia syndrome in Huntington's chorea: (1) a slowly progressive dilapidation of all cognitive powers; (2) a prominent psychic apathy and inertia that worsens to an akinetic mute state; and (3) an *absence* of aphasia, alexia, cortical blindness, or Korsakov-type amnesia.

We want to point out that, although symptoms that resemble portions of this syndrome can appear with localized cerebral pathologies such as the apathetic state in patients with frontal lobe disease, the combination of the three features that form this syndrome is distinctive and is found in disorders with prominent subcortical pathology such as Parkinsonism,[13] hydrocephalus,[15] and Huntington's chorea. The syndrome defined by these features is not found in disorders with prominent cortical pathology such as Alzheimer's disease or Jakob–Creutzfeldt disease. We thus have referred to this[16] as the ''subcortical dementia syndrome'' and distinguished it from ''cortical dementia syndrome.''

There are advantages to making these clinical distinctions, although it is agreed that mental function is an outcome of the integrative activity of the whole brain and many of these disorders including Huntington's chorea have both cortical and subcortical pathology. The most obvious is the drawing of attention in human illness to the role of other parts of the brain than the cortex in cognitive activities and another is that the distinctions between dementia syndromes should help us recognize clinically conditions with different pathologies.

SYNDROMES THAT RESEMBLE THE "FUNCTIONAL PSYCHOSES"

Although a dementia syndrome is so characteristic of Huntington's chorea that Hallock[8] suggested that the eponymous title of the disorder be replaced in favor of the term dementia choreica, patients may suffer dramatic mental changes that in every way mimic one of the two "functional" endogenous psychoses, affective disorders or schizophrenia, during the first few years of the illness when the dementia symptoms may be minimal and the movement disorder inapparent. In considerations of Huntington's chorea, the symptoms of these psychoses are frequently lumped together as paranoid features or schizophrenia-like symptoms[2,7] in a fashion little more descriptive than Huntington's original statement that the patients have a tendency to "that form of insanity which leads to suicide." It is possible to improve on this considerably and distinguish in the earliest years of the illness two different forms of mental disorder, one an episodic mood disorder resembling the manic-depressive psychosis and the other a delusionary hallucinatory state resembling an acute schizophrenic illness.

Mood Disorder

The disturbance in mood that resembles the manic–depressive disorder is the easier to delimit and define and was the more common of the two psychotic pictures in our group of patients, appearing in five of the eight (B.U., L.M., E.Z., B.B., and H.P.).

It usually appears in a depressive guise as episodes of depression associated with an attitude of hopelessness and guilt and the appearance of delusions of sinfulness, blameworthiness, poverty, or disease. Several of our patients showed these delusions. L.M. believed that he had cancer, that he was improverished, and that he was "ruining the lives of my family." E.Z. believed she had committed unpardonable offenses. B.B. said that she felt Satan was dwelling within her and that she acted in accordance with his wishes. H.P. believed that he had a reputation of homosexuality. If at the onset of the mood disorder the patient has established choreic movements, he may believe that he is ridiculed because of these movements or that they are the stigmata of some sin.

As Huntington implied,[10] ideas of suicide and suicidal attempts spring directly out of this mental state. Two of our patients, L.M. and E.Z., had frequent suicidal thoughts. Reed and Chandler[21] found that suicide was the cause of death in 7% of nonhospitalized Huntington patients. The delusions of blameworthiness and sinfulness also probably explain some of the reports of family homicide and bizarre suicidal acts in some patients with Huntington's chorea.[4,6] B.U. had threatened her children with a knife and for this reason was separated from her family. It is undoubtedly true that similar delusions led to the willingness of early English and New England patients with Huntington's chorea to cooperate with those who accused them of witchcraft. Vessie[29] describes one Elizabeth Wanne, a progenitrix of a long line of choreics, who confessed during her interrogation for witchcraft in Suffolk England in the 1600's that "she had the devil in her body" and should be punished. Her delusion was identical to that of our patient B.B.

Along with the change in mood and delusions, the patients may show psychomotor retardation, with both verbal productivity and motor activity being very slow. L.M. was so hesitant in thinking, sometimes taking between 30 seconds and 1 minute between words, that it often took him 3–5 minutes to complete a sentence during his depressions. B.B. was also noted to be slow in her responses. E.Z. provided us a potentially important observation relating the mood and the degree of abnormal movements in that her choreiform movement disorder, which was quite severe, was greatly suppressed during her depressive phases when she was slow in thoughts and actions.

These episodes of depression can last from weeks to months and may persist for several years and then spontaneously resolve. They are responsive to antidepressant treatment, and all three of our patients who received electroconvulsive treatment (L.M., B.U., and E.Z.), recovered temporarily from their mood disorder. Brothers and Meadows[2] also pointed out that the depression in Huntington's chorea will improve with ECT.

Although depression is the more common affective state, it can reverse into mania, and such episodes of mania were seen in two of our patients, H.P. and E.Z. The symptoms are those typical of mania: the patient is elated, expansive, and garrulous, he takes on ideas of grandeur and self-importance and will often overspend, overeat, and be overactive. When manic, patient E.Z. thought that despite her movement disorder she was well enough to walk many miles to visit relatives. She would go to her local shops and spend beyond her means and when in the hospital would often tell the doctors that she could treat and cure other patients. H.P. believed that he was a great inventor of gyroscopes and the complications of his beliefs in his behavior and tractability were described above.

Overactivity in the manic stages can affect the movement disorder just as the psychomotor retardation can modify it. E.Z. showed a greatly exaggerated choreic movement disorder during her manic stage so that she could not walk down a corridor without striking the walls. Increases in psychomotor activity were also reflected in a "flight of ideas" during the manic stages. This feature was prominent in both H.P. and E.Z.

The manic state can persist for weeks and like the depressive episodes spontaneously resolve often with a return to depression. We attempted to treat E.Z. with lithium, without success, during her manic stages but phenothiazines were effective in relieving them.

As can be recognized from this description, there is little, if anything, to distinguish this state from the manic–depressive psychosis. As so often happens, and in fact occurred in patients B.U. and B.B., if the mood disorder appears before any firm evidence of motor disturbance or dementia, it may be impossible to make the distinction by symptoms alone. Only a family history of Huntington's chorea will suggest that this is not the usual idiopathic manic-depressive disorder but rather a psychosis symptomatic of Huntington's chorea.

If a mood disorder, particularly a depressive one, appears after the establishment of the diagnosis or after the appearance of motor symptoms, there is a tendency to consider it a psychologic reaction akin to discouragement and sadness engendered by the patient's appreciation of the implication of his illness. Such a diagnostic decision might lead a physician to fail to explore the mental status of the patient for evidence of delusionary and suicidal elements. This is a clinical error. Patients may well be sad and discouraged when they recognize the fact or prognosis of their illness and, as Pearson reported,[20] they may also show these symptoms when they first learn of the diagnosis and its hereditary nature. It is stretching an interpretation, however, to make such understandable attitudes explain (1) the episodic nature of the mood changes, (2) the manic as well as the depressive features, (3) the psychomotor retardation or overactivity that can alter the chorea itself and (4) the delusionary beliefs, all of which can appear prior to any knowledge by the patient of his disease. Since these psychotic states can be treated and suicide or even homicide avoided, depressive changes in Huntington's chorea should be of serious concern, prompting thorough examination, early recognition, and early treatment.

Delusionary–Hallucinatory State

The other psychotic state occurring in the early years of the course of Huntington's chorea is the one most often mentioned as schizophrenic-like,[7,18] but as discussed below, we think that such labeling may be misleading and hence prefer the term delusionary–hallucinatory disturbance. As with the mood disorder, this disturbance can appear early in the course of the illness prior to the motor disability.

In its most characteristic guise, the patient is taken over by a vague but all-pervasive impression of a change in reality of the world and of himself, an uncanny change laden with some meaning of an uncertain nature, perhaps foreboding, perhaps enlightening, but often with a sense of supernatural importance. All the patient's experiences and perceptions will be colored by this inner feeling. This is the state called delusionary mood (Wahnstimmung) by continental psychiatrists. The patient describes the uncanny quality as different from his ordinary state of consciousness, as though he were drugged or hypnotized. Although the patient seems preoccupied and inaccessible, consciousness to formal examination is unimpaired and orientation and other cognitive functions are unchanged.

From out of this state come vague delusions of influence and control, persecution or grandiosity, as well as equally vague hallucinations and illusions. K.M. felt that she was controlled by extraplanetary creatures for good and also for evil purposes. She also had auditory hallucinations in which the creatures spoke to and about her and tactile hallucinations in which she felt they sexually abused her.

The patients are convinced of the reality of these hallucinations and delusions and may act upon them as K.M. did when she called the police.

This state can come on suddenly and, as with the mood disorder, it can appear before the motor and intellectual disturbances. It is reported to last longer than the mood changes, and K.M. suffered two attacks lasting 4 months separated by a remission of several months' duration. Treatment with phenothiazines can be helpful, but K.M. also needed amitriptyline to relieve her symptoms. One of K.M.'s attacks seemed to be precipitated by a diagnostic trial of L-Dopa.

The schizophrenic-like features of this condition are obvious enough but are quite different from those of chronic schizophrenia of insidious onset in which a patient is not so vague and inaccessible to examination nor taken up by an inner sense of foreboding change. However, as with K.M., a diagnosis of acute schizophrenia with paranoid and catatonic features will commonly be made and the diagnosis of Huntington's chorea not considered.

It seems to us that these symptoms should not be viewed confidently as typical schizophrenia symptoms. Some acute affective psychoses or the "schizophrenics of good prognosis" that are so like affective disorders can show identical symptoms, and K.M. clearly responded to antidepressant medication. A decision on classification depends on the vexed question of just what symptoms are to be called schizophrenic. In order to keep the question of the relationship of this state to other psychiatric disorders an open one, it could be referred to nonspecifically and nonprejudicially as a delusionary–hallucinatory state in Huntington's chorea.

Summary

The terms to be given these disorders and the issues of what they resemble are of less practical importance than the fact that they can be hard to distinguish from the standard "functional psychosis" and can appear before any choreic movements signal the diagnosis. Our experience confirms that of Streletzki.[28] The first symptoms of Huntington's chorea can present problems of differentiation from the endogenous psychoses, affective disorder, and schizophrenia. As shown in Table 13-1, such diagnoses were entertained or temporarily given before the diagnosis of Huntington's chorea was established in six of our eight patients.

DISTURBANCES DERIVED FROM THE FUNDAMENTAL SYNDROMES

In the first 4–6 years of the illness before the apathy, mutism and the cognitive disturbances of the progressing dementia syndrome come to predominate, features of both the "functional" and dementia syndromes are often seen mixed together. In fact, patient L.M. was given the diagnosis of both manic–depressive disorder and Alzheimer's disease before the diagnosis became clear, and as can be seen from our psychometric tests in Table 13-1, E.Z. and B.B., although thought possibly to be manic–depressive, already had intellectual difficulty. We believe that the two aspects of Huntington's chorea that are so frequently referred to in textbooks as paranoid features and personality changes derive from the various individual mixtures of the "functional" and dementia syndromes that the patients can show in the disease. We will discuss the paranoid features and personality changes separately to make this point clear.

Paranoid Features

The term "paranoid," as has been pointed out by Lewis,[12] is one so burdened with a history of changing meanings that it has lost much of its power of definitiveness. It is not our purpose to elaborate on what paranoid means but to point out that many psychologic symptoms, such as delusions, hallucinations, or even changing attitudes, tend to be clumped together under the term paranoid as if they belonged to some category related to schizophrenia. We use "paranoid" only as a descriptive term for any mental experience or persisting trait that provokes feelings of fear, suspiciousness, resentment, or hatred in the patient. If such experiences or traits are searched for in Huntington's chorea, they will be found in abundance, but in multiple forms and settings, and with assorted companion symptoms. It is from these features that the symptoms will take their particular significance, diagnosis, treatment, and prognosis, and not from any common "paranoid" quality. Defined in this fashion, it is apparent that symptoms that could be called "paranoid features" can emerge from the psychotic states, from the dementia syndrome, or from a mixture of both in Huntington's chorea.

The mood disorder with its change in self-attitude can prompt ideas of reference or persecution, as when the patients believe that because of some failing or transgression they are discussed in the news as notorious and that punishments or restrictions are planned for them. H.P., for instance, believed that he was to be arrested and persecuted because he had a reputation for homosexuality. In the manic stage, the patients can become resentful because they feel they are being held unfairly from their grandiose plans, and H.P., in this state, believed that all the hospital rules were being made to restrict him. Likewise, the delusionary–hallucinatory form of the psychosis can produce beliefs of personal danger, as in K.M., who believed she was being assaulted and sought police help.

In any dementia syndrome, regardless of cause, the tendency to false impressions can prompt severe and uninhibited fears and hatreds. These may be impulsively developed and express themselves in violent form. Patient A.S. developed a morbid jealousy because she misinterpreted her husband's casual conversations with women. She arrived at our hospital with a diagnosis of schizophrenia, paranoid type, solely on the basis of this symptom that, on closer examination, could be seen to be derived from her cognitive uncertainties.

The management of the paranoid features will depend on the condition from which they emerge. Those that derive from affective change, as in patients L.M. and E.Z., respond to antidepressant treatment. Those that derive from misunderstanding require efforts to clarify and reinterpret for the patient situations that have provoked the difficulty.

Personality Changes

The literature on Huntington's chorea often describes alterations of personality as an early symptom of the illness.[6,9,18] Since the term personality is a descriptive concept intended to gather up into one category the prominent but abiding feelings, moods, and attitudes that constitute an individual's potential to respond to circumstances in particular ways, changes can be expected that derive from the fundamental psychologic syndromes of Huntington's chorea.

We think that two kinds of changes can be derived in this way and are particularly prominent in Huntington's chorea. One is the apathetic, slow and slovenly attitude that leads a patient to neglect himself, his duties, his former interests, and his friends, which we have described as a part of the dementia syndrome. Both K.M. and J.M. showed this change giving up their school and professional work, their interest in world affairs, and their concern for their own appearance. The other is a change toward a growing irritability and oversensitivity expressed often as a moody discontent with frequent outbursts of anger and violence. Patient B.U. is a good example of this feature. She gradually changed from a sympathetic, well-controlled, efficient nurse and mother to a person with such an explosive temperament that she could no longer work, became miserably discontent over the details of household management, and frightened her children with threats of violence. It seemed that this change can be at least in part ascribed to a mixture of the dementia features with depressive elements. B.U. was suffering from depressive delusions of bodily decay and a moderate dementia. Her personality change was considerably relieved by electroconvulsive treatment.

These personality changes could be considered more specific and not derived as we have interpreted them from the other psychologic syndromes of Huntington's chorea. They do after all resemble some of the changes associated with frontal lobe pathology. But some evidence for our point of view is that these two changes in personality are not mutually exclusive categories. Even the patient examples we have chosen here as prototypes can show aspects of the other features at other times. Thus, J.M., whose apathy and indolence was prominent, often had periods of irritation and oversensitivity. All of our other patients show elements of both these changes in less dramatic form and in changing fashion as the illness progresses.

Although we are emphasizing the symptomatic changes in the patient's personality, we do not intend to imply that the patients's emotional reactions to their changing circumstances, changing appearance, and changing capabilities are not also important in altering their abiding feelings, moods, and attitudes. Persistent discouragement and anxiety arising after the illness had been diagnosed and the disabilities established were common. Patient B.U., between her attacks of depression and the delusions that preoccupied her, would then speak of her sadness over her lost abilities as a nurse and mother. J.M. was lonely for her family when in the hospital and spoke often of her dread that she would not be able to return home. L.M. grieved when he learned of his daughter K.M. becoming ill and hoped that her illness was misdiagnosed. These features intermingled with the symptomatic features and it was sometimes difficult to be sure where understandable feelings left off and were replaced by symptoms of a recurring affective disorder. B.U. was a good example of this, her sadness often worsening just before delusions reappeared.

Finally, we saw a change in one of our patients that could not be readily explained as a result of the cardinal syndromes or as a reaction to her illness and its implications. Patient J.M. was hospitalized primarily because of an obsessional disorder that developed 5 years after the appearance of her choreic movements. The content of the obsessions (related to knives and danger to her family) could be interpreted as a reaction of fear prompted by her awareness of illness, but such an interpretation would not explain the obsessional form. Since depressive disorder is known to prompt obsessional symptoms, it seemed possible that such was the explanation in J.M., but treatment with antidepressant medication produced little improvement and the symptom was never completely relieved.

DISCUSSION

We have reported our clinical experience with patients seen at one mental hospital. Our intentions were to define the psychiatric features of this disorder, relieve some of the persisting disagreements on matters of clinical fact and analyze what psychiatric syndromes seem to be fundamental in the illness.

From this work, we can say that two psychiatric syndromes are found in patients with Huntington's chorea: (1) a dementia syndrome that afflicts all the patients, and (2) an affective disorder that afflicts a considerable proportion and can mimic in every way manic–depressive illness. A delusionary-hallucinatory state is seen in a few patients, but whether it is a distinct syndrome or a form of affective disorder is uncertain.

Most of the other symptoms that are reported and we have seen can be derived from these, are understandable as aspects of discouragement and disability, or appear as individual idiosyncracies. Important as these features may be in the day-to-day management of particular patients, they are much less helpful to a consideration of neurobiologic mechanisms in psychiatric symptom formation. Only the established and fundamental syndromes will do for that.

It must be admitted that our knowledge of symptom formation in Huntington's chorea is meager not only for the psychiatric disorders but for the neurologic ones as well. Bruyn's chapter[3] can be consulted as a repository of facts on Huntington's chorea derived from observations in many disciplines including neuropathology, biochemistry, and pharmacology. But few of these facts have been successfully related to one another, or developed into an appreciation of the mechanisms that are failing when symptoms appear. In the same way it is difficult for us to relate the psychiatric syndromes to one another or to point to their pathologic mechanisms.

Some new unifying observation and conception is awaited here that will bring together the disconnected facts produced by the application of established methods. A likely source of such a hypothesis is an appreciation of the newly discovered ascending cholinergic and monoaminergic neural pathways in the brain.[24] A degenerative disorder in one of them (the dopamine pathway) is probably the explanation of Parkinsonism. A degeneration of an ascending cholinergic system may be the explanation of Huntington's chorea.

Such a degeneration could affect neo-cortical structure and function, since this system is distributed throughout the cortex.[11] The role of this system in the cortex has been thought by Shute and Lewis[24] to be arousing, alerting one (a similar function has been ascribed to the norepinephrine system, however), and so the suggestion that its degeneration might produce a dementia with a prominent apathetic feature such as is found in Huntington's chorea is plausible. The degeneration of the cholinergic system could lead to disruption of the caudate–putamen structure that is a pathologic characteristic of Huntington's chorea, since a high concentration of acetylcholine neurons are found there.[14] Since this cholinergic system is also distributed in limbic and hypothalamic regions, its degeneration could lead to mood disorder. Huntington's chorea thus could reveal a role for the cholinergic system in the regulation of mood, a function usually left to the monoamine systems.

Degeneration of this diffusely distributed system should provide the very kind of diffuse neuropathology that has hindered previous attempts at regional neuropathologic analysis of symptom formation. Some evidence rendering this suggestion at least plausible is found in the occasional amelioration of neurologic symptoms in Huntington's chorea by treatment with physostigmine,[1] and a reduction in enzymes for acetylcholine synthesis in the brains of Huntington's chorea patients.[14] That a disorder that is presumably produced by one gene should result in a degeneration of one discrete neural system has the pleasing feature of conforming to the one-gene-one-enzyme-one-protein hypothesis.

Finally, if degeneration of any one of these diffusely distributed neuronal systems could be established as the fundamental defect in Huntington's chorea, it would help explain why two apparently unrelated psychiatric syndromes, dementia and affective disorder, should occur together in an illness. Thus, the potential of knowledge of these neural systems is not limited for psychiatry to an appreciation of the disturbances in Huntington's chorea but may come to answer some of the most fundamental questions of the discipline.

ACKNOWLEDGMENTS

We thank Drs. James Gibbs and Phillip Slavney for their most helpful suggestions.

REFERENCES

1. Aquilonius SM, Sjostrom R: Cholinergic and dopaminergic mechanisms in Huntington's chorea. Life Sci 10:405–414, 1971
2. Brothers CRD, Meadows AW: An investigation of Huntington's chorea in Victoria. Ment Sci 101:548–563, 1955
3. Bruyn GW: Huntington's chorea: Historical, clinical and laboratory synopsis, in Vinken PJ, Bruyn GW (eds): Handbook of Clinical Neurology, vol 6, 1968, Amsterdam, North-Holland, pp 298–378
4. Critchley M: Huntington's chorea: Historical and geographical considerations, in The Black Hole and Other Essays. London, Pittman, 1964
5. Curran D: Huntington's chorea without choreiform movements. J Neurol Psychopathol 10:305–310, 1930
6. Dewhurst K, Oliver J, Trick KLK, McKnight AL: Neuropsychiatric aspects of Huntington's chorea. Confin Neurol 31:258–268, 1969
7. Garron DC: Huntington's chorea and schizophrenia, in Barbeau A, Chase TN, Paulson GW (eds): Advances in Neurology, vol 1, Huntington's Chorea. New York, Raven, 1973
8. Hallock FK: A case of Huntington's chorea with remarks upon the propriety of naming the disorder "dementia choreics." J Nerv Ment Dis 25:851–864, 1898
9. Heathfield KWC: Huntington's chorea, investigation into the prevalence of this disease in the area covered by the Northeast Metropolitan Regional Hospital Board. Brain 90:203–232, 1967
10. Huntington G: On Chorea. Med Surg Rep 26:317–321, 1872
11. Krnjevic K, Silver A: A histological study of cholinergic fibers in the cerebral cortex. J Anat 99:711–759, 1965
12. Lewis AJ: Paranoia and paranoid: A historical perspective. Psychol Med 1:2–12, 1970
13. Loranger AW, Goodell H, Lee JE, McDowell F: Levo-dopa treatment in Parkinson's syndrome. Arch Gen Psychiatry 26:163–168, 1972
14. McGeer PL, McGeer EG, Fibiger HC: Choline acetylase and glutamic acid decarboxylase in Huntington's chorea. Neurology 23:912–917, 1973
15. McHugh PR: Occult hydrocephalus. Quart J Med 33:297–308, 1964
16. McHugh PR, and Folstein MF: Address to the American Academy of Neurology, Recent Advances in Dementia, April, 1973 (unpublished)
17. Minski L, Guttmann E: Huntington's chorea. J Ment Sci 84:21–96, 1938
18. Myrianthopoulous MC: Huntington's chorea. J Med Genet 3:298–314, 1966
19. Oscar-Berman M, Sax DS, Opoliner L: Effects of memory aids on hypothesis behavior and focusing in patients with Huntington's chorea, in Barbeau A, Chase TN, Paulson GW (eds): Advances in Neurology, vol 1, Huntington's Chorea. New York, Raven 1973
20. Pearson JS: Behavioral aspects of Huntington's chorea, in Barbeau A, Chase TN, Paulson GW (eds): Advances in Neurology, vol 1, Huntington's Chorea. New York, Raven, 1973
21. Reed TE, Chandler JR: Huntington's chorea in Michigan. I. Demography and genetics. Am J Hum Genet 10:201–225, 1958

22. Roos R, Gajousek DC, Gibbs CJ: The clinical characteristics of transmissible Creutzfeldt-Jakob disease. Brain 97:1–20, 1973
23. Shternberg RF: Certain aspects of the mental changes in Huntington's chorea. Z Neuropat Psikhiat Korsakoff 61:400–410, 1961
24. Shute CCD, Lewis FR: Cholinergic and monoazinergic pathways in the hypothalamus. Br. Med Bull 22:221–226, 1966
25. Sjogren T, Sjogren E, Lindgren AGH: Morbus Alzheimer and Morbus Pick. Acta Psychiat Neurol Scand Suppl 82, 1952
26. Slater E, Roth M: Clinical Psychiatry (ed 3). London, Baillière, Tindall, & Cassell, 1969
27. Spillane J, Phillips R: Huntington's chorea in South Wales. Quart J Med 6:403–423, 1937
28. Streletzki F: Psychosen in Verlauf der Huntingtonschen Chorea unter besonderer Berücksichtigung der Wahnbildungen. Arch Psychiat Nerv 202:202–214, 1961
29. Vassie RP: On the transmission of Huntington's chorea for 300 years—The Bures family group. J Nerv Ment Dis 76:553–573, 1932
30. Wilson SAK: Neurology. Williams & Wilkins, Baltimore, 1955

Commentary

With this careful longitudinal study, the authors have provided more useful information than can be found in many, far larger, cross-sectional studies. For instance, the fact that the serious manic–depressive problems subside with the increasing indifference characteristic of the ''apathetic'' stage is not demonstrated by the lists of symptoms usually presented. The manic-depressive episodes of Huntington's chorea can be treated successfully, but competent management demands this type of longitudinal information. Long lists of signs and symptoms are available for many organic mental disorders but only in a few do we possess enlightening longitudinal studies of this type. From the anatomical viewpoint, whether the behavioral changes of Huntington's chorea reflect frontal deterioration, subcortical pathology or a combination cannot presently be answered but studies of this type will offer excellent background information for future pathologic correlation.

Finally, the editors feel that there should be a chapter discussing the psychiatric aspects of neurologic disease as seen from the autopsy table. Pathology is not a major topic in most current psychiatric training, but, as forcefully demonstrated in the following chapter, primary neurologic pathology often produces psychiatric symptomatology that masks the underlying disorder. The psychodynamically oriented psychiatrist is at a particular disadvantage when seeing such a patient, since it is perfectly possible to demonstrate significant psychodynamic factors in individuals suffering from a progressive organic brain disorder. An awareness that neurologic disorders may present with purely psychiatric symptomatology must be recognized by every psychiatrist. The following chapter will emphasize this point by presenting a representative selection of incorrectly diagnosed cases.

Nathan Malamud, M.D.

14

Organic Brain Disease Mistaken for Psychiatric Disorder: A Clinicopathologic Study

The masking of an underlying organic brain disease by psychiatric symptoms is demonstrated through case illustrations from inflammatory and metabolic disorders of childhood, presenile dementias, convulsive disorders and brain tumors. The diagnostic difficulties stem from (1) inadequate neurologic evaluation and (2) lack of recognition of the role of disturbances of the limbic system in the production of psychiatric symptoms. The latter is especially evident in temporal lobe epilepsy and in tumors involving various limbic structures.

The neuropathologist is not infrequently confronted with cases clinically diagnosed as psychiatric disorders only to find postmortem evidence of one or another type of organic brain disease. Although such misdiagnosis can often be attributed to errors in clinical judgment or to incomplete neurologic examination, it is likely that, at least in some instances, the mental symptoms may be the only or predominant expressions of the organic condition.

The close association between some neurologic and psychiatric disorders has long been known, although its interpretation has remained controversial. Some have argued that the organic disease merely precipitates an underlying personality disorder, while others have maintained that the latter may be more directly related to structural changes occurring in the specific anatomical locations of the brain. In any case, the correct evaluation under such circumstances, presents a clinical challenge with respect to diagnosis, pathogenesis, and therapy.

The incidence of such misdiagnosis is difficult to estimate, since it ultimately depends on adequate necropsy studies that are often lacking. It has been the experience of this author to have discovered a number of such cases at autopsy, some of which have been the subject of previous publications.

It is the purpose of this presentation to elaborate further on this theme through illustrations from the following conditions: (1) chronic encephalitis; (2) metabolic disorders of childhood; (3) presenile dementias; (4) psychomotor epilepsy; and (5) brain tumors.

CHRONIC ENCEPHALITIS

Observations during the early part of this century regarding the prominent psychiatric manifestations in chronic lethargic encephalitis marked a historic landmark in psychiatry. In this disease, the combination of psychiatric, neurologic and vegetative symptoms formed the basis for a complex interplay between organic and dynamic factors. According to Wilson[22] mental signs remained as sequelae in over 50 percent of patients who showed them during the acute phase of the illness and were present in about one third of all survivors below age 16. When occurring in children, the disease was especially prone to manifest itself as a behavior disorder, masking the less obvious neurologic signs, until later when symptoms of Parkinsonism became established. Under the circumstances, errors in diagnosis were apt to occur, resulting in confusion with psychopathic, neurotic and psychotic states. The following case illustrates the diagnostic problem.

CASE LPNI 4957

A 42-year-old white man had a normal birth and early development. In 1915, at the age of 3 years, he is said to have had an attack of influenza, but there were no further details. A change in behavior was noted at age 7, when he began running away from school and home and tended to sleep a lot. He was committed to a state school because of increasing delinquent behavior. At the age of 13, he was admitted to a state hospital for the mentally retarded, where his I.Q. was 71, but was soon discharged. He continued to show disturbed behavior and slept most of the time. At age 20, a diagnosis of hysteria was made in an outpatient clinic. Subsequently, he began complaining that people were talking about him, saying "that his eyes were going up and down." He was then committed to a state hospital for the mentally ill, where a diagnosis of schizophrenia was entertained. During this hospitalization, a neurologic examination revealed indistinct speech, anisocoria with the right pupil being larger than the left, and sluggish reaction of both pupils. He was soon discharged. At age 36, he was again committed to a state hospital for the retarded. At this time, it was noted that he was dragging his right leg, walking stiff-legged, speaking indistinctly, and fixing his eyes on something above his head for periods of time. He would sleep all day and be awake during the night. Later, a tremor of his hands, lips, and eyelids, masked facies, and drooling became apparent. It was then that a diagnosis of postencephalitic Parkinsonism was made, and he was started on Artane with some improvement. During the following 4 years, he had an occasional seizure and died in 1955 during one of these attacks.

At autopsy, the brain showed the gross features of depigmentation of the substantia nigra (Fig. 14-1A) that was confirmed microscopically by a marked paucity of the melanin-bearing neurons in the compact zone (Fig. 14-1B); similar changes were present in the periaqueductal area.

Comment.   It is obvious that this case was a classic example of lethargic encephalitis, in which the vague history of an acute febrile illness, followed by a behavior disorder after a free interval of several years, were misleading early features, resulting in a diagnosis of either a neurotic or psychotic state, despite such symptoms as sleep reversal and oculogyric crises. The correct diagnosis was ultimately established when the Parkinsonian manifestations became prominent, and only then was treatment with antiparkinsonian drugs instituted.

METABOLIC DISORDERS OF CHILDHOOD

The concept of childhood schizophrenia or infantile autism developed historically in close association with that of infantile dementia of Heller. The latter condition was described by its author[10] as having an onset at about the age of 3–4 years with initial changes in mood, marked by anxiety, rage, and negativism, progressing to loss of speech, tics, grimaces, and cataleptic posturing, ultimately leading to an end-stage of emotional blunting and intellectual deterioration. Heller's disease came to be regarded by some as essentially an organic disorder[12] but by others as indistinguishable from infantile autism and schizophrenia. Because of the blurring of the clinical features, as between an organic or functional basis, the diagnosis in any given case has continued to present a challenge to the psychiatrist.

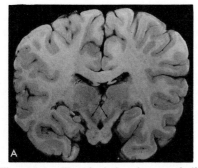 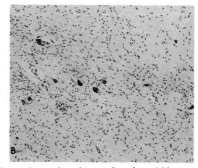

Fig. 14-1. Chronic lethargic encephalitis: substantia nigra, showing (A) gross depigmentation and (B) reduction in melanin-bearing cells. Nissl method, × 130.

There have been few postmortem reports in such cases.[3,13] Of those reported, the underlying organic disease has not been uniform, varying from neurolipidosis to various degenerative or inflammatory conditions, as illustrated below.

Neurolipidosis

It has been well documented in the literature that in four cases of clinically diagnosed Heller's disease, Corberi[4] in 1926 found histologic evidence of neurolipidosis on examination of cortical biopsies. I[13] reported in 1959 the necropsy findings of three pairs of siblings diagnosed as schizophrenics. In two of these, the changes in the brain were characteristic of neurolipidosis, while in the third pair of siblings the findings pointed to an unclassified heredofamilial degenerative disease. The following report concerns one of the cases of neurolipidosis.

CASE LPNI 279

A 7-year-old white girl had a normal birth and early development. At about the age of 3 years, she was said to have been frightened at a Halloween party, which precipitated a marked fear reaction and a period of nocturnal screaming continued unabated for the next 6 weeks. She gradually became more withdrawn, negativistic, and mute, was unable to adjust in kindergarten, and later developed incontinence of urine and feces. At the age of 5, she was examined in a pediatric clinic where no physical or neurologic abnormalities were found. Mentally she was described by the psychologist as showing "essentially marked instability in emotional reactions, varying between apathy, unmotivated laughing and crying, and between mutism and outbursts of unintelligible words and songs." A diagnosis of infantile autism was made. She was committed to a hospital for the mentally retarded where she progressively deteriorated and expired.

The autopsy revealed grossly diffuse atrophy of the cerebral and cerebrellar cortex (Fig. 14-2A) that on microscopic examination showed widespread ballooning of the neurons that contained large amounts of stored lipid (Fig. 14-2B).

After the autopsy findings confirmed the diagnosis of neurolipidosis, clinical examination of the patient's younger sister disclosed evidence of a similar condition. However, a more careful evaluation of the neurologic status revealed ataxia, dysarthria, mental deterioration, and EEG abnormalities.

Comment. It was of interest that these instances represented a form of "amaurotic family idiocy sine amaurosis," in which the retinal changes, diagnostic of other forms of lipidosis, were absent. In the experience of this author, these negative retinal findings appear to be an almost consistent feature of the late infantile or Jansky–Bielschowsky form of neurolipidosis. Therefore, the clinical picture usually is characterized by nonspecific mental and motor deterioration, in which emotional and personality changes may be overemphasized at the expense of an adequate neurologic examination. Creak,[5] who reported two cases of neurolipidosis in which there was no evidence of neurologic

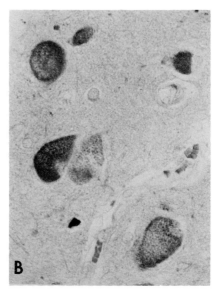

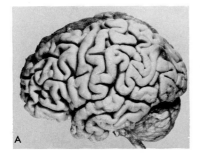

Fig. 14-2. Neurolipidosis, late infantile form: (A) Diffuse cerebral and cerebellar atrophy and (B) ballooning of neurons with deposits of granular lipid material. Nile blue sulfate stain, × 475.

disability, was of the opinion that ''the distinction between a psychosis and an organic disorder may be possible only on a long-term basis.''

Wilson's Disease

In cases of Wilson's disease, it is not uncommon to encounter prominent personality disturbance and signs of emotional instability along with the rigidity and involuntary movements of choreoathetosis, dystonia, and tremor. Such mental changes are probably determined by the frequent location of the lesions in the thalamus and cerebral cortex, in addition to the more common involvement of the lenticular area. Confusion with psychiatric disorders may thus result, as illustrated by the following example.

CASE LPNI 10278

An 11-year-old white girl was admitted to a general hospital with a history of emotional difficulties in school along with slight evidence of incoordination of movement of 2 years duration prior to admission. She was then transferred to the child psychiatric unit where for about a year she underwent treatment for what was considered to be childhood schizophrenia. However, because of increasing evidence of a dystonic movement disorder, an ophthalmologic examination was recommended and led to the discovery of a Kayser-Fleischer corneal ring and to a diagnosis of Wilson's disease. Laboratory studies further confirmed the diagnosis, revealing a low level of ceruloplasmin (6 mg/100 ml) and of globulin-bound copper in the serum (35 ug/100 ml); a liver biopsy was positive for copper. The patient was then started on penicillamine therapy. However, by now her condition was too far advanced for favorable response, and she expired approximately 1 month following institution of therapy.

The brain showed a characteristic spongy type of degneration in the lenticular region (Fig. 14-3A) and in the thalamus. Microscopically, pathognomonic giant astrocytes, known as Alzheimer glia and Opalski cells (Fig. 14-3B) were observed.

Comment. The brains of two other young adults with Wilson's disease, in whom the initial diagnosis was schizophrenia, were examined by the author. It was evident retrospectively that the misdiagnosis in each of the three cases resulted from insufficient attention paid to the neurologic signs and symptoms.

PRESENILE DEMENTIAS

Alzheimer's, Pick's, and Jakob–Creutzfeldt's diseases are generally included in the category of presenile dementias. The prominent signs of an organic brain syndrome, in all these conditions, should theoretically present no diagnostic difficulties. Yet, ever since the early accounts of the psychopathology of dementia paralytica, various organic cerebral disorders, acute or

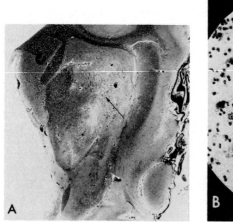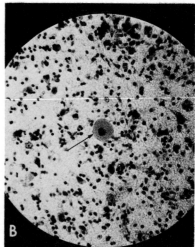

Fig. 14-3. Wilson's disease: (A) Spongy degeneration of lenticular region and (B) giant glial cell (Opalski form) in center of field. Hematoxylin–van Gieson stain, × 350.

chronic, have been known to mimic functional disorders, whether released by previous personality deviations, or as direct expressions of the disease in question. In many instances, depressive, paranoid, and schizophrenic reactions were diagnosed. This is borne out by the following data collected by the author, in the group of presenile dementias.

It may be seen from Table 14-1 that diagnostic errors are more apt to occur in cases of Pick's disease than in either of the two other conditions. This is understandable, since the prominent and early impairment of the memory function in Alzheimer's disease on the one hand and the conspicuous neurologic signs in Jakob–Creutzfeldt's disease on the other tend to preclude such misdiagnoses. Such is not the case in Pick's disease, where memory is preserved for a long time; the dementia concerns many more abstract than concrete functions and sensorimotor neurologic signs are virtually absent. The impairment of the highest associative functions in Pick's disease may be correlated with the tendency of the lesions to be restricted to the phylogenetically youngest regions of the brain.[14] Initial symptoms of loss of initiative and impoverishment of speech may also contribute to confusion with psychiatric conditions, as illustrated by the following case.

CASE LPNI 1833

A 39-year-old white man had a history of a normal prepsychotic personality, but at about the age of 34, while in the Army, he became withdrawn and slovenly in his personal appearance and was discharged from the service with a diagnosis of chronic schizophrenia. Three years later, he was admitted to a V.A. hospital because he had become increasingly mute and negativistic. Examination revealed negative neurologic and laboratory studies, a clear sensorium, but emotional apathy, tendency to perseveration and incontinence. The diagnosis of schizophrenia was maintained and he received electroshock therapy without benefit. Prefrontal leucotomy was then recommended. When this was attempted, bilateral organized subdural hematomas were found compressing the brain. These were evacuated and the leucotomy was not performed. The patient's condition remained unchanged and he finally expired of bronchopneumonia.

The brain showed gross evidence of cerebral compression (by the old subdural

Table 14-1

Incidence of Diagnosis of Functional Disorder in Presenile Dementias

Type of Disorder	No. of Cases	No. with Diagnosis of Functional Disorder
Alzheimer's disease	103	9 (9%)
Pick's disease	35	8 (23%)
Jakob–Creutzfeldt's disease	32	3 (10%)

hematomas) superimposed on the classic features of lobar atrophy, in which the involvement of the frontal, inferior temporal and posterior parietal regions was sharply demarcated from the well-preserved postcentral, superior temporal and occipital gyri (Fig. 14-4A). Microscopically, a diffuse loss of pyramidal cells especially in the third cortical layer (Fig. 14-4B) was associated with scattered inflated neurons with argyrophilic inclusions, or so-called Pick cells (Fig. 14-4C), but without evidence of senile plaques or neurofibrillary tangles of Alzheimer.

Comment. It is obvious that the primary diagnosis in this case is Pick's disease and that the subdural hematomas are incidental complications of minor head injuries. The diagnosis of schizophrenia was made despite the apparently normal prepsychotic personality. The misdiagnosis appeared to derive from the absence of the usual features of an organic brain syndrome, a characteristic feature of Pick's disease, as pointed out previously.

PSYCHOMOTOR EPILEPSY

Much has been written about ictal psychic phenomena and interseizure personality changes of psychomotor or temporal lobe epilepsy. The high incidence of ictal or interictal states of aggressive and at times violent behavior, fugues, fear, and depressive emotional reactions, sensory illusions or hallucinations, and feelings of depersonalization are sufficient grounds for confusion with psychoneurotic or psychotic states. Thus, Gibbs[8] observed that psychiatric disorders were three times as common in patients with psychomotor seizures and temporal lobe EEG foci than among individuals with normal EEGs. Mulder and Daly[17] analyzed 100 patients with lesions of the temporal lobe in whom the presenting complaints were psychiatric; paroxysmal symptoms characteristic of temporal discharges were present in 95 percent, while in 72 percent of cases there were also nonparoxysmal mental symptoms of anxiety, depression, or schizoid reaction. Hill[11] noted EEG evidence of epilepsy in 18 among 80 patients with schizophrenia. Ervin et al.[6] found that 81 percent of 42 patients with EEG foci in the temporal lobes had a diagnosis of schizophrenia. Similar findings were reported by Rodin et al.[19] Bartlett[2] reported 11 instances of psychosis, 8 of schizophrenia, and 3 of affective disorder in a large series of epileptic patients, noting that 8 of the 11 cases were associated with temporal epilepsy. Slater and Beard[21] were impressed with a relatively high incidence of association between epilepsy and schizophrenia; it was their contention that the psychosis could be regarded as a "symptomatic form of purely epileptic causation."

From a pathoanatomical standpoint,[15,20] wide acceptance has been given to the occurrence of mesial temporal sclerosis as one of the more common pathologic substrates in psychomotor epilepsy, although its precise pathogenesis has remained controversial. This has been confirmed to a large

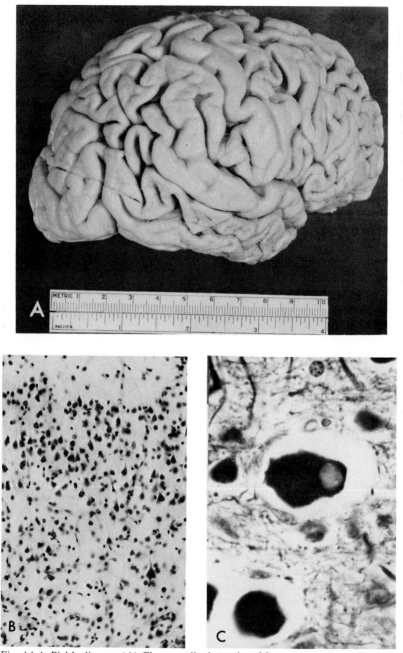

Fig. 14-4. Pick's disease: (A) Circumscribed atrophy of frontal, posterior parietal, and infero-temporal regions and (B) loss of neurons in lamina III of the cerebral cortex. Nissl method, × 200. (C) Inflated cortical neurons with argyrophilic inclusions. × 720.

extent by the experience of neurosurgeons, notably Falconer et al.,[7] in the course of performing temporal lobectomies. Attention is drawn to the location of this lesion in an important part of the limbic system. By way of illustration, the following two cases are presented.

CASE LPNI 7887.

A 12-year-old boy with a negative family history, normal birth, and early development, had the onset, at the age of 2½ years, of grand-mal seizures associated with an upper respiratory infection and high fever. Subsequently the convulsions continued with increasing frequency despite treatment with Dilantin and phenobarbital. Some of his seizures were later characterized as running fits, during which "he would suddenly scream, start to run, fall, kick and writhe, and would be very weak when the seizure was over." He became increasingly subject to "temper tantrums" and at the age of 10 was brought to the attention of the juvenile court after he had made overt threats with a loaded rifle. Commitment to a state hospital for the retarded was recommended, although tests revealed a normal intelligence. In the hospital, repeated EEGs disclosed a spike and wave focus in the middle and anterior regions of the left temporal lobe. His condition was diagnosed as mixed grand-mal and psychomotor epilepsy. Death occurred when, on a hike near the hospital reservoir, he had one of his running seizures, ran into the lake and drowned.

The brain was edematous but otherwise grossly normal, with the exception of sclerosis of the left cornu Ammonis (Fig. 14-5A).

CASE LPNI 6607.

A 65-year-old man had a history of "fits" in childhood that stopped at age 15. In 1918, at age 30, while serving in the Army, he was hospitalized for 6 weeks with a diagnosis of "neurasthenia" and was discharged. Soon afterwards he had an episode, for which he claimed amnesia, during which he castrated himself and was committed to a state hospital, but was discharged after 6 months. In 1933, he was committed to another state hospital because he developed delusions of persecution, was threatening and destructive of personal property. A diagnosis of schizophrenia, hebephrenic type, was made. While in the hospital he had one grand-mal seizure accompanied by incontinence and was given phenobarbital. His behavior was characterized as noisy and combative. In 1940, he was transferred to a V.A. hospital where neurologic and laboratory examinations were negative, but there was a hyperactive and delusional mental state. While there he had a number of seizures. Some of his attacks were described as brief episodes of jerking of the left extremities with eyes turned to the left, followed by stupor, aphasia, and immobility of the left side with bilateral Babinski signs; others were described by the patient as "sensations of electricity" in the left hand or feelings that he was "going to strike out." Repeated EEGs showed generalized dysrhythmia with a focus of spiking in the right temporal region. His seizures were partially controlled with Dilantin and phenobarbital. The clinical diagnosis was schizophrenia and epilepsy of grand-mal and psychomotor type. He died suddenly in 1953 of arteriosclerotic heart disease.

The brain showed no gross abnormalities, with the exception of sclerosis of the right cornu Ammonis (Fig. 14-5B).

In both of the above cases, the microscopic appearance of the hippocampal lesion was similar. It disclosed virtually complete loss of neurons (Fig. 14-5C), with reactive dense gliosis (Fig. 14-5D), restricted to Sommer's sector (hl) and end plate (h 3-5) of the hippocampal formation. This lesion is considered to be the most consistent manifestation of so-called mesial temporal sclerosis in cases of temporal lobe epilepsy.

Comment. It can be seen that an identical unilateral Ammon's horn sclerosis, in one case on the left and in the other on the right side, correlated exactly with the EEG findings. Clinically, although epilepsy was diagnosed in both instances, the behavior disorder in the one and the psychosis in the other were considered to be merely coincidental and not an integral part of the convulsive disorder. From the previous survey of the literature, however, it appears more likely that a direct cause and effect relationship exists between the epilepsy and the psychiatric disorder. Indeed, it may be argued that the latter represent ictal and interictal psychic phenomena, reflecting both episodic discharges and interseizure electrical abnormalities.

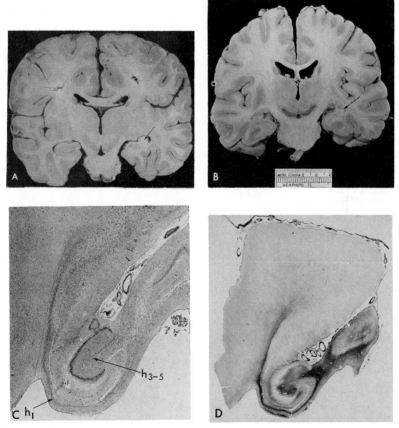

Fig. 14-5. Temporal lobe epilepsy: Sclerosis of cornu Ammonis in (A) case 7887, left side (sides reversed); (B) case 6607, right side; (C) loss of neurons in hl and h 3–5. Nissl method × 5. (D) reactive gliosis in corresponding areas. Holzer method × 5.

BRAIN TUMORS

Closely related to the clinical manifestations of cases with mesial temporal sclerosis are those observed in brain tumors that have a predilection for various parts of the limbic system. The experience with temporal lobectomy has also directed attention to cases of psychomotor epilepsy in which the tumor is located in the uncus–amygdaloid–hippocampal region. The same might apply to tumor involvement of such other components of the limbic system as the orbital–frontal, cingulate, septal and hypothalamic–thalamic regions.

It has long been demonstrated in the literature that intracranial tumors have a high incidence of mental symptoms that for a long time were considered to be of no localizing value but depended more on such factors as increased intracranial pressure, rapidity of growth, and previous personality structure. However, following Bard's experimental production of sham rage through stimulation of the hypothalamus in decorticate animals, Alpers[1] drew attention to the occurrence of mental symptoms, including psychotic states, in cases with tumors of the hypothalamus. But with the exception of isolated examples, the frequency of a frank psychosis as the predominant manifestation of a brain tumor had not been determined.

Recently, Remington and Rubert[18] found, among 34 cases of psychosis with brain tumor admitted to a psychiatric hospital, 24 instances in which the tumors were unrecognized and a diagnosis of a functional disorder was entertained until or unless overt neurologic symptoms had developed. In a recent survey, I[16] found that of 245 cases of intracranial tumor, proven by necropsy, 155 showed various mental symptoms. Out of this number, 18 (11.5%) were diagnosed as purely functional disorders throughout their clinical course, as noted in Table 14-2.

It can be seen in Table 14-2 that the location of the lesions, in all cases diagnosed as functional disorders, involved one or another part of the limbic

Table 14-2
Eighteen Cases of Intracranial Tumor With Clinical Diagnosis of Functional Disorder

Location	Clinical Diagnosis			
	No. of Cases	Schizophrenia	Affective Disorder	Psychoneurosis
Uncus–amygdaloid– hippocampal region	8	4	3	1
Cingulate region	2	2		
Third ventricle region	8	5	1	2
Total	18	11	4	3

system. The tumor types comprised gliomas, craniopharyngiomas, colloid cysts, and hemangiomas, varying from small hamartomatous lesions to large neoplasms of differing malignancy, although fairly restricted to the above regions.

By way of illustration, the following examples are presented.

CASE LPNI 7120: TUMOR OF UNCUS-AMYGDALOID REGION

A 26-year-old white male university student developed, at the age of 13 years, spells that were variously manifested by feelings of numbness, hallucinations of smell, taste, hearing, or vision but without apparent loss of consciousness.

When first hospitalized at the age of 15, a neurologic examination, including a pneumoencephalogram, was normal but several EEGs revealed generalized paroxysmal dysrhythmia with focal activity, initially in the left occipital and subsequently in the left temporal–parietal region. He was treated with anticonvulsant medication for what was diagnosed as petit-mal epilepsy. In the following 10 years, the patient's condition was dominated by a psychiatric disorder. At first, it was characterized by seclusiveness and ideas of reference. At the age of 18, he had an acute psychotic episode, manifested by auditory hallucinations and delusions of persecution. He was admitted to a psychiatric institute where a diagnosis of schizophrenia, catatonic form, was made. A course of combined electroshock and insulin therapy led to apparent improvement and he was discharged. Subsequently, he had a number of readmissions to the same psychiatric institute, each time receiving shock, psychotherapy, or both. Psychologic tests revealed a normal intelligence but evidence of a schizophrenic disorder. The psychiatrists attributed his condition to environmental factors, namely, ''cold and distant family relationships with ambivalence toward his mother and intense sibling rivalry toward his brother.'' At the same time, it was noted that when anticonvulsant medication was stopped, the patient would have either a petit-mal or grand-mal attack. In one of his spells, he described a sensation of micropsia; in another he left the house undressed, for which he was amnesic. His condition followed a progressive decompensating course. Toward the end of his hospitalization, a pneumoencephalogram and a carotid arteriogram were interpreted as normal (no further EEGs were performed). He was ultimately transferred to a state hospital where he died from a pulmonary embolism complicating a thrombophelebitis. The final clinical diagnosis was schizophrenia, undifferentiated form, and epilepsy of mixed petit-mal, grand-mal, and psychomotor forms. At autopsy, a small ill-defined and partly cystic tumor was found in the left anterior hippocampal region, largely involving the uncus–amygdaloid area and diminishing toward the hippocampus (Fig. 14-6A); histologically, it showed an admixture of proliferating well-differentiated ganglion and glial cells (Fig. 6B) diagnostic of a ganglio–glioma that had the appearance of an indolent hamartomatous lesion.

CASE LPNI 10640: TUMOR OF HIPPOCAMPAL REGION

A 19-year-old white male had a history of several episodes of febrile convulsions in early childhood but without apparent residuals. At the age of 9 years, he developed a chronic convulsive disorder. The seizures were initially described as ''of a brief staring, petit-mal type.'' Later, he also experienced grand-mal attacks that were initiated by jerking of the left extremities and inability to speak, and were followed by right-sided headaches and occasional vomiting. At the age of 13, his seizures became more complex semipurposeful acts that were characterized as automatisms and were regarded as psychomotor, for which he received a variety of anticonvulsant medications. At the same time, personality changes developed with increasing withdrawal and emotional tension, aggressive behavior, and negativism. These were considered by psychiatrists to be reactions to a difficult environmental situation manifested by chronic alcoholism and criminal behavior on the part of his father, friction between the parents, and ambivalent

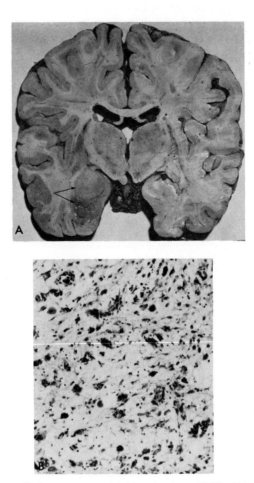

Fig. 14-6. Tumor of left uncus–amygdaloid region (case 7120): (A) Gross appearance and (B) microscopic structure of ganglioglioma, with a mixture of large ganglion cells and small fibrillary astrocytes. Nissl method × 200.

reactions by the patient toward them. At the age of 17, a neurologic examination, including that of the spinal fluid, was normal. However, several EEGs were interpreted as abnormal, with generalized paroxysmal dysrhythmia and right-sided foci of decreased voltage with spike and slow wave bursts that were centered about the right temporal region. It was recommended that the patient have depth electrode studies for possible stereotactic surgery. However, examination by psychiatrists stressed symptoms of depression, anxiety, suicidal, and paranoid tendencies, which in their opinion contraindicated surgery, since it was feared that it might precipitate an overt psychosis. The patient was then committed to a state hospital, where he remained for the next 2 years. Toward the end, he suddenly developed a state of coma and died within 48 hours. The clinical diagnosis was schizophrenic reaction with epilepsy of mixed petit-mal, grand-mal, and psychomotor forms. Autopsy revealed a very small multicystic tumor occupying the right hippocampal gyrus, that compressed the hippocampal formation and was associated on its lateral side with a massive acute hemorrhage (Fig. 14-7A). Histologically, the tumor was for the most part a slowly growing and well-differentiated fibrillary astrocytoma (Fig. 14-7B) but showed recent evidence of anaplasia with areas of bizarre large cells and increased vasularity that terminated in the hemorrhage (Fig. 14-7C).

CASE LPNI 7872: TUMOR OF CINGULATE-CALLOSAL REGION

A 33-year-old white man had a history of an "unstable" personality and an indefinite onset, about 5 years before his death, of episodes of assaultiveness and convulsions. The latter were characterized by momentary loss of consciousness followed by prolonged confusion or states in which he was unable to express himself in words. In between attacks he became increasingly more irritable and abusive. When admitted to a state hospital a year after the onset, the results of the neurologic examination were normal. His behavior was characterized by periods of hostility and aggressiveness, alternating with quiet, cooperative periods. He was treated with electroshock and psychotherapy. The seizures increased in frequency and an EEG showed a slow wave focus in the left frontal–temporal region. Toward the end, he suddenly lapsed into coma and died. The clinical diagnosis was schizophrenia and epilepsy. Pathologically, an avascular tumor that blended imperceptibly with the adjacent normal nervous tissue involved the gray and white matter of the gyrus cinguli of the left frontal lobe with extension into the genu of the corpus callosum (Fig. 14-8A). Microscopically, it showed the structure of a well-differentiated astrocytoma, consisting of uniform plump astrocytes (Fig. 14-8B).

CASE LPNI 5098: TUMOR OF THIRD VENTRICLE REGION

A 43-year-old white woman who had a somewhat "eccentric" personality make-up, experienced, about 9 months before her death, several episodes of prolonged coma, lasting many hours to a few days. In the hospital she expressed delusions of unreality, hypnotism, and depersonalization and made many suicidal attempts. There was evidence of impairment of memory with a tendency to confabulation. The results of the

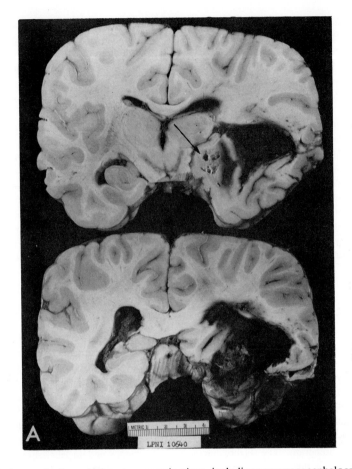

physical, neurologic, and laboratory examinations, including pneumoencephalography, were essentially normal. She died during an episode of prolonged coma. The clinical diagnosis was schizophrenic reaction and epilepsy of unknown etiology. Autopsy disclosed a tumor that involved the walls, floor, and roof of the third ventricle, virtually occluding it, and extending into the body of the fornix (Fig. 14-9A). Histologically, it showed the characteristic features of a pleomorphic and necrotic glioblastoma multiforme (Fig. 14-9B).

   Comment.   In each of the above four cases the clinical diagnosis was schizophrenia and epilepsy, implying coincidental independent disorders. Although the effects of previous personality structure and environmental stress on the development of the psychosis could not be ruled out, many if not all, of the clinical features of the latter suggested ictal psychic phenomena with related interseizure personality disorder. Since the neoplasms were not recognized, thereapy in all the cases was primarily directed at the psychiatric disorder.

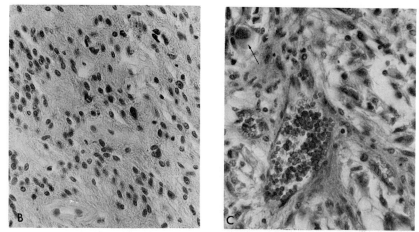

Fig. 14-7. Tumor of right hippocampal region (case 10640): (A) Gross appearance. Note small size and avascular multicystic nature of tumor and adjacent massive hemorrhage. (B) Microscopic structure of astrocytoma with uniform fibrillary astrocytes in avascular portion. Hematoxylin–eosin stain, × 200. (C) Pleomorphic cellular structure with scattered giant cells in vascular hemorrhagic portion of tumor. Hematoxylin–eosin stain × 200.

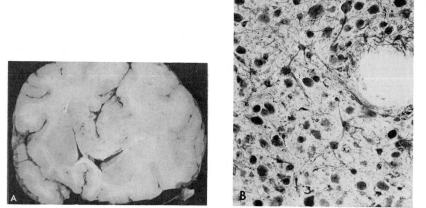

Fig. 14-8. Tumor of left cingulate–callosal region (case 7872, sides reversed): (A) Gross appearance and (B) microscopic structure of astrocytoma, with uniform plump astrocytes. Cajal gold chloride method × 200.

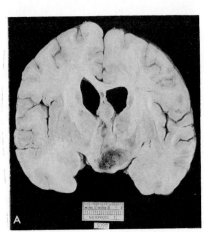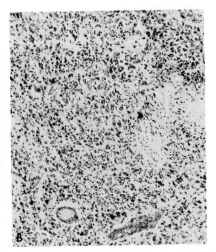

Fig. 14-9. Tumor of third ventricle region (case 5098): (A) gross appearance, and (B) microscopic structure of glioblastoma multiforme, with pleomorphic cells and focal necrosis. Hematoxylin–van Stain × 75.

SUMMARY AND CONCLUSIONS

The masking of an underlying organic brain disease by psychiatric symptoms has been demonstrated above through case illustrations from a variety of disorders. These ranged from inflammatory and metabolic disorders of childhood to presenile dementias, convulsive disorders, and brain tumors. Although each of these conditions presents its own individual problems, the diagnostic difficulties appear to stem from two general considerations: (1) inadequate neurologic evaluation with consequent overemphasis of the psychiatric condition and (2) failure to recognize the role of the neural–anatomical basis of some psychiatric symptomatology in such conditions as temporal lobe epilepsy and in brain tumors involving various limbic structures. It is possible, although less clearly demonstrable, that more diffuse diseases of the central nervous system may also owe their psychiatric symptomatology to involvement of such areas. It is obvious that failure to recognize these implications can lead to errors in diagnosis and failure to utilize appropriate therapy.

REFERENCES

1.   Alpers BJ: Personality and emotional disorders associated with hypothalamic lesions, in Fulton JF, Ranson SW, Frantz AM (eds): Assn. Res. Nerv. & Ment. Dis., vol 20. Baltimore, Williams & Wilkins, 1940, pp 725–748

2. Bartlett JEA: Chronic Psychosis following epilepsy. Am J Psychiatry 114:338–343, 1957
3. Benda CE, Melchior JC: Childhood schizophrenia, childhood autism and Heller's disease. Intern Rec Med 172:137–154, 1959
4. Corberi G: Sindromi di regressione mentale infantogiovanile. Riv Patol Nerv Ment 31:6–45, 1926
5. Creak M: Childhood psychosis: A review of 100 cases. Br J Psychiatry 109:84–89, 1963
6. Ervin F, Epstein AA, King HE: Behavior of epileptic and non-epileptic patients with temporal spikes. Arch Neurol Psychiatry 74:488–496, 1955
7. Falconer MA, Serafetinides EA, Corsellis JAN: Etiology and pathogenesis of temporal lobe epilepsy. Arch Neurol 10:233–248, 1964
8. Gibbs FA: Ictal and non-ictal psychiatric disorders in temporal lobe epilepsy. J Nerv Ment Dis 113:522–528, 1951
9. Glaser GH: The problem of psychosis in psychomotor temporal lobe epileptics. Epilepsia 5:271–278, 1964
10. Heller T: Über Dementia infantilis. Z Kinderforsch 37:661–667, 1930
11. Hill D: The relationship between epilepsy and schizophrenia: EEG studies. Folia Psychiat Neurol Neurochir Neerlandicn 51:95–111, 1948
12. Kanner L: Child Psychiatry (ed 4). Springfield, Ill, Thomas, 1972, pp 267–269
13. Malamud N: Heller's disease and childhood schizophrenia. Am J Psychiatry 116:215–218, 1959
14. Malamud N, Waggoner RW: Genealogic and clinicopathologic study of Pick's disease. Arch Neurol Psychiatry 50:288–303, 1943
15. Malamud N: The epileptogenic focus in temporal lobe epilepsy from a pathological standpoint. Arch Neurol 14:190–195, 1966
16. Malamud N: Psychiatric disorder with intracranial tumors of limbic system. Arch Neurol 17:113–123, 1967
17. Mulder DW, Daly D: Psychiatric symptoms associated with lesions of the temporal lobe. JAMA 150:173–176, 1952
18. Remington FB, Rubert SL: Why patients with brain tumors come to a psychiatric hospital. Am J Psychiatry 119:256–257, 1962
19. Rodin EA, DeJong RN, Waggoner RW, Bagchi BK: Relationship between certain forms of psychomotor epilepsy and schizophrenia. Arch Neurol Psychiatry 77:449–463, 1957
20. Sano K, Malamud N: Clinical significance of sclerosis of the cornu Ammonis. Arch Neurol Psychiatry 70:40–53, 1953
21. Slater E, Beard AW: The schizophrenia-like psychoses of epilepsy. Br J Psychiatry 109:95–150, 1963
22. Wilson SAK: Neurology. Baltimore, Williams & Wilkins, 1940, p 131

Commentary

No attempt will be made to summarize the articles in this volume. The topics discussed are too varied and the information offered too specific to handle in a simple summary. We would, however, like to emphasize that these articles have, in one way or another, directed the clinician toward recognition and treatment of organic mental problems. This has been accomplished through sharper focus on neuropsychiatric syndromes, improved diagnostic techniques, and by direct suggestion for therapy including some fairly novel methods. Without specific diagnosis, the therapy of psychiatric disorders has not been successful, but improved diagnostic methods now allow more specific and more successful therapy. Therapy of organic mental problems has received far too little emphasis for several decades; it is the editors' hope that these articles will convince the reader that there is a real potential for active therapy.

The lack of diagnostic specificity has not only hampered therapy, but it has also curtailed scientific and academic research in the organic mental syndromes. In dealing with neuropsychiatric disorders without specific and accurate diagnostic criteria the researcher has had to apply his techniques to a rather random patient group. Thus, much of the careful psychologic, physiologic, and even psychoanalytic research of the past three or more decades has been performed on mixed disorders, a point that weakens any conclusions that have been drawn. Again, it is hoped that improvements in the diagnosis of neuropsychiatric disorders will lead to increased research interest in the field.

Let us close with a comment on a little-known item from the history of neuropsychiatry. Sigmund Freud was originally a neurologist, trained well in the neuroanatomy and neurophysiology of his time and devoted to the investigation of brain function. Even after his early studies in hysteria he still desired to correlate psychologic processes with the physiology of the nervous system. Thus, in 1895 he wrote a "Project for a Scientific Psychology" and in the introduction stated: "The intention is to furnish a psychology that shall be a natural science; that is, to represent mental processes as quantitatively determinate states of specifiable material particles . . . ."[1] Kris[2] has described this project as "a determined attempt to describe the function of the mental apparatus as functions of a neuronal system and to comprehend all processes ultimately as quantitative changes." Within the next few years, however, Freud developed the method of psychoanalysis, a new approach to understanding the mental apparatus, and was never able to return to his original attempt. Szondi[3] has reviewed indirect but compelling evidence that the life-long inability to return to this early idea represented a bitter disappointment to Freud.

At the present time, based in part on Freud's works, much more is understood about mental processes; similarly, a great deal more is known about brain function. Nonetheless, there is still no shortcut to the understanding of how brain function correlates with mental activity. Neither by ignoring the complexity of the mind or brain nor by relying on exact but narrow methods of explanation can this most difficult quest be furthered, and, at present, only partial and tentative conclusions can be made. This imperfect state is reflected in our book. It is our firm belief, however, that the careful pursuit of clinical neuropsychiatric studies will ultimately allow more definite correlation of brain function and mental activity.

REFERENCES

1. Freud S: Project for a scientific psychology, in Strachey J (ed): The Standard Edition of the Complete Psychological Works of Sigmund Freud, vol I. London, Hogarth Press, 1966
2. Bonaparte M, Freud A, Kris E (eds): Aus den Anfangen der Psychoanalyse. London, Imago, 1950
3. Szondi L: Freud als Wissenschafter. Neue Zürcher Zeitung, Nr. 13:432, 1964

Index